PSYCHIATRIC NEUROIMAGING RESEARCH

Contemporary Strategies

PSYCHIATRIC NEUROIMAGING RESEARCH

Contemporary Strategies

EDITED BY

Darin D. Dougherty, M.D., M.Sc.
Scott L. Rauch, M.D.

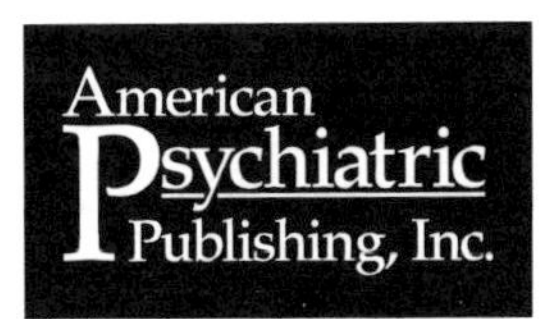

Washington, DC
London, England

Manufactured in the United States of America on acid-free paper

04 03 02 01 4 3 2 1
First Edition

American Psychiatric Press, Inc.
1400 K Street, N.W.
Washington, DC 20005
www.appi.org

Library of Congress Cataloging-in-Publication Data
Psychiatric neuroimaging research : contemporary strategies / edited by Darin D. Dougherty, Scott L. Rauch.
p. ; cm.
Includes bibliographical references and index.
ISBN 0-88048-844-1 (alk. paper)
1. Brain—Imaging. 2. Neuropsychiatry—Research. 3. Mental illness—Diagnosis. I. Dougherty, Darin D. II. Rauch, Scott L.
[DNLM 1. Diagnostic Imaging. 2. Mental Disorders—diagnosis. 3. Magnetic Resonance Imaging. WM 141 P9738 2001]
RC473.B7 P78 2001
616.8'04754—dc21

00-061073

British Library Cataloguing in Publication Data
A CIP record is available from the British Library.

To my wife, Christina, and our daughter, Emma

DDD

CONTENTS

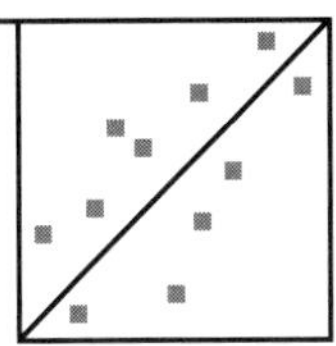

CONTRIBUTORS

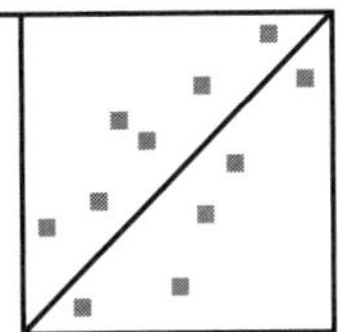

Anissa Abi-Dargham, M.D.
Associate Professor, Departments of Psychiatry and Radiology, Columbia University College of Physicians and Surgeons, New York State Psychiatric Institute, New York, New York

Nathaniel M. Alpert, Ph.D.
Division of Nuclear Medicine, Massachusetts General Hospital, Boston, Massachusetts

George W. Arana, M.D.
Director, Mental Health Services, Ralph H. Johnson Veterans Affairs Medical Center; Professor, Department of Psychiatry, Vice Dean for Graduate Affairs, Medical University of South Carolina, Charleston, South Carolina

James C. Ballenger, M.D.
Professor, Department of Psychiatry, Medical University of South Carolina, Charleston, South Carolina

Daryl E. Bohning, Ph.D.
Professor, Department of Radiology, Director, Advanced Magnetic Resonance Physics Research, Medical University of South Carolina, Charleston, South Carolina

Tim Curran, Ph.D.
Assistant Professor, Department of Psychology, University of Colorado, Boulder, Colorado

Chandlee Dickey, M.D.
Associate Psychiatrist, Department of Psychiatry, Associate Physician, Department of Neurology, Brigham and Women's Hospital; Instructor, Department of Psychiatry, Harvard Medical School, Boston, Massachusetts

Darin D. Dougherty, M.D., M.Sc.
Clinical Associate, Department of Psychiatry, Massachusetts General Hospital; Assistant Professor, Department of Psychiatry, Harvard Medical School, Boston, Massachusetts; Visiting Scientist, Massachusetts Institute of Technology, Cambridge, Massachusetts

Wayne C. Drevets, M.D.
Associate Professor, Departments of Psychiatry and Radiology, Western Psychiatric Institute, University of Pittsburgh School of Medicine, Pittsburgh, Pennsylvania

Craig F. Ferris, Ph.D.
Professor, Departments of Psychiatry and Physiology, Director of Neuroimaging, Department of Psychiatry, University of Massachusetts Medical School, Worchester, Massachusetts

Iris A. Fischer, A.B.
Research Assistant, Department of Psychiatry, VA Boston Healthcare System, Brockton, Massachusetts

Alan J. Fischman, M.D., Ph.D.
Director, Division of Nuclear Medicine, Massachusetts General Hospital; Associate Professor, Department of Radiology, Harvard Medical School, Boston, Massachusetts

Blaise deB. Frederick, Ph.D.
Assistant Biophysicist, Brain Imaging Center, McLean Hospital; Assistant Professor (proposed), Department of Psychiatry, Harvard Medical School, Belmont, Massachusetts

Melissa Frumin, M.D.
Psychiatrist, Departments of Psychiatry and Neurology, Brigham and Women's Hospital; Instructor, Department of Psychiatry, Harvard Medical School, Boston, Massachusetts

Mark S. George, M.D.
Professor, Departments of Psychiatry, Radiology, and Neurology, Director, Functional Neuroimaging Division, Department of Psychiatry, and Director, Brain Research Stimulation Laboratory, Medical University of South Carolina; Director, Psychiatric Neuroimaging, Ralph H. Johnson Veterans Affairs Medical Center, Charleston, South Carolina

Joseph Grun, B.S.
Research Scientist, Department of Child and Adolescent Psychiatry, Columbia University College of Physicians and Surgeons, New York, New York

Stephan Heckers, M.D.
Clinical Associate, Department of Psychiatry, Assistant Director, Psychiatric Neuroimaging Research, Massachusetts General Hospital; Assistant Professor, Department of Psychiatry, Harvard Medical School, Boston, Massachusetts

Michael E. Henry, M.D.
Director of Electroconvulsive Therapy, McLean Hospital; Instructor, Department of Psychiatry, Harvard Medical School, Belmont, Massachusetts

Lawrence Kegeles, M.D., Ph.D.
Assistant Professor, Department of Psychiatry, Columbia University College of Physicians and Surgeons, New York State Psychiatric Institute, New York, New York

Charles H. Kellner, M.D.
Electroconvulsive Therapy Professor, Departments of Psychiatry and Neurology, Director, ECT Services, Medical University of South Carolina, Charleston, South Carolina

Ron Kikinis, M.D.

Director, Surgical Planning Laboratory, MRI Division, Department of Radiology, Brigham and Women's Hospital; Associate Professor, Department of Radiology, Harvard Medical School, Boston, Massachusetts

Jean A. King, Ph.D.

Associate Professor, Department of Psychiatry, University of Massachusetts Medical School, Worchester, Massachusetts

Stephen M. Kosslyn, Ph.D.

Professor of Psychology, Department of Psychology, Harvard University, Cambridge, Massachusetts; Associate Psychologist in Neurology, Department of Neurology, Massachusetts General Hospital, Boston, Massachusetts

Marc Laruelle, M.D.

Associate Professor, Departments of Psychiatry and Radiology, Columbia University College of Physicians and Surgeons, New York State Psychiatric Institute, New York, New York

Ilise Lombardo, M.D.

Research Fellow, Department of Psychiatry, Columbia University, College of Physicians and Surgeons, New York State Psychiatric Institute, New York, New York

Stephan E. Maier, M.D., Ph.D.

Research Associate, MRI Division, Department of Radiology, Brigham and Women's Hospital; Assistant Professor, Harvard Medical School, Boston, Massachusetts

Andrea L. Malizia, M.D., M.R.C.Psych., M.B.B.S., B.A.

Honorary Senior Lecturer in Clinical Psychopharmacology, Psychopharmacology Unit, University of Bristol, Bristol, United Kingdom

Helen S. Mayberg, M.D., F.R.C.P.C.
Sandra A. Rotman Chair in Neuropsychiatry and Professor, Departments of Psychiatry and Neurology, Rotman Research Institute, University of Toronto, Toronto, Ontario, Canada

Robert W. McCarley, M.D.
Professor and Chair, Harvard Medical School, Department of Psychiatry; Director, Laboratory of Neuroscience, VA Boston Healthcare System, Brockton, Massachusetts

Constance M. Moore, Ph.D.
Assistant Physicist, Brain Imaging Center, McLean Hospital; Instructor, Department of Psychiatry, Harvard Medical School, Belmont, Massachusetts

David P. Olson, M.D., Ph.D.
Assistant Professor, Department of Psychiatry, University of Massachusetts Medical School, Worchester, Massachusetts

Bradley S. Peterson, M.D.
House Jameson Associate Professor of Child Psychiatry and Director of Neuroimaging, Yale Child Study Center, New Haven, Connecticut

Daniel S. Pine, M.D.
Intramural Research Program, National Insitute of Mental Health, Bethesda, Maryland

Roger K. Pitman, M.D.
Coordinator, Research and Development, Veterans Affairs Medical Center, Manchester, New Hampshire; Associate Professor, Department of Psychiatry, Harvard Medical School, Boston, Massachusetts

Robert Plomin, Ph.D.
MRC Research Professor, Social, Genetic and Developmental Psychiatry Research Centre, Institute of Psychiatry, King's College, London, United Kingdom

Scott L. Rauch, M.D.
Director, Psychiatric Neuroimaging Research, Massachusetts General Hospital; Associate Professor, Department of Psychiatry, Harvard Medical School, Boston, Massachusetts

Perry F. Renshaw, M.D., Ph.D.
Director, Brain Imaging Center, McLean Hospital; Associate Professor, Department of Psychiatry, Harvard Medical School, Belmont, Massachusetts

S. Craig Risch, M.D.
Professor, Department of Psychiatry, Medical University of South Carolina, Charleston, South Carolina

Martha E. Shenton, Ph.D.
Professor and Director, Clinical Neuroscience Division, Laboratory of Neuroscience, Department of Psychiatry, Harvard Medical School, VA Boston Healthcare System, Brockton, Massachusetts; Director, Psychiatry and Behavioral Studies, Surgical Planning Laboratory, MRI Division, Department of Radiology, Brigham and Women's Hospital, Harvard Medical School, Boston, Massachusetts

Lisa M. Shin, Ph.D.
Assistant Professor, Department of Psychology, Tufts University, Medford, Massachusetts; Instructor, Department of Psychiatry, Harvard Medical School, Boston, Massachusetts

David A. Silbersweig, M.D.
Codirector, Functional Neuroimaging Laboratory, Department of Psychiatry, Weill Medical College of Cornell University, New York, New York

Andrew M. Speer, M.D.
Senior Staff Fellow, Biological Psychiatry Branch, Division of Intramural Research Programs, National Institute of Mental Health, Bethesda, Maryland

Laurie Stallings, Pharm.D.
Research Fellow, Department of Nuclear Medicine, Medical University of South Carolina, Charleston, South Carolina

Emily Stern, M.D.
Codirector, Functional Neuroimaging Laboratory, Department of Psychiatry, Weill Medical College of Cornell University, New York, New York

Eve Stoddard
Research Assistant, Brain Imaging Center, McLean Hospital, Belmont, Massachusetts

Vidya Upadhyaya, M.D.
Research Fellow, Department of Psychiatry, Medical University of South Carolina, Charleston, South Carolina

Diana J. Vincent, Ph.D.
Associate Professor, Department of Radiology, Medical University of South Carolina, Charleston, South Carolina

Carl-Fredrik Westin, Ph.D.
Research Associate, Department of Radiology, Brigham and Women's Hospital; Instructor, Department of Radiology, Harvard Medical School, Boston, Massachusetts

Paul J. Whalen, Ph.D.
Assistant Professor, Departments of Psychiatry and Psychology, University of Wisconsin, Madison, Wisconsin

INTRODUCTION

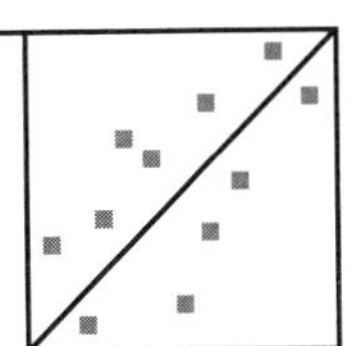

Psychiatric neuroimaging research has progressed considerably in the past decade. In tandem with impressive advances in imaging technology, innovative strategies have been developed for exploiting the awesome potential of these new tools. Presented in this volume are myriad experimental designs; in each chapter, the authors use accounts of their own research as vehicles for illustrating the power of particular paradigmatic approaches. Thus, we hope to demonstrate the wealth of ways by which neuroimaging can contribute to the field of psychiatry. These techniques not only hold promise for delineating pathophysiology and advancing basic neuroscience but also may yield findings of direct clinical significance—from diagnostic tests, to predictors of treatment response, to new medications. In this introduction, we briefly outline the range of methodology and psychopathology addressed by the authors.

Some of the earliest psychiatric imaging studies involved systematic qualitative analysis of routine clinical computed tomography scans or magnetic resonance images. Often relying on a radiologist's subjective judgment, these initial investigations emphasized global atrophy, ventricular size, or the presence of discrete lesions such as infarcts and masses. Subsequently, morphometric techniques emerged for quantifying regional brain volumes. With state-of-the-art morphometric magnetic resonance imaging (MRI), subtle abnormalities that may be imperceptible to the clinical neuroradiologist can be detected and characterized. **Shenton and colleagues** describe contemporary morphometric techniques in the context of their research pertaining to schizophrenia.

Cognitive activation studies of psychiatric disease entail validation of experimental tasks in the service of tapping designated cognitive domains or reliably recruiting brain regions of interest. In this way, such paradigms can serve to test specific hypotheses regarding the functional integrity of implicated neural systems. **Heckers and Rauch** provide examples of this approach from their studies of schizophrenia and obsessive-compulsive disorder.

Continuing the theme of cognitive activation paradigms, **Whalen and colleagues** describe methods for probing nonconscious information processing systems. Specifically, by using masked stimuli and other task manipulations, these investigators have been able to assay brain activity that occurs outside the realm of conscious awareness. The authors suggest that this approach may be particularly germane to studies of anxiety disorders. Recent findings involving the amygdala and striatum are highlighted.

Symptom provocation paradigms provide a means for experimentally manipulating study conditions to identify the neural correlates of psychiatric symptoms. This capability is particularly valuable in psychiatry, given that the current diagnostic scheme is symptom based in its criteria. A variety of specific strategies have been employed to induce states of interest. **Shin and colleagues** describe the use of script-driven imagery and in vivo exposure methods, while reviewing findings from symptom provocation studies across anxiety disorders against the backdrop of the normal emotional state induction literature.

Some psychiatric symptoms are not easily induced because they occur spontaneously, and some are not easily imaged because they occur sporadically. **Stern and Silbersweig** describe symptom capture paradigms and explain the innovative imaging techniques that they derived to study hallucinations and psychomotor tics.

With the advent of human brain mapping methods and the proliferation of activation studies, investigators have highlighted the importance of state-related considerations. **George and colleagues** describe new methods for experimentally manipulating the state of the central nervous system in a safe and noninvasive manner. Specifically, they describe the ability to induce or inhibit cortical activity in select brain regions with repetitive transcranial magnetic stimulation (TMS), with measurement of the accompanying neural behavior being performed using serial perfusion MRI. These paradigms have been designed to explore how various brain systems interact to regulate complex processes such as mood. Using TMS, researchers can induce "reversible lesions" that have the unprecedented potential for permitting delineation of the role of various brain regions across functional domains.

Continuing the theme of major depression, **Dougherty and Mayberg** describe neutral-state pretreatment-posttreatment positron emission tomography (PET) studies. By employing a longitudinal design in conjunction with a pharmacologic manipulation, such paradigms are intended to provide information about therapeutic mechanisms of psychotropic medications as well as possible predictors of treatment response. The authors synthesize findings across numerous neuroimaging studies and present an original neurobiologic model of major depression.

Beyond their role in elucidating the neural underpinnings of psychiatric diseases, neuroimaging techniques also play a part in the development of psychotropic medication. **Dougherty and colleagues** provide an overview of imaging strategies to be applied in pharmaceutical development. PET and single photon emission computed tomography (SPECT) methods for characterizing the in vivo behavior of candidate drugs are emphasized.

Lombardo and colleagues describe SPECT receptor characterization methods for studying the dopaminergic system. In addition to measuring receptor binding capacity at rest in health and disease, the authors have explored new avenues for quantifying endogenous transmitter release in response to pharmacologic manipulations.

Malizia describes methods for imaging benzodiazepine receptors. He presents a review of recent findings on this topic and suggests a future role for these strategies in the study of psychiatric diseases and their treatments.

Classic functional neuroimaging studies employ neutral-state paradigms to contrast brain activity profiles between groups during a nominal resting state. Such neutral-state studies yield invaluable information, providing initial clues to the pathophysiology of various psychiatric illnesses. By integrating structural and functional imaging data from the same subjects, researchers may attain insights that could not have been possible with either modality alone. For example, a subtle functional abnormality may prompt detailed morphometric analysis of the corresponding structure; conversely, quantification of regional volumetric abnormalities can be used to generate volume-adjusted factors for interpreting the corresponding functional data. Furthermore, fused structural and functional renderings provide an enriched view of the brain, with representations of more than three dimensions. **Drevets** discusses the integration of structural and functional neuroimaging techniques in the context of his group's research on major depression.

Henry and colleagues explain the gamut of applications afforded by magnetic resonance spectroscopy (MRS). The authors review studies in which MRS was used to quantify brain concentrations of exogenous compounds, as well as research based on the measurement of endogenous products as neuronal markers and indices of cellular energy metabolism.

Until recently, psychiatric imaging research was largely restricted to adult populations. However, with the evolution of modern morphometric techniques, as well as the invention of noncontrast functional MRI, the potential to study children and adolescents has been realized. **Pine and colleagues** have taken a leading role in child psychiatric neuroimaging research. They present examples from their own work in Tourette's syndrome and anxiety disorders, while reviewing special considerations in the study of developmental phenomena.

Although the emphasis of this volume is on human studies, a chapter is included on the power of imaging animals. **Ferris and colleagues** present data from research in nonhuman primate preparations, demonstrating how this work can contribute to models of emotion.

Finally, **Kosslyn and Plomin** explore how neuroimaging methods can be employed to investigate genetic contributions to normal cognitive function. Ultimately, neuroimaging is likely to be used for characterizing endophenotypes in genetic research of psychiatric diseases. Consequently, there is much excitement about the paradigmatic aspects of neuroimaging studies designed to delineate heritable factors.

ACKNOWLEDGMENTS

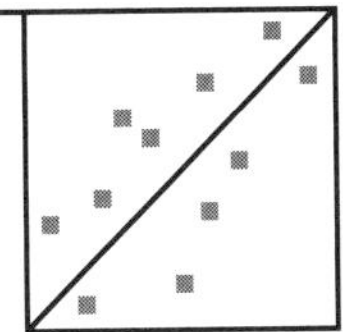

This volume is largely the by-product of a seminar series conducted in conjunction with the Psychopharmacology Unit of Massachusetts General Hospital, under the supervision of Jerrold F. Rosenbaum, M.D. We express our thanks to Dr. Rosenbaum for his thoughtful guidance and generosity in fostering the completion of this work. In addition, we acknowledge our mentors and collaborators; in particular, we express our appreciation to Michael A. Jenike, M.D., Nathaniel M. Alpert, Ph.D., Alan J. Fischman, M.D., Ph.D., Robert H. Rubin, M.D., and Ned Cassem, M.D. We thank Yong Ke, Ph.D., of McLean Hospital and Harvard Medical School, and Steve Weise of the Department of Nuclear Medicine of Massachusetts General Hospital for their contributions to the cover art. Finally, we thank the editorial and production staff of American Psychiatric Publishing, Inc., for their expertise, support, and patience.

1

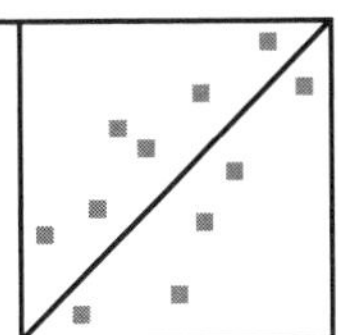

MORPHOMETRIC MAGNETIC RESONANCE IMAGING STUDIES

Findings in Schizophrenia

Martha E. Shenton, Ph.D.
Melissa Frumin, M.D.
Robert W. McCarley, M.D.
Stephan E. Maier, M.D., Ph.D.
Carl-Fredrik Westin, Ph.D.
Iris A. Fischer, A.B.
Chandlee Dickey, M.D.
Ron Kikinis, M.D.

Schizophrenia affects close to 1% of the general population and is often psychologically and financially devastating to patients, their families, and the community. The onset generally occurs in early adulthood, when individuals are entering what are considered to be the most productive and formative years of life. Symptoms of the disorder may include auditory hallucinations, disor-

---

Portions of this chapter are adapted from previous publications, including Shenton ME: "Temporal Lobe Structural Abnormalities in Schizophrenia: A Selective Review and Presentation of New MR Findings," in *Psychopathology: The Evolving Science of Mental Disorders.* Edited by Matthysse S, Levy D, Kagan J, et al. New York, Cambridge University Press, 1996, pp. 51–99; Shenton ME, Wible CG, McCarley RW: "A Review of Magnetic Resonance Imaging Studies of Brain Abnormalities in Schizophrenia," in *Brain Imaging in Clinical Psychiatry.* Edited by Krishnan KRR, Doraiswamy PM. New York, Marcel Dekker, 1997, pp. 297–380; Anderson JE, O'Donnell BF, McCarley RW, et al.: "Progressive Changes in Schizophrenia: Do They Exist and What Do They Mean?" *Restorative Neurology and Neuroscience* 12:1–10, 1998; and McCarley RW, Wible CG, Frumin M, et al.: "MRI Anatomy of Schizophrenia." *Biological Psychiatry* 45:1099–1119, 1999.

dered thinking, and delusions as well as avolition, anhedonia, and apathy. Not all symptoms are observed in every patient, nor are the same symptoms necessarily observed in a given patient over time. The course of the illness is also variable, and there are often exacerbations and remissions. Although some patients show progressive deterioration, it is not unusual for some patients to remain stable and for others to improve (for example, see M. Bleuler 1971; Ciompi 1980; Huber et al. 1975, 1980; Tsuang et al. 1979, 1981). Additionally, broad areas of functioning are frequently disturbed, including attention, memory, emotion, motivation, thought and language processes, and social functioning (see, for instance, Nestor et al. 1993; Park and Holzman 1992; Saykin et al. 1994; Shenton et al. 1987, 1992).

The etiology of schizophrenia is currently unknown, although it is likely that there are several interactive biological factors (e.g., genetic factors, fetal anomalies) and environmental factors (e.g., viral infection, fetal insult) that predispose individuals to schizophrenia (see, for example, Arndt et al. 1995; Crow 1990a, 1990b; Kendler et al. 1993). In addition, subtypes of schizophrenia may result from different interactions among these presumed causative factors.

This multitude of symptoms, courses, and outcomes, as well as etiologies, has led some to argue that schizophrenia is a complex disorder best conceptualized as a syndrome rather than a single entity. The distinction, though heuristic, has not helped to further our understanding of the etiology of schizophrenia. Any theory about schizophrenia must, however, account for the variety of symptoms, courses, and outcomes observed in this patient population.

During the past two decades, one of the most promising areas of research in schizophrenia has been brain abnormalities. The notion that brain abnormalities may be implicated in the pathophysiology of schizophrenia can be traced back to Kraepelin (1919/1971) and Bleuler (1911/1950), who first described this disorder. However, results of early efforts to identify brain abnor-

---

We thank our collaborators at Harvard Medical School, especially Ferenc A. Jolesz, M.D., James Levitt, M.D., and Yoshio Hirayasu, M.D., Ph.D. We also thank Lawrence P. Panych, Ph.D., Stephanie Fraone, B.A., Marianna Jakab, M.S., and William M. Wells III, Ph.D., for their technical assistance and Alaka Pellock, A.B., Christopher Dodd, B.A., and Marie Fairbanks for their administrative assistance. Additionally, we gratefully acknowledge the support of the National Institute of Mental Health (grants MH 50740 and MH 01110 to M.E.S. and grant MH 40799 to R.W.M.), National Institutes of Health (grants NIH P41 RR13218 and R01 RR11747 to R.K.), Department of Veterans Affairs Center for Clinical and Basic Neuroscience Studies of Schizophrenia (R.W.M.), and Department of Veterans Affairs (Merit Review Awards to M.E.S. and to R.W.M.).

malities were inconsistent, primarily because of a lack of sophisticated measurement tools (see, for example, Alzheimer 1897; Crichton-Browne 1879; Jacobi et al. 1927; Kahlbaum 1874). Consequently, progress, as well as interest, in this area came to a near standstill (for reviews of early postmortem and imaging studies, see Benes 1995; Bogerts et al. 1993b; Chua and McKenna 1995; Gur and Pearlson 1993; Kirch and Weinberger 1986; McCarley et al. 1999; Pearlson and Marsh 1993; Rauch and Renshaw 1995; Seidman 1983; Shenton 1996; Shenton et al. 1997). In fact, as recently as 1972, Plum discouraged research in this area, stating that "schizophrenia is the graveyard of neuropathologists." Although some researchers continued to believe that studying the brain and its functions was critical to understanding schizophrenia (see, for example, Kety 1959; MacLean 1952; Stevens 1973; Torrey and Peterson 1974), it was not until the first computed tomography (CT) study of lateral ventricles in schizophrenic patients (Johnstone et al. 1976) that there was a renewed interest and belief that brain abnormalities in schizophrenia could be identified and understood. This seminal study led to a proliferation of CT and magnetic resonance imaging (MRI) studies of schizophrenia. The newer imaging techniques encompass both in vivo structural brain imaging (for instance, see Andreasen et al. 1986; Barta et al. 1990; Johnstone et al. 1976; Shenton et al. 1992; Weinberger et al. 1979) and postmortem neurochemical and cellular studies (see, for example, Benes 1995; Bogerts et al. 1985, 1993b; Brown et al. 1986; Stevens 1973). There is now evidence to suggest that brain abnormalities are present in schizophrenia and that at least some structural brain changes may originate from neurodevelopmental anomalies (for example, see Akbarian et al. 1993a, 1993b; Benes 1989; Heyman and Murray 1992; Jakob and Beckmann 1986, 1989; Kikinis et al. 1994; Murray and Lewis 1987; see also reviews by Shenton et al. 1992, 1997; Weinberger 1987).

In this chapter we review the evidence regarding morphometric MRI–detected brain abnormalities in schizophrenia. We begin with a description and review of some of the technological advances in MRI that have made it possible to address heretofore unanswerable questions concerning brain abnormalities in schizophrenia. These questions are listed in Table 1–1.

We then review morphometric MRI findings in schizophrenia, including findings from our laboratory, where studies have focused on the temporal lobe, a region of the brain linked to many of the symptoms observed in schizophrenia, including verbal and memory problems, delusions, hallucinations, and formal thought disorder. We conclude with a synthesis of MRI findings and a discussion of the direction of future imaging studies.

TABLE 1–1. Questions that we can now begin to address

Are there brain abnormalities in schizophrenia?
- Where are these abnormalities?
- Are the abnormalities focal or diffuse?

Are brain abnormalities related to the symptoms observed in schizophrenia?
- Are some brain abnormalities specific to schizophrenia and others nonspecific concomitants of psychosis?

What is the time course of these abnormalities?
- At what stage of development do these brain abnormalities occur? Do some occur early (i.e., prenatally and/or perinatally) and others occur over the course of development?

What are the etiologies of brain abnormalities in schizophrenia?
- Is an abnormality in one region linked functionally or anatomically to an abnormality in another?

Are there potential neuroprotective treatments?
- If so, will the brain abnormalities change?

■ ADVANCES IN MRI TECHNOLOGY

An extensive review of the basic principles of MRI is not possible here. However, nuclear MRI in medicine and psychiatry is described in several reviews (see, for example, Bradley et al. 1985; Callaghan 1991; Ernst et al. 1987; Krishnan and MacFall 1997; Slichter 1990; Young 1984). Available through the Internet is a review of basic imaging techniques that includes many examples of high spatial resolution images as well as different pulse sequences with representative images (Hornak 1996 [Web site: http://www.cis.rit.edu/htbooks/mri]).

Our goal in this section is to provide a context for understanding MRI findings in schizophrenia. We begin, therefore, with a description of early magnetic resonance (MR) scans and the advantages of MR scans over CT scans, followed by a summary of MR scan parameters and image-quality trade-offs that must be considered when selecting specific MRI parameters (see also Bradley et al. 1985; Horowitz 1991). Next we provide an example and a description of the double spin-echo MRI pulse sequence selected for our MRI studies of schizophrenia, followed by a description of the segmentation procedures used to identify different tissue classes. This is followed by an example and a description of the three-dimensional (3D) MRI pulse sequence that we use to evaluate temporal lobe regions of interest (ROIs). Additionally, we discuss the development of a brain atlas based on images derived from this 3D MRI pulse sequence. We then describe 3D visualization techniques and future plans for model-based segmentation using the brain atlas to identify automatically the shape and volume of brain structures in new MRI data sets. Finally, we describe a new protocol for diffusion tensor MRI of the brain that we will be using to evaluate more closely white matter abnormalities in schizophrenia.

The First Magnetic Resonance Images

Computed tomograms, or CT scans, were introduced into medicine in the early 1970s, and the introduction of nuclear MR quickly followed. In 1982, the first MR image of a human hand, based on Fourier encoding, was produced (Bradley et al. 1985). The term *nuclear magnetic resonance* lost favor because of its potential negative connotations, and *magnetic resonance imaging* was coined to describe this new noninvasive imaging technique that uses radiofrequency waves (i.e., electromagnetic radiation in the radiofrequency range and magnetic fields) to produce images. In 1984, Smith and colleagues conducted the first MRI study of schizophrenia.

The history of CT and MRI technology is thus relatively short, although advances in MRI technology since the early 1980s have been remarkable. MRI offers several advantages over CT scans. For example, MR images, unlike CT, provide excellent gray and white matter contrast. Additionally, MR images are not prone to "bone hardening" artifact (streak artifacts that appear in the part of the image closest to bone) as CT scans are. On CT scans, this kind of artifact is also visible in the medial temporal lobe, a region surrounding the temporal bone. Given that this brain region is important in studies of schizophrenia, MRI offers a significant advantage over CT in such studies. MRI also is noninvasive and involves no radiation, and the physics of MRI are based on more complex and more versatile contrast mechanisms than the physics of CT (i.e., T1, T2, proton density, and blood flow in the case of MRI, and tissue absorption in the case of CT). Further, longitudinal studies of progressive disorders such as multiple sclerosis, and perhaps schizophrenia, as well as tracking of tumor growth after resection, to give just a few examples, can be performed using MRI without undue concern about repeated exposure to radiation, as would be the case with CT.

Early MR images, however, were inferior to present-day MR images because of limited spatial resolution, restrictions with regard to the area scanned (the entire brain could not be scanned), weak magnetic field strength, patient motion, inhomogeneity in the magnetic field, and the acquisition of thick slices (i.e., thicker than 1.0 cm). Additionally, there were often gaps of up to 7 mm between slices. All these factors compromised the quality of early MR images, and it was not until the late 1980s that the signal-to-noise ratio (SNR) improved sufficiently to make it possible to extract objective, quantitative information from MR scans (Gerig et al. 1989, 1990; Höhne et al. 1990). In addition, measurements of neuroanatomy all too often relied on crude and imprecise methods such as one-dimensional linear and two-dimensional planimetric analyses of cross sections of brain regions (for further details, see Filipek et al. 1988; Pfefferbaum et al. 1990; Wyper et al. 1979). Such measurements not only were less than accurate but also did not take full advantage of the information contained in MR images.

Today, many improvements in MR image acquisition and processing have made it possible to exploit more fully information contained in MR images. Such improvements have also resulted in more precise and accurate measurements, factors particularly important in the study of schizophrenia, in which brain abnormalities are often subtle and thus harder to detect than in other disorders. The application of these tools to schizophrenia is thus promising. We have used these newer MR image acquisition and processing techniques in our MRI studies of schizophrenia, described in this chapter.

Factors Influencing Magnetic Resonance Image Quality

Multiple factors influence MR image quality. One such factor is magnetic field strength. In general, the stronger the magnetic field, the faster the precession rate and resonant frequency of protons and the higher the image quality. Today, it is common to use magnets with field strengths of 1.5 teslas (T), and some research centers use high-field magnets of 3 or 4 T. Most of the parameters that determine image quality are selected before imaging and are dependent on the available hardware and software. The goal is to select scan parameters that both optimize the tissue contrast of interest and provide the highest spatial resolution possible. However, the quality of images is dependent on a combination of factors as well as on a number of possible trade-offs, summarized in Table 1–2.

In reviewing Table 1–2, it becomes clear that, although increasing the SNR is important for increasing image quality, factors that increase SNR, such as increased slice thickness and field of view (FOV), also decrease spatial resolution. At the bottom of Table 1–2 is information pertaining to patient time in the magnet and pulse sequences. In general, it is clinically optimal to reduce the amount of time patients are in the magnet, although this, too, is a trade-off. The choice of a specific pulse sequence is also important because

TABLE 1–2. Magnetic resonance imaging parameters: optimization and associated trade-offs

Parameter	How to optimize parameter	Trade-offs and considerations
Magnetic field strength	Increase number of tesla.	Monetary cost
Signal-to-noise ratio (SNR)	Increase NEX, TR, slice thickness, and FOV and decrease TE, AM, and bandwidth.	Increasing NEX results in longer scan time. Increasing TR alters image contrast and increases scan time Increasing slice thickness and FOV decreases spatial resolution, thereby possibly missing small tissue abnormalities. Decreasing TE alters image contrast. Decreasing AM decreases spatial resolution. Decreasing bandwidth increases chemical shift artifact.
Acquisition matrix (AM)	Increase AM to increase spatial resolution.	Decreasing AM decreases spatial resolution (e.g., 512×512 to 256×256 to 128×128). Increasing AM increases spatial resolution but decreases SNR. Increasing AM may increase scan time.
Receiver bandwidth	Decrease bandwidth to increase SNR.	Decreasing bandwidth increases chemical shift artifact.
Number of excitations (NEX)	Increase NEX to increase SNR.	Increasing NEX increases scan time. Decreasing NEX reduces SNR.
Slice thickness	Decrease slice thickness to increase spatial resolution.	Increasing slice thickness decreases spatial resolution. Decreasing slice thickness (i.e., acquiring thin slices) increases spatial resolution but decreases SNR.
Number of slices	Increase number of slices.	Increasing number of slices *may* increase scan time for 2DFT imaging and *will* increase scan time for 3DFT imaging.

TABLE 1–2. Magnetic resonance imaging parameters: optimization and associated trade-offs *(continued)*

Parameter	How to optimize parameter	Trade-offs and considerations
Interslice gap	Avoid interslice gap.	Increasing interslice gap reduces cross-talk between slices, but this may exclude important information not sampled, which could further result in measurements of ROIs being less informative than contiguous slices.
Imaging plane (axial, sagittal, coronal)	Select imaging plane perpendicular to region or structure of interest.	Axial, coronal, and sagittal planes are conventional planes; oblique plane can be used. Optimal plane for evaluating one structure of interest may not be optimal plane for evaluating second or third structure of interest. For example, plane that is perpendicular to hippocampus, and therefore optimal, is coronal plane. In this plane, slicing of hippocampus is similar to cutting a sausage from front to back. In axial plane, slicing would be similar to cutting a sausage from top to bottom. With isotropic voxels, imaging plane is less important because images can be acquired and then reformatted in any plane.
Field of view (FOV)	Decrease FOV to increase spatial resolution.	SNR is decreased with smaller FOV.
Patient artifact	Decrease patient artifact.	Patient artifact includes movement (e.g., Maier et al. 1994), metal, and chemical shift. Techniques have been developed to reduce these artifacts, including cardiac gating, flow compensation, and presaturation. Chemical shift artifacts can also be reduced by using stronger frequency-encoding gradients (i.e., by increasing bandwidth).

TABLE 1–2. Magnetic resonance imaging parameters: optimization and associated trade-offs *(continued)*

Parameter	How to optimize parameter	Trade-offs and considerations
Scanner artifact	Decrease scanner artifact.	Inhomogeneities in magnetic field lead to distortion artifacts in images. Solution is to perform daily tests on scanner to adjust inhomogeneities in magnetic field. Inhomogeneities in transmit-receive RF field may lead to differences in pixel intensity of same tissue. For example, white matter in one part of image may have different signal intensity than white matter in another part of image. Solution is to use segmentation algorithms that correct for these inhomogeneities. Another possible artifact is wraparound, which occurs when FOV is too small for area being imaged, resulting in area outside FOV being placed on opposite end of area being imaged. Two other artifacts are cross-talk between slices and partial voluming. Latter occurs when structure is close to same size as voxel and information that includes low-signal intensity is obscured. Solution is to decrease slice thickness. Other artifacts include shim, gradient, and RF artifacts.
Time in magnet	Decrease amount of time in magnet.	To optimize some parameters, amount of time in magnet must be increased.
Pulse sequence	Select pulse sequence to produce desired tissue contrast (i.e., adjust TE and TR, along with other MRI factors, to optimize tissue contrast).	Often, optimizing contrast for one tissue does not optimize contrast for another tissue class. It is difficult, for example, to optimize contrast between gray matter, white matter, and CSF, although a pulse sequence can be selected that optimizes contrast between gray and white matter in one sequence and brain (gray and white together) and CSF in another sequence.

Note. 2DFT = two-dimensional Fourier transform; 3DFT = three-dimensional Fourier transform; AM = acquisition matrix; CSF = cerebrospinal fluid; FOV = field of view; MRI = magnetic resonance imaging; NEX = number of excitations; RF = radio frequency; SNR = signal-to-noise ratio; TE = echo time; TR = repetition time.

sequences determine tissue contrast, and the sequence should therefore be selected on the basis of considerations such as the tissue contrast needed to discern an abnormality, the optimal plane for visualizing the ROI, and patient time in the scanner. All these factors must be balanced in the final selection of an image acquisition protocol.

In the next section, we describe the double spin-echo pulse sequence used for our MRI studies of schizophrenia, whereby two echoes of the same neuroanatomical region are acquired to obtain excellent contrast between gray and white matter in the first echo and excellent contrast between brain (gray and white matter) and cerebrospinal fluid (CSF) in the second echo (i.e., proton density–weighted image and T2-weighted image, respectively).

We then describe tissue classification, or segmentation, which is the process of identifying and classifying image voxels[1] (i.e., gray matter, white matter, or CSF). Next we describe a 3D Fourier transform spoiled gradient-recalled acquisition in steady state (3DFT SPGR) sequence, selected for our manually guided segmentation of ROIs within the temporal lobe. We also provide an example of the visualization capabilities derived from 3D surface renderings of segmented ROIs, and we discuss our work with model-based segmentation using a 3D digitized brain atlas as a template. Lastly, we present a brain diffusion tensor MRI sequence, line-scan diffusion imaging, developed at Brigham and Women's Hospital, that we will be using to examine white matter abnormalities in schizophrenic patients.

Double Spin-Echo Sequence

As noted previously, MRI pulse sequences are selected to optimize different tissue contrasts. We have been interested in quantifying gray matter, white matter, and CSF in the entire brain and wanted to develop an automated segmentation algorithm that would separate these tissue classes (see, for example, Shenton et al. 1992), particularly because manual segmentation of all three tissue classes in the entire brain is neither practical nor feasible.

We selected a double spin-echo acquisition sequence because that sequence provides different contrast information (a proton density–weighted image and a T2-weighted image) at each neuroanatomical level throughout the entire brain. We were interested in highlighting the contrast between gray and white matter in the first echo and in highlighting the contrast between

---

[1]The term *pixel* is used to refer to a picture element, and *voxel* is used to refer to a 3D pixel, or volume element.

CSF and brain tissue in the second echo. We thus selected a proton density–weighted image, or T1-weighted image (first echo), in which CSF and fluid appear darker (lower signal intensity) relative to gray and white matter (higher signal intensity), thus optimizing the contrast between gray and white matter (Figure 1–1, A). We then selected a T2-weighted image (second echo), in which CSF appears brighter (higher signal intensity) relative to gray and white matter (lower signal intensity), thus optimizing the contrast between CSF and brain tissue (Figure 1–1, B). The MRI parameters selected were the following: echo times (TEs), 30 and 80 milliseconds (ms); repetition time (TR), 3,000 ms; axial plane; 3-mm-thick interleaved slices with no gaps between slices; FOV, 24 cm; and bandwidth, ±12.8 kHz (for both echoes), resulting in 108 slices 3 mm thick at 54 brain levels.

Segmentation of Tissue Classes

A number of image processing tools have been developed to segment tissue into distinct tissue classes (see, for example, Cline et al. 1988, 1990; Kikinis et al. 1992; Wells et al. 1996). Our approach begins with a user-guided classification of tissue using seed points. *Seed points* refer to the selection of a small set of pixels that are representative of the signal intensities for the different tissue classes. We chose this approach because a user can readily see beyond nonuniformities in images to select the most representative points for tissue classification. Additionally, knowledge of neuroanatomy can be used to select the initial seed points used for the multivariate classification derived from each of the two images of the double spin-echo MRI data set (described earlier).[2]

These user-guided seed points are selected from areas of high contrast in tissue classes, such as a slice through the largest body of the lateral ventricles where the contrast between CSF and gray and white matter is clearly visible. Information from seed points can then be used from the first echo, which shows good contrast between gray matter and white matter, and from the second echo, which shows good contrast between brain tissue and CSF. Once multiple seed points (generally 12–15 per tissue class) are selected, a two-dimensional map of their intensity distribution can be constructed using the signal intensity from each echo as the axes of the map. In Figure 1–1, E, the two-dimensional feature map is displayed with the first echo on the X axis and

---

[2]The segmentation algorithms described can be applied to both spin-echo and 3DFT SPGR images. Here, for the purpose of illustration, we describe their application to double spin-echo images.

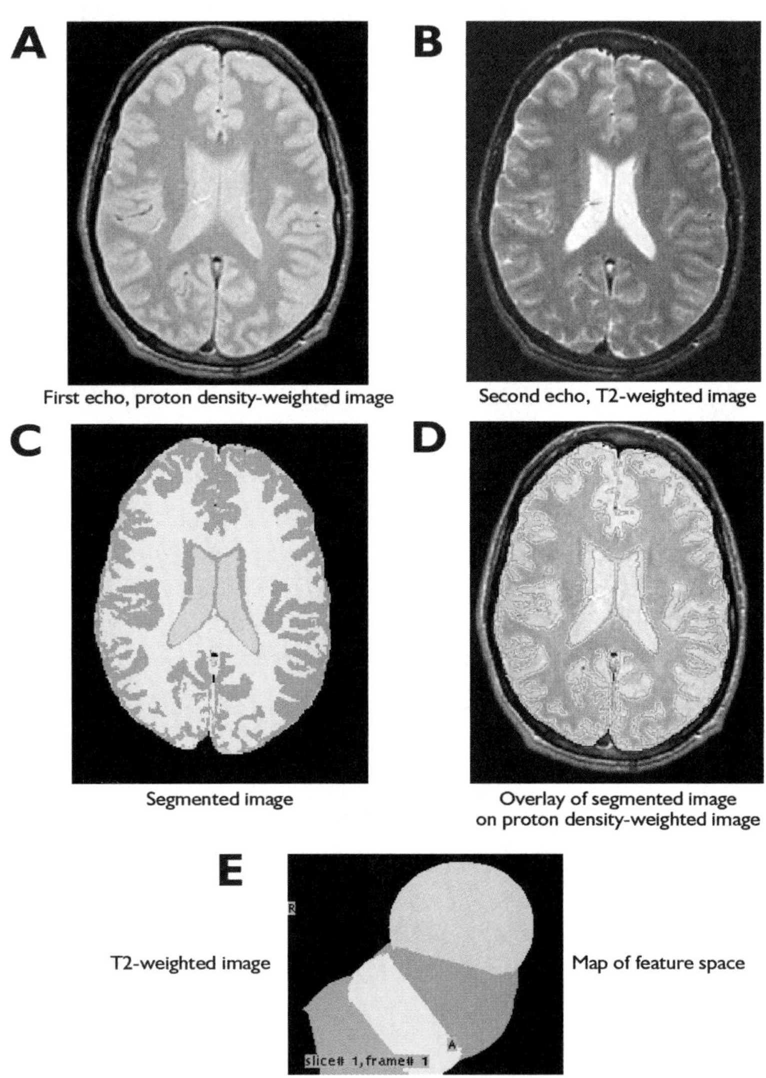

FIGURE 1–1. Double spin-echo pulse sequence images and maps.
First *(A)* and second *(B)* echo images for one axial slice at the level of the lateral ventricles. *(C)* Display map showing the classification of pixels into three tissue classes, with gray matter (gray), white matter (yellow), and cerebrospinal fluid (CSF) (blue) visible. *(D)* Overlay of the segmented tissue classes on the proton density–weighted image. *(E)* Map of feature space for the four tissue classes: gray matter (gray), white matter (yellow), CSF (blue), and skin (beige). Skin is classified in the first step of our segmentation process, when brain is separated from the intracranial cavity.

the second echo on the Y axis. The classification of tissue into gray matter, white matter, and CSF can be seen in Figure 1–1, C. An overlay of the segmented tissue map on the proton density–weighted image is also shown (Figure 1–1, D). Images at one neuroanatomical level (i.e., two slices at the same neuroanatomical level) are displayed in Figure 1–1, but it should be mentioned that initial seed points are used to classify all voxels throughout all slices in the entire brain. A histogram program is then used to sum the volume for each voxel, over each slice of the brain, for each tissue class.

To classify brain tissue, we have used segmentation algorithms based on a nonparametric nearest-neighbor cluster analysis (Cline et al. 1988, 1990). We now also use an iterative expectation-maximization (EM) algorithm that combines both the statistical classification of tissue classes with the automatic identification of pixel intensity inhomogeneities in the images (see, for instance, Wells et al. 1996). Accurate segmentation of tissue classes from MR images is difficult because of the spatial inhomogeneities in pixel intensity (see also the description in Table 1–2). For example, a pixel representing white matter in the upper left side of an image is often much brighter than a pixel representing white matter in the lower right side of the same slice, because of inhomogeneities in the transmit-receive radiofrequency field.

The EM segmenter alternates two computational steps to solve this problem. In one step, the spatial intensity inhomogeneities are estimated, and in a second step, this estimate is used to improve the accuracy of the tissue classification. More specifically, an initial semiautomated segmentation algorithm, used in our previous studies (Cline et al. 1988, 1990), is used as the input to the EM segmenter, and then the EM algorithm improves the segmentation in several iterations (see Wells et al. 1996 for further details).

The EM segmenter uses the same statistical model, or semiautomated segmentation as the input, or label map, for all the scans in a given acquisition type, thus eliminating any error that might result from different users creating individual label maps for each individual subject. Previously, a label map was used for each subject, an approach that was labor-intensive and more prone to error because label maps were created by multiple trained users. With the EM segmenter, one single statistical model, based on one label map (created from seed points containing information about the signal intensities for the three tissue classes), is used for all subjects in a given study. Additionally, estimating inhomogeneities in the MR images allows for a more consistent segmentation of scans across magnet upgrades and/or different imaging sites. Finally, the EM segmenter is more consistent in estimating tissue classes than were previous semiautomated segmentation procedures used by our group (Wells et al. 1996).

In summary, we selected a double spin-echo acquisition for our MRI schizophrenia studies in order to optimize the tissue contrast between gray matter, white matter, and CSF. We use the EM segmenter to classify gray matter, white matter, and CSF automatically. We plan to replace the double spin-echo pulse sequence with a fast spin-echo sequence or rapid acquisition with relaxation enhancement sequence. The fast spin echo will reduce the scan time of the conventional spin echo by a factor of four, and such time savings will allow us to reduce slice thickness to 2 mm. We will thus image the entire brain in approximately the same time as with a conventional spin-echo protocol, but with much higher spatial resolution.

3DFT SPGR Sequence

Three-dimensional Fourier transform spoiled gradient-recalled acquisition (3DFT SPGR) in a steady state sequence is a newer pulse sequence that affords excellent gray and white matter contrast. Spin-echo sequences use frequency and phase encoding in two dimensions to determine spatial information for each slice, and this sequence involves "the use of two-dimensional Fourier transform to decode information into a recognizable image for each slice" (Horowitz 1991, p. 128). With 3DFT imaging, a slab covering all slices of interest is selected, instead of individual slices, and "then each of three orthogonal axes is encoded: frequency along x axis and phase along the y and the z axis" (Horowitz 1991, p. 128). 3DFT imaging is thus needed to encode information because there are three axes involved.

A major advantage of 3DFT over two-dimensional Fourier transform (2DFT) is that the SNR is improved when thinner slices are used, and therefore images can be more easily reformatted along any direction. Also, thin slices are inherently contiguous, whereas in 2DFT imaging, the interslice gap must be adjusted. Further, the SNR is improved with 3DFT imaging because the signal comes from the whole volume rather than from the individual slice (Kumar et al. 1975). With 3DFT imaging, it is thus possible to obtain nearly isotropic voxels (i.e., $0.9 \times 0.9 \times 1.5$ mm^3) in a relatively short period. One disadvantage of 3DFT compared with 2DFT is that scan time is longer (see also Table 1–3).

Taken together, these improvements in image quality make it possible to use 3D segmentation and visualization techniques to obtain detailed 3D anatomical information. Moreover, these techniques can be used to develop a 3D digitized atlas of the human brain (see the next section).

We have used 3DFT imaging to investigate temporal lobe morphometric abnormalities in schizophrenia. We use a 3DFT SPGR pulse sequence with

TABLE 1–3. Magnetic resonance imaging studies with positive or negative findings in schizophrenia

Brain region	Total no. of studies	Studies with positive findings (%)	Studies with negative findings (%)	Reference[a]
Whole brain	32	19	81	+ (Andreasen 1990, 1994a; Gur 1994, 1998; Jernigan 1991; Nasrallah 1990) – (Barta 1990; Bilder 1994; Blackwood 1991; Breier 1992; Buchanan 1993; Colombo 1993; Dauphinais 1990; DeLisi 1991, 1992; Flaum 1995; Harvey 1993; Hirayasu 1998; Johnstone 1989; Kawasaki 1993; Kelsoe 1988; Marsh 1994; Nopoulos 1995; Reite 1997; Rossi 1990, 1994a; Schlaepfer 1994; Shenton 1992; Sullivan 1998; Vita 1995; Zipursky 1992, 1997)
Ventricles				
Lateral ventricles	43	77	23	+ (Andreasen 1990, 1994a; Barr 1997; Becker 1990[b]; Bogerts 1990[b]; Bornstein 1992; Buchsbaum 1997; Corey-Bloom 1995; Dauphinais 1990; Degreef 1990, 1992c; DeLisi 1991, 1992; Egan 1994; Flaum 1995; Gur 1994; Harvey 1993; Johnstone 1989; Kawasaki 1993; Kelsoe 1988; Lauriello 1997; Lim 1996; Marsh 1994, 1997; Nasrallah 1990; Nopoulos 1995; Rossi 1988; Stratta 1989; Suddath 1989, 1990; Sullivan 1998; Vita 1995; Zipursky 1992) – (Blackwood 1991; Colombo 1993; Hoff 1992; Jernigan 1991; Rossi 1990, 1994a; Schwartz 1992; Schwarzkopf 1990; Shenton 1991, 1992)
Third ventricles	24	67	33	+ (Becker 1996; Bornstein 1992; Dauphinais 1990; Degreef 1990, 1992c; Egan 1994; Flaum 1995; Kelsoe 1988; Lim 1996; Marsh 1994, 1997; Nasrallah 1990; Rossi 1994a; Schwarzkopf 1990; Sullivan 1998; Woodruff 1997b) – (Andreasen 1990; Barta 1990; Colombo 1993; DeLisi 1991; Schwartz 1992; Shenton 1992; Suddath 1990; Zipursky 1992)
Fourth ventricles	3	0	100	– (Rossi 1988; Shenton 1992; Stratta 1989)

TABLE 1–3. Magnetic resonance imaging studies with positive or negative findings in schizophrenia *(continued)*

Brain region	Total no. of studies	Studies with positive findings (%)	Studies with negative findings (%)	Reference[a]
Temporal lobe	90	—	—	
Whole temporal lobe	37	62	38	+ (Andreasen 1994a; Barta 1990; Becker 1996; Bogerts 1990; Dauphinais 1990; DeLisi 1991; Di Michele 1992; Egan 1994; Gur 1998; Harvey 1993; Jernigan 1991; Johnstone 1989; Marsh 1997; Rossi 1988, 1989b, 1990, 1991; Suddath 1989, 1990; Sullivan 1998; Woodruff 1997b; Woods 1996; Zipursky 1992) – (Becker 1990; Bilder 1994[c]; Blackwood 1991; Colombo 1993; DeLisi 1992; Flaum 1995; Hoff 1992; Kawasaki 1993; Kelsoe 1988; Nopoulos 1995; Raine 1992; Shenton 1992; Swayze 1992; Vita 1995)
Medial temporal lobe	30	77	23	+ (Barta 1990, 1997b; Becker 1990, 1996; Blackwood 1991; Bogerts 1990, 1993a; Breier 1992; Buchanan 1993; Dauphinais 1990; DeLisi 1988; Egan 1994; Flaum 1995; Hirayasu 1998; Jernigan 1991; Kawasaki 1993; Marsh 1994; Ohnuma 1997; Rossi 1994a; Shenton 1992; Suddath 1989, 1990; Woodruff 1997b) – (Colombo 1993; Corey-Bloom 1995; DeLisi 1991; Harvey 1993; Marsh 1997; Swayze 1992; Zipursky 1994)
Superior temporal gyrus gray matter	7	100	0	+ (Hajek 1997; Hirayasu 1998; Menon 1995; Schlaepfer 1994; Shenton 1992; Sullivan 1998; Zipursky 1994) – (None)
Superior temporal gyrus gray and white matter	8	63	37	+ (Barta 1990, 1997b; Flaum 1995; Marsh 1997; Reite 1997) – (Kulynych 1996; Vita 1995; Woodruff 1997b)
Planum temporale	7	57	43	+ (Barta 1997a; DeLisi 1994; Petty 1995; Rossi 1992) – (Kleinschmidt 1994; Kulynych 1995; Rossi 1994b)

TABLE 1–3. Magnetic resonance imaging studies with positive or negative findings in schizophrenia *(continued)*

Brain region	Total no. of studies	Studies with positive findings (%)	Studies with negative findings (%)	Reference[a]
Frontal lobe	33	55	45	+ (Andreasen 1994a; Bilder 1994[c]; Breier 1992; Buchanan 1993; Gur 1998; Harvey 1993; Jernigan 1991; Nopoulos 1995; Ohnuma 1997; Raine 1992; Rossi 1988; Schlaepfer 1994; Stratta 1989; Sullivan 1998; Woodruff 1997b; Woods 1996; Zipursky 1992, 1994) – (Andreasen 1990; Blackwood 1991; Corey-Bloom 1995; DeLisi 1991; Egan 1994; Kawasaki 1993; Kelsoe 1988; Kikinis 1994[d]; Nasrallah 1990; Rossi 1990; Shenton 1992; Suddath 1989, 1990; Vita 1995; Wible 1995)
Parietal lobe	10	50	50	+ (Andreasen 1994a; Bilder 1994[c]; Jernigan 1991; Schlaepfer 1994; Zipursky 1994) – (Egan 1994; Jernigan 1991; Nopoulos 1995; Sullivan 1998; Zipursky 1992)
Occipital lobe	7	43	57	+ (Andreasen 1994a; Bilder 1994[c]; Zipursky 1992) – (Jernigan 1991; Nopoulos 1995; Schlaepfer 1994; Sullivan 1998)
Other sites	58	—	—	
Basal ganglia	17	65	35	+ [Breier 1992; Buchanan 1993; Chakos 1994, 1995; Elkashef 1994; Hokama 1995; Jernigan 1991; Keshavan 1995; Mion 1991; Ohnuma 1997; Swayze 1992] – [Blackwood 1991; Corey-Bloom 1995; DeLisi 1991; Flaum 1995; Kelsoe 1988; Rossi 1994a]
Thalamus	6	67	33	+ [Andreasen 1990, 1994b; Buchsbaum 1996; Flaum 1995] – [Corey-Bloom 1995; Portas 1998]

TABLE 1–3. Magnetic resonance imaging studies with positive or negative findings in schizophrenia *(continued)*

Brain region	Total no. of studies	Studies with positive findings (%)	Studies with negative findings (%)	Reference[a]
Corpus callosum	18	61	39	+ [Casanova 1990; DeLisi 1997; Gunther 1991; Hoff 1994; Lewine 1990; Raine 1990; Rossi 1988, 1989a; Stratta 1989; Uematsu and Kaiya 1988; Woodruff 1993] – [Blackwood 1991; Colombo 1994; Guenther 1989; Hauser 1989; Kawasaki 1993; Kelsoe 1988; Woodruff 1997a]
Cerebellum	7	29	71	+ [Andreasen 1994a; Breier 1992] – [Coffman 1989; Flaum 1995; Mathew and Partain 1985; Rossi 1993; Uematsu and Kaiya 1989]
Cavum septi pellucidi[c]	10	90	10	+ [Degreef 1992a, 1992b; DeLisi 1993; Jurjus 1993; Kwon 1998; Mathew et al. 1985; Nopoulos 1996, 1997; Scott 1993; Uematsu and Kaiya 1989] – [Fukuzako 1996]

Note. For numbers of subjects per diagnosis, see McCarley et al. 1999.
[a]Studies are cited by first author or first and second authors and year.
[b]Temporal horn only.
[c]Findings were of asymmetry differences only; planum temporale study findings were mainly of asymmetry differences and therefore citations in those rows are not followed by "[c]."
[d]Findings not based on area, length, or volume measures.
Source. Adapted from Shenton ME, Wible CG, McCarley RW: "A Review of Magnetic Resonance Imaging Studies of Brain Abnormalities in Schizophrenia," in *Brain Imaging in Clinical Psychiatry.* Edited by Krishnan KRR, Doraiswamy PM. New York, Marcel Dekker, 1997, pp. 297–380, by courtesy of Marcel Dekker, Inc.; and adapted by permission of Elsevier Science from "MRI Anatomy of Schizophrenia," by McCarley RW, Wible CG, Frumin M, et al. *Biological Psychiatry* 45:1099–1119, 1999. Copyright by The Society of Biological Psychiatry.

the following imaging parameters: TE, 5 ms; TR, 35 ms; 45-degree flip angle; FOV, 24 cm; number of excitations (NEX), 1; bandwidth, ±16 kHz; and acquisition matrix, 256 (frequency x)×192 (phase-y)×128 (phase-z), resulting in 124 contiguous coronal images with voxel dimensions of 0.9 mm (x)×0.9 mm (y)×1.5 mm (z).

Examples of 3DFT SPGR images are shown in Figure 1–2. On the left is a gray-scale image at the level of the amygdala, and on the right is a gray-scale image at the level of the hippocampus. An overlay of manually drawn outlines for the ROIs can be seen on the right (subject's left), with the caudate and amygdala displayed in Figure 1–2, A, and the caudate and hippocampus displayed in Figure 1–2, B. Additionally, both the left and right lateral ventricles are outlined on the two gray-scale images. Thus, ROIs are identified on two different slices at two different neuroanatomical locations in the brain. However, it is important to keep in mind that the volume for specific brain regions is calculated by summing the voxels across all slices containing the ROIs. We have used these manual segmentations to investigate specific morphometric brain abnormalities in schizophrenia, and these segmentations have served as the basis for our brain atlas (discussed in the next section).

Visualization of Tissue Classes and Use of an Atlas for Model-Based Segmentations

We have also used 3DFT imaging both to visualize complex brain regions and to create a 3D digitized brain atlas (Anderson et al. 1998a; Kikinis et al. 1996; Shenton et al. 1995). We developed the brain atlas, derived from 3DFT SPGR images, to teach neuroanatomy in three dimensions, to visualize complex brain structures for surgical planning (Kikinis et al. 1996; Shenton et al. 1995), and to provide a model-based segmentation for new MRI data sets.

We have identified more than 150 structures in the brain atlas, derived from MR images of one psychiatrically healthy 25-year-old man. To define individual ROIs, we used several brain atlases (see, for example, Crosby et al. 1962; Radamacher et al. 1992) and we (neuroradiologists, neurosurgeons, psychiatrists, and psychologists) met on numerous occasions to determine the best landmarks for defining each ROI. The 3D Slicer, a computer program, developed in the Surgical Planning Laboratory, enabled us to reformat the images into coronal, axial, and sagittal planes, which facilitated the editing process (for instance, see Kikinis et al. 1996; Shenton et al. 1995). To visualize each ROI, we used both the dividing cubes and the marching cubes algorithms to create 3D surface renderings (Cline et al. 1988; Lorensen and Cline

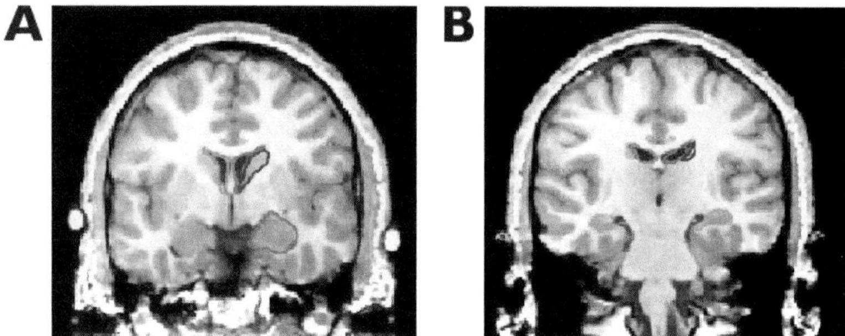

FIGURE 1–2. Coronal slices (1.5 mm) at two neuroanatomical levels.
Gray-scale images at the levels of the *(A)* amygdala and *(B)* hippocampus. Regions of interest, including the caudate (chestnut brown), amygdala (golden brown), hippocampus (green), and left (silver) and right (silver blue) lateral ventricles, are manually outlined.

1987). An example of 3D surface reconstructions of the lateral ventricles, caudate, amygdala, and hippocampus (seen in Figure 1–2, B) is shown in Figure 1–3. There, structures are displayed in different rotations so that one can more readily appreciate the 3D nature of neuroanatomical structures. (For reviews of atlases developed by other groups, see Kikinis et al. 1996; Shenton et al. 1995.)

Our brain atlas, which can be accessed on the Internet with a personal computer (Java applet), can be used as an educational tool. We created a neuroanatomy browser whereby brain structures can be readily grouped, viewed, and rotated (Anderson et al. 1998a [Web site: http://ej.rsna.org/ej2/0050-97.fin/index.html]; see also our Web site: http://splweb.bwh.harvard.edu:8000). Because neuroanatomy is spatially complex and best appreciated in 3D space, we think it important for a student to be able to manipulate brain structures and to view them in juxtaposition. The neuroanatomy browser makes this possible. Additionally, the ROIs are labeled hierarchically so that the student can learn about different brain systems as well as identify specific brain structures. Our use of the brain atlas as a tool in surgical planning has been described in detail (Kikinis et al. 1996).

Lastly, we used the brain atlas for model-based segmentation of neuroanatomical structures in new MRI data sets. We used elastic registration, a warping technique that can deform the 3D brain atlas to fit the geometry of new MRI data sets. For example, we used elastic registration to investigate the topology of white matter lesions in multiple sclerosis, and we found that white matter topology is not maintained (Warfield et al. 1995). We also used

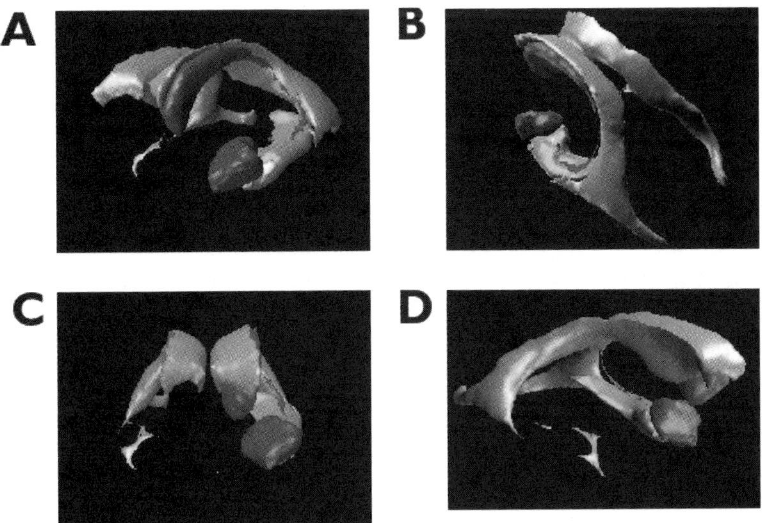

FIGURE 1–3. Three-dimensional reconstructions of the left caudate (chestnut brown), left amygdala (golden brown), left hippocampus (green), and left (silver) and right (silver blue) lateral ventricles in different rotations.
(A) A view from the subject's left; *(B)* a slightly posterior view from the subject's left, with the left side facing the viewer; *(C)* a view from the front; and *(D)* a view from the subject's right. These reconstructions were generated using the marching cubes algorithm and were further processed to reduce complexity and to improve appearance. The final rendering was done using Visualization Toolkit (VTK) (Kitware, Inc., Clifton Park, NY).

elastic registration to segment total brain, deep gray matter, and neocortical gray matter (see, for example, Iosifescu et al. 1997). More specifically, we identified basal ganglia structures and reported a high correspondence between measurements of basal ganglia structures obtained using warping techniques and manual measurements of these same structures (Iosifescu et al. 1997).

We plan to combine model-based segmentation of both volume and shape, derived from the 3D digitized brain atlas, to segment automatically brain structures in multiple MRI data sets automatically, in a matter of seconds. Fitting neuroanatomical templates such as a brain atlas to new MRI data sets has greatly increased the number of structures that can be segmented at the same time in a large number of subjects. We predict that this type of model-based segmentation will replace the labor-intensive manual tracing of brain structures to visualize and to quantify individual brain ROIs.

Diffusion Tensor MRI of the Brain

Many studies have found gray matter abnormalities in schizophrenia (see the review of MRI findings in schizophrenia later in this chapter), but few have found white matter abnormalities. One problem with investigating white matter is that white matter appears uniform and homogeneous on conventional MR images. However, a new imaging technique, diffusion tensor MRI of the brain, makes it possible to investigate white matter more closely. This technique has been used to evaluate tissue changes after acute stroke in humans (for instance, see Le Bihan et al. 1986, 1987; Maier et al. 1998; Moseley et al. 1990; Warach et al. 1992), to evaluate brain tumors (see, for example, Hajnal et al. 1991; Le Bihan et al. 1986), and to evaluate normal and abnormal white matter via diffusion anisotropy (Chien et al. 1990; Doran et al. 1990; Douek et al. 1991; Le Bihan 1995; Peled et al. 1998). Diffusion tensor MRI of the brain is well suited for evaluating white matter because water diffusion is restricted by the physical characteristics of the fiber tracts.[3] There is currently one published study involving schizophrenic patients: Buchsbaum and colleagues (1998) reported diminished anisotropic diffusion in the right inferior prefrontal region in six schizophrenic patients.

In physics and engineering, the term *tensor* is used to describe vector systems in multiple directions. The particular tensors used to describe diffusion can be further conceptualized and visualized as an ellipsoid. The three main directions of the ellipsoid describe an orthogonal coordinate system with three axes, the axes being the so-called eigenvectors of the tensor. In diffusion tensor MRI, a tensor that describes diffusion is acquired for each voxel (3D pixel) and contains information about diffusion in all directions. Its three eigenvectors describe the three main axes of the diffusion ellipsoid (i.e., a direction of maximum diffusion, a direction of minimum diffusion, and a direction orthogonal to the first two directions). The lengths of the vectors, or eigenvalues, further describe the amount of diffusion in the vectors' directions. If the three eigenvalues are equal, then the diffusion is said to be isotropic and the diffusion tensor can be visualized as a sphere.

Thus, if water diffusion is not limited—for example, in the case of fluid—the mathematical description of the diffusion tensor is best characterized by spherical, or isotropic, diffusion.[4] In all other cases, the diffusion is said to be anisotropic. For example, if tissue characteristics (i.e., density of white matter

---

[3]Anisotropic diffusion is a mathematical description of restricted water motion and, as noted by Westin and co-workers (1997), it is the perfect model for white matter.

fibers, amount of myelination, average diameter of white matter fibers, or similarity or dissimilarity of fibers) restrict the mobility of water, then diffusion is best characterized by a measure of linearity, or anisotropy. Mathematically, such restriction of water motility is characterized by high linearity when diffusion is restricted primarily to one direction and by low linearity when diffusion is not restricted and occurs in more than one direction (e.g., 1 = high linearity and 0 = no linearity) (Peled et al. 1998). Thus in any given voxel, a measure of linearity can be described as being between high and low, and such measurements reflect the mobility of water in the tissue, with white matter fibers having the highest linearity and fluid the lowest. Westin and colleagues (1997) further classified geometric types of diffusion (e.g., anisotropic diffusion is classified into linear and planar diffusion). For example, in white matter tracts in which one of the three vectors is much larger than the other two, the direction of diffusion is along the orientation of the fibers, corresponding to linear diffusion.

A major problem with diffusion tensor MRI techniques is motion artifact. This problem has been so severe that the use of such techniques in humans has been hindered, although with more recent advances in technology such as single-shot echo planar diffusion imaging and line-scan diffusion imaging (see the discussion that follows) there may be more clinical applications, including evaluation of stroke (see, for example, Maier et al. 1998; Warach et al. 1992), normal and abnormal white matter (Chien et al. 1990; Doran et al. 1990; Douek et al. 1991), and brain tumors (Hajnal et al. 1991; Le Bihan et al. 1986).

We plan to use line-scan diffusion imaging as our diffusion tensor MRI technique. This single-shot diffusion imaging technique was developed at Brigham and Women's Hospital and can be implemented with conventional MR scanners using existing hardware (Gudbjartsson et al. 1996; Maier and Jolesz 1998; Maier et al. 1998). More than 600 routine patient scans have been performed at Brigham and Women's Hospital over a 1-year period, and these scans provide supporting evidence for the remarkable robustness of this technique. Line-scan diffusion imaging offers distinct advantages over single-shot echo planar imaging methods, which are more commonly used for diffusion imaging. More specifically, single-shot echo planar imaging methods are very sensitive to susceptibility variations and chemical shift and, in conjunction with inadequate shimming, can result in ghost artifacts, image distortions, and/or complete signal loss. In contrast, line-scan diffusion images do not

---

[4]The decomposition into spherical, linear, and planar diffusion is based on properties of the diffusion ellipsoid (see Le Bihan 1995; Westin et al. 1997).

have such artifacts. Moreover, the superior quality of line-scan diffusion images is particularly evident in areas near large bone structures, such as the orbitae, the maxillary cavities, the temporal lobes, and the inferior fossa. Further, eddy currents, mainly due to diffusion gradients, may result in a mismatch of the images obtained with diffusion weighting along different directions. Consequently, the determination of fiber direction may be unreliable. We have found, however, that eddy current–related mismatches of images obtained with line-scan diffusion imaging are minimal, unlike such mismatches of images obtained with single-shot echo planar diffusion imaging. Additionally, line-scan diffusion imaging requires no electrocardiographic gating or head restraints, which facilitates patient handling considerably. The lack of a need for head restraints is particularly important in the case of psychiatric patients, who often find it difficult to lie still in the magnet for long periods.

Examples of diffusion tensor MR scans of the brain can be seen in Figure 1–4. A 1.5-T GE Echospeed system (General Electric Medical Systems, Milwaukee, Wisconsin) was used, which permits maximum gradient amplitudes of 22 millitesla/m. For each brain section, six images were obtained with high diffusion weighting (750 seconds/mm^2) along six noncollinear directions (e.g., relative amplitudes [gradients Gx, Gy, Gz] of [1, 1, 0], [0, 1, 1], [1, 0, 1], [–1, 1, 0], [0, –1, 1], and [1, 0, –1]). With low diffusion weighting (5 seconds/mm^2), we obtained two images, an adequate number because diffusion-related signal changes are minimal. The following scan parameters were used: rectangular FOV, 220×165 mm; scan matrix, 128×96 (image matrix, 256×192); effective slice thickness, 4.4 mm; interslice distance, 5.0 mm; receiver bandwidth, ±6 kHz; TE, 70 ms; TR, 80 ms (effective TR, 2,500 ms); and scan time, 60 seconds per section. After reconstruction, diffusion-weighted images are transferred to a Sun Microsystems workstation (Sun Microsystems, Palo Alto, California), where eigenvalue and eigenvector maps of the diffusion tensor are calculated (for details, see Maier and Jolesz 1998; Peled et al. 1998). In addition, we can compute average apparent diffusion coefficient maps, average diffusion-weighted images, and average T2-weighted images, as well as anisotropy maps based on the standard deviation of the apparent diffusion coefficient along the six different directions (for specific details, see Maier and Jolesz 1998).

■ APPLICATION OF MRI IN MORPHOMETRIC STUDIES OF SCHIZOPHRENIA

Although the first MRI study of schizophrenia was conducted in 1984 (Smith et al. 1984), it was not until 1987 and 1988 that second-generation MR scan-

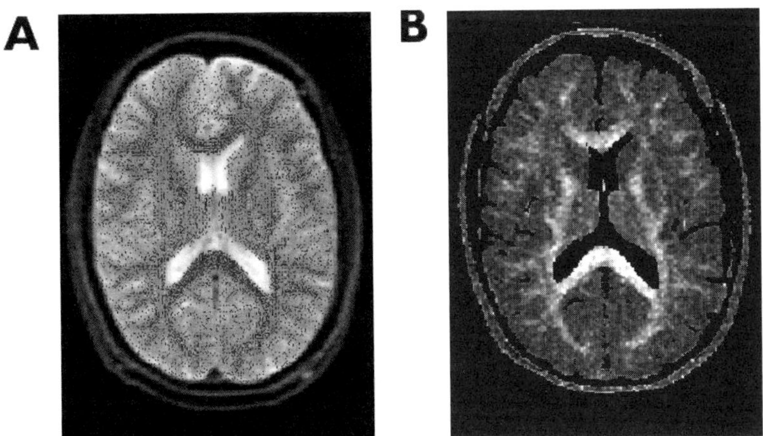

FIGURE 1–4. Brain diffusion tensor map and anistropy map for a psychiatrically healthy control subject.
(A) This diffusion tensor map is displayed as eigenvectors, with blue lines representing the direction of the in-plane components of each eigenvector that correspond to the largest eigenvalue. Anisotropy is represented by the length of the blue lines. Note the length of the lines in the corpus callosum and the orientation of the fibers there. In gray matter, where spherical diffusion symmetry is predominant, the eigenvector of the largest eigenvalue points in a random direction (there are always at least signal-to-noise-ratio–related differences in diffusion). However, because anisotropy is very low in gray matter regions, the displayed lines are very short and thus we reduce the disturbing impression of vectors pointing in random directions. Harder to visualize here are the out-of-plane components (blue and yellow dots), where yellow denotes the largest out-of-plane eigenvector. *(B)* Anisotropy measures are displayed. White matter appears brightest. A main direction of the fibers gives a high anisotropy value (more linearity brighter on display), here best observed in the corpus callosum. The longest blue lines (i.e., the most anisotropy) in A are the same areas that are bright on the anisotropy map.

ners and more sophisticated MR image acquisition and postprocessing techniques became available. Accordingly, our review of morphometric MRI studies in schizophrenia begins with studies published in 1988. However, such a cutoff is arbitrary and results in the exclusion of the pioneering study by Andreasen and co-workers (1986).

The MRI data presented here are drawn from our most recent review (McCarley et al. 1999), which is an update of our more extensive earlier review (Shenton et al. 1997). The scope of the review is broad, although we chose to exclude from our summary table (Table 1–3) studies that involved fewer than 10 subjects, focused primarily on relaxation times as opposed to area or volume measures, did not include a control group, or focused on family members. Additionally, we counted studies only once in the summary table, even if the data set was presented in more than one study. Finally, although we considered using a meta-analysis for tabulating the positive and negative findings for each ROI, we rejected this approach because we realized that most of the 170 MRI studies cited were not comparable in terms of magnetic field strength, slice thickness, postprocessing analyses, or the number of slices used to measure the ROIs (see Rosenthal 1987 for a thoughtful discussion of the use of meta-analysis). Here, we summarize morphometric MRI findings in schizophrenia (for more details, refer to our previous MRI reviews: McCarley et al. 1999; Shenton et al. 1997).

Our primary goal here is to begin to address some of the questions listed in Table 1–1, including the following: Are there brain abnormalities in schizophrenia? Which brain regions are affected? Are brain abnormalities diffuse or localized? Are brain abnormalities in schizophrenia related to symptom clusters? Are these abnormalities neurodevelopmental, progressive, or a combination of the two?

For heuristic reasons, and because many MRI studies have focused on specific structures within the frontal, temporal, parietal, or occipital lobe, the studies reviewed are grouped by specific lobe. We also have included the category "Other Sites," into which we have placed basal ganglia, thalamus, corpus callosum, cerebellum, and cavum septi pellucidi (CSP) studies.[5]

Whole Brain

Consideration of the role of overall brain size in mental illness dates back to Pinel (1801) and to the presumed association between brain size and intelligence, socioeconomic status, and cognitive deficits (see, for example, Kretschmer 1925; Pinel 1801). Brain size, or volume, is an important consideration in schizophrenia because it may be an indicator of neurodevelopmental abnormalities. Surprisingly, however, the findings of MRI studies of whole brain volume in schizophrenia have been largely negative (negative findings in 81% of studies [Table 1–3]). We think it premature, however, to conclude that the findings reflect a lack of difference in overall brain volumes between

[5]The "Other" category includes two studies from 1985. Because there are so few published studies, we did not want to exclude these two. Additionally, with regard to the corpus callosum, we may not have included all studies published, given that we searched *MEDLINE* using terms and abbreviations such as *MRI, MR,* and *magnetic resonance imaging,* which were not consistently used for the corpus callosum studies.

patients with schizophrenia and control subjects. The high percentage of studies with negative findings might be due to variable methods used across studies (i.e., the use of different magnetic field strengths, different slice thicknesses [1 mm to 1 cm for a slab], or contiguous slices versus gaps between slices). Such methodological differences may prevent the detection of very small differences between groups, particularly when the structure being evaluated is relatively large (e.g., large relative to the hippocampus). In addition, very small differences in brain volume between groups may not be inconsequential. For example, small brain volume has been reported in childhood-onset schizophrenia, suggesting that small differences in overall brain volume may reflect a more severe form of the disorder (Jacobsen et al. 1996). Finally, there is a need for more careful selection of comparison subjects and of well-defined and well-delineated subgroups of patients; such selection might lead to the detection and clarification of very small volume differences.

Ventricles

Lateral Ventricles

Interest in measuring the lateral ventricles in schizophrenia dates back to the creation of early casts and molds from postmortem brains and to early pneumoencephalographic studies (see, for example, Haug 1962; Jacobi et al. 1927; Southard 1910, 1915). This interest continued with the advent of CT, which permitted easy viewing of the lateral ventricles and by which planimetric and area measures were made, usually from one slice showing the largest body of the lateral ventricles. These CT studies are well summarized by Shelton and Weinberger (1986), who documented that 75% of CT studies of schizophrenia found lateral ventricular enlargement. Given that high percentage, this finding is one of the most robust findings in schizophrenia.

Lateral ventricular enlargement is not specific to schizophrenia, however, as such enlargement is also observed in many other illnesses, including Alzheimer's disease and Huntington's disease. Furthermore, chemotherapy and steroid treatment can result in lateral ventricular enlargement. Nevertheless, lateral ventricular enlargement may be indicative of tissue loss or reduction in brain regions surrounding the lateral ventricles (e.g., medial temporal lobe structures). Such enlargement may also suggest a failure of normal brain development.

In 77% of the 43 MRI studies reviewed (Table 1–3), lateral ventricular enlargement was found, a percentage similar to that for CT studies. The evidence for lateral ventricular enlargement is thus compelling.

An increase in the temporal horn of the lateral ventricles has also been reported by several investigators (e.g., Barta et al. 1990; Bogerts et al. 1990; Dauphinais et al. 1990; Degreef et al. 1990; Johnstone et al. 1989; Kawasaki et al. 1993; Shenton et al. 1991, 1992). This CSF increase is in the region of medial temporal lobe structures. Of note, this increase in CSF in the temporal horn tends to be lateralized to the left, and this finding is consistent with postmortem study findings of tissue loss within the medial temporal lobe, including the amygdala-hippocampal complex and parahippocampal gyrus (see, for example, Bogerts et al. 1985; Brown et al. 1986; Colter et al. 1987; Crow 1989; Falkai and Bogerts 1986; Falkai et al. 1988; Jakob and Beckmann 1989; Jeste and Lohr 1989; Kovelman and Scheibel 1984). This latter finding is also consistent with MRI findings of medial temporal lobe volume reductions in schizophrenia.

In summary, lateral ventricular enlargement is one of the most robust findings in schizophrenia, and the finding of an increase in CSF in the temporal horn of the lateral ventricles suggests that reduced volume in medial temporal lobe structures may account for this increase in CSF.

Third and Fourth Ventricles

Fewer MRI studies have evaluated the third ventricle, but in two-thirds of these studies (67%), findings were positive. With regard to the fourth ventricle, findings were uniformly negative (Table 1–3).

Temporal Lobe

Anatomy and Function

The temporal lobe has three major gyri: the superior temporal gyrus (STG), the middle temporal gyrus, and the inferior temporal gyrus (Figure 1–5). The STG lies along the Sylvian fissure of the temporal lobe, and the middle and inferior temporal gyri are inferior and parallel to this gyrus. The STG includes the temporal pole, Heschl's gyri, and the planum temporale. The latter two are located on the superior-posterior surface of the STG. (Because Heschl's gyri and the planum temporale lie on the surface of the temporal lobe, they are not visible in Figure 1–5, which is a lateral view of the brain.) The STG includes both primary auditory cortex (Heschl's gyri) and secondary auditory cortex (planum temporale). Primary auditory cortex is important for the initial processing of auditory information, whereas the secondary auditory cortex is associated with the processing of environmental sounds, on the right, and language, on the left.

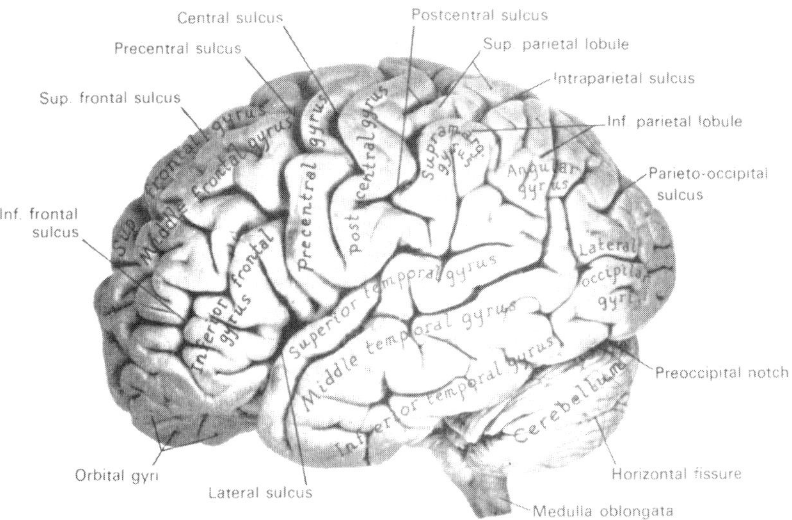

FIGURE 1–5. Lateral view of the brain.
Source. Reprinted with permission from Carpenter MB: *Core Text of Human Neuroanatomy,* 4th Edition. Baltimore, MD, Williams & Wilkins, 1991.

The planum temporale, in fact, is highly asymmetric in humans, with the left planum temporale larger than the right planum temporale in two-thirds of humans (Galaburda 1984; Galaburda et al. 1987; Geschwind and Levitsky 1968). This asymmetry has also been observed in postmortem studies of human fetuses (Witelson and Pallie 1973). Moreover, phylogenetically planum temporale asymmetry first appears in chimpanzees, suggesting a further link with the evolution of language (Gannon et al. 1997). Additionally, the left planum temporale is within Wernicke's area, which is critical for language and speech production, leading to the speculation that the planum temporale is an important biological substrate of language (see, for example, Galaburda 1984; Galaburda et al. 1987; Penfield and Roberts 1959; Wernicke 1874) and thus may play an important role in both formal thought disorder and language abnormalities observed in schizophrenia.

The middle and inferior temporal gyri are important for processing sensory stimuli, including complex stimuli such as faces. Medial temporal lobe structures include the amygdala-hippocampal complex and the parahippocampal gyrus. These structures, particularly the hippocampus and the parahippocampal gyrus, play important roles in verbal and spatial memory processing (see, for instance, Corkin 1984; Milner 1972; Ojemann 1991;

Ojemann et al. 1988; Penfield and Perot 1963; Squire 1992; Squire and Zola-Morgan 1991), whereas the amygdala has a more important role in the emotional strength attached to stimuli (see, for example, Gloor 1986; Whalen et al. 1998). Shown in Figure 1–6 is a 3DFT SPGR coronal 1.5-mm-thick slice with the entire temporal lobe outlined on the left (subject's right) and the STG and amygdala outlined on the right (subject's left).

Whole Temporal Lobe

In 62% of MRI investigations of whole temporal lobe volume, in which all structures are grouped together, findings were positive (Table 1–3).

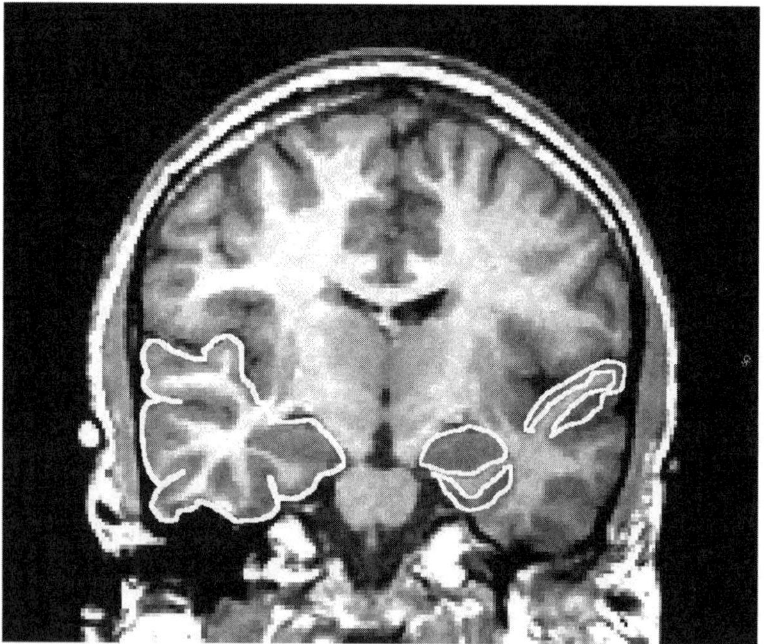

FIGURE 1–6. Coronal 1.5-mm slice showing medial temporal and neocortical structures.
The region bordering the Sylvian fissure on the right (subject's left) is the superior temporal gyrus. The almond-shaped region in the medial portion of the temporal lobe is the amygdala, and the region demarcated beneath is the parahippocampal gyrus. The whole temporal lobe is outlined on the left (subject's right).
Source. Reprinted from Shenton ME, Kikinis R, Jolesz FA, et al.: "Abnormalities of the Left Temporal Lobe and Thought Disorder in Schizophrenia: A Quantitative Magnetic Resonance Imaging Study." *New England Journal of Medicine* 327:604–612, 1992.

Medial Temporal Lobe

Compared with findings of MRI studies focusing on the whole temporal lobe, findings of MRI studies of medial temporal lobe structures, which include the amygdala-hippocampal complex and the parahippocampus, were more striking, with findings of 77% of these studies positive with regard to one or more of these structures. Thus, medial temporal lobe findings are among the most robust positive findings in schizophrenia.

Most of the MRI studies of the medial temporal lobe found more anterior amygdala-hippocampal volume reduction, although three studies found more prominent posterior amygdala-hippocampal volume reduction (Bogerts et al. 1990, 1993a; Flaum et al. 1995). Moreover, most found more prominent volume reduction on the left, and more frequently in male schizophrenic patients (Barta et al. 1990; Becker et al. 1990; Bogerts et al. 1990, 1993a; Kawasaki et al. 1993; Rossi et al. 1994a; Shenton et al. 1992). Of the studies with negative findings, two studies used only three or four slices to estimate volume (Colombo et al. 1993; Swayze et al. 1992), one excluded portions of the posterior temporal lobe (DeLisi et al. 1991), one had different proportions of males and females in the patient and control groups (Harvey et al. 1993), one evaluated medial temporal lobe gray matter but did not delineate individual structures (Corey-Bloom et al. 1995), and one evaluated a portion of the amygdala-hippocampal complex (the hippocampus only) (Zipursky et al. 1994).

The volume reduction noted in medial temporal lobe structures also appears to be correlated with increased CSF in the lateral ventricles, particularly the left temporal horn, as noted previously (for instance, see Barta et al. 1990; Becker et al. 1990; Bogerts et al. 1990, 1993a; Dauphinais et al. 1990; Kawasaki et al. 1993; Shenton et al. 1992). Medial temporal lobe volume reduction is also correlated with prefrontal white matter volume (see, for example, Breier et al. 1992; Buchanan et al. 1993). Suddath and co-workers (1989, 1990) also reported a correlation, during the Wisconsin Card Sorting Test, between left hippocampal volume reduction and decreased regional blood flow in the dorsolateral prefrontal cortex in the affected twin of monozygotic twins discordant for schizophrenia. Moreover, a study in our laboratory found a correlation between left amygdala-hippocampal, left parahippocampal, and left STG volume reduction and reduced volume in left prefrontal gray matter in patients with chronic schizophrenia (Wible et al. 1995). These findings, taken together, suggest that neural connections between prefrontal cortex and medial temporal lobe structures may be disrupted in schizophrenia. This finding is also consistent with the postmortem findings of Selemon and co-workers (1995), who reported an 8% reduction in the cortical ribbon of the dorsolateral prefrontal cortex in schizophrenic patients compared with control subjects. An 8% difference is close to the threshold for detecting differences using current MRI methods, which may explain, in part, the lack of consistency in MRI findings regarding the frontal lobe in schizophrenia (discussed later in this chapter).

Provided in Figure 1–7, B, is an example of left lateralized medial temporal lobe abnormalities, enlarged lateral ventricles, increased CSF in the left Sylvian fissure (viewer's right), and reduced volume in the STG in a schizophrenic patient. The fact that the MR scan of the patient was considered by a clinical neuroradiologist not to show abnormalities highlights the subtlety of brain changes in schizophrenia and the importance of using a finer template and measurement to detect small differences.

Several interesting correlations between medial temporal lobe volume reduction and clinical symptoms have also been observed. For example, Bogerts and co-workers (1993a) reported a correlation between bilateral reduction of medial temporal lobe structures (grouped together) and the psychotic factor, measured by the Brief Psychiatric Rating Scale. Additionally, in investigations involving the same subject group as that studied by Suddath et al. (1989), Goldberg and co-workers (Goldberg et al. 1990; Weinberger et al. 1992) found a correlation between left hippocampal volume reduction and increased positive symptoms, along with disruptions in logical memory, in the affected compared with the nonaffected monozygotic twin. These findings are consistent with what is known about the function of the hippocampus in associative memory. Nestor et al. (1993), in our laboratory, also noted a correlation between parahippocampal gyrus volume reduction, STG volume reduction, and poor scores on tests of verbal memory, abstraction, and categorization. Nestor and colleagues (1993) interpreted these data as being consistent with a disruption in the semantic system in patients with schizophrenia. Our laboratory also reported a correlation between the auditory P300 (an event-related potential that is involved in detecting novelty and discerning relevant from irrelevant stimuli) and reduced left STG volume in patients with schizophrenia compared with control subjects (McCarley et al. 1993).

Superior Temporal Gyrus

Interest in the STG and its role in schizophrenia can be traced to early studies by Southard (1910, 1915), who described a "suprasylvian atrophy" of the entire left Sylvian fissure and a "withering away" of the left STG in the postmortem brains of schizophrenic patients. These patients were characterized

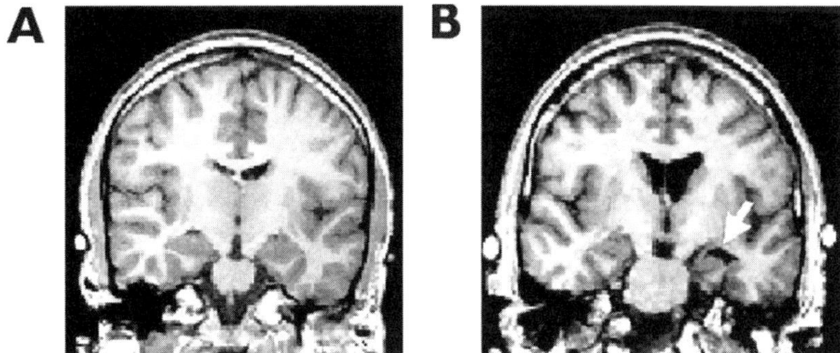

FIGURE 1–7. Coronal 1.5-mm slices from a psychiatrically healthy subject and a patient with schizophrenia, acquired at approximately the same neuroanatomical level.
(A) Control subject. *(B)* Schizophrenic patient. The patient has enlarged lateral ventricles (viewer's right; the black region in the center is cerebrospinal fluid [CSF]), increased CSF (black) in the left Sylvian fissure (viewer's right), and reduced tissue in the left superior temporal gyrus (viewer's right). The volume reduction in the left amygdala (viewer's right) is accompanied by an increase in CSF (black) in the temporal horn (see white arrow).
Source. Reprinted from Shenton ME, Kikinis R, Jolesz FA, et al.: "Abnormalities of the Left Temporal Lobe and Thought Disorder in Schizophrenia: A Quantitative Magnetic Resonance Imaging Study." *New England Journal of Medicine* 327:604–612, 1992.

clinically as having prominent auditory hallucinations. Southard (1910, 1915) also noted a striking disruption in the sulco-gyral pattern in the left temporal lobe, which led him to conclude that the temporal lobe was importantly implicated in the pathophysiology of schizophrenia. This latter finding was followed up in more recent postmortem studies of schizophrenia (Bruton et al. 1990; Jakob and Beckmann 1986) and in an MRI investigation of the sulco-gyral pattern in schizophrenia. In the latter study, Kikinis and co-workers (1994) found a disruption in the sulco-gyral pattern of the left temporal lobe, which was not observed in the right temporal lobe or in the left or right frontal lobes. Such findings suggest a neurodevelopmental origin in at least a subset of patients with schizophrenia, because the sulco-gyral pattern is determined prenatally.

Barta and co-workers (1990), the first to investigate the STG using MRI technology, reported an 11% volume reduction in anterior STG that was associated with auditory hallucinations. Our group further investigated the STG in schizophrenic patients and reported a 15% volume reduction in the posterior STG that was associated with formal thought disorder (Shenton et al. 1992). More specifically, left posterior STG volume reduction was associated with greater severity of formal thought disorder (Figure 1–8). We thought this finding was intriguing because the posterior STG includes the planum temporale, a brain region long implicated as a neuroanatomical substrate of language. We also reported intercorrelations between left posterior STG, left amygdala-hippocampal complex, and left parahippocampal gyrus volumes in schizophrenic patients but not in control subjects. We further speculated that these correlations among neuroanatomically interconnected structures might reflect damage to an interconnected network that is functionally important for associative links in memory (see, for example, Ojemann et al. 1988; Penfield and Perot 1963; Squire and Zola-Morgan 1991), which, in turn, is manifested by formal thought disorder and what Bleuler (1911/1950) described as "incidental" linkages.

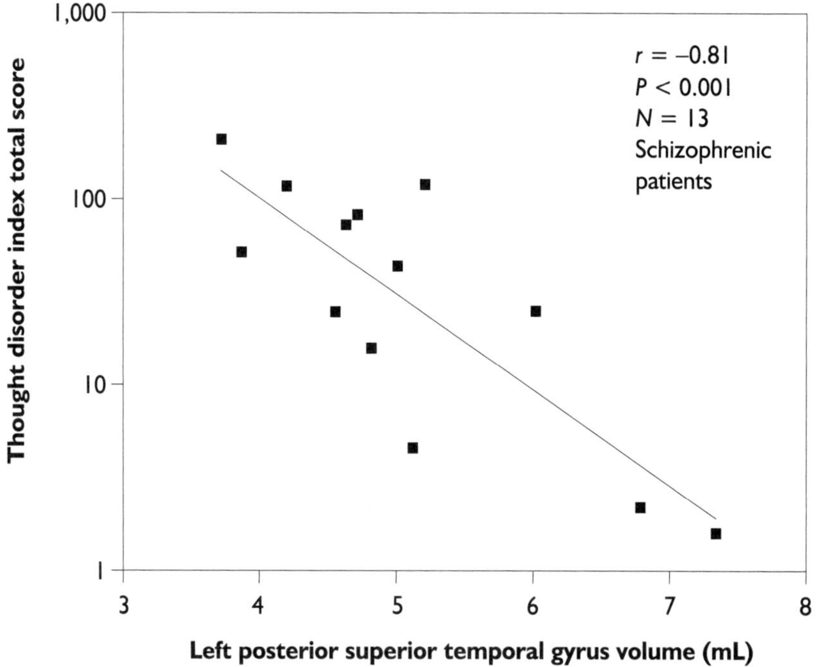

FIGURE 1–8. Volume of the left posterior superior temporal gyrus correlated with total score on the Thought Disorder Index (Johnston and Holzman 1979) in 13 patients with schizophrenia.

Source. Reprinted from Shenton ME, Kikinis R, Jolesz FA, et al.: "Abnormalities of the Left Temporal Lobe and Thought Disorder in Schizophrenia: A Quantitative Magnetic Resonance Imaging Study." *New England Journal of Medicine* 327:604–612, 1992.

The studies by Barta et al. (1990) and Shenton et al. (1992) led to a further focus on the STG and planum temporale in schizophrenia. Most informative is the difference in findings when STG gray and white matter are grouped together versus when they are separated. Seven studies examined gray matter (separated from white matter), and all found reduced STG volume in schizophrenic patients (Table 1–3). In contrast, in only 63% of the eight studies that combined gray and white matter were findings positive. In one recent study, patients with first-episode schizophrenia had reduced left STG gray matter volume compared with patients with first-episode affective disorder and control subjects (Hirayasu et al. 1998).

We thus conclude that STG abnormalities are evident in schizophrenia when gray matter alone is evaluated but when gray and white matter are combined in the analyses, this finding is less robust. Overall, these findings suggest that brain regions important for language function may be disrupted in schizophrenia.

Planum Temporale

MRI investigations of the planum temporale have been hampered by tremendous variation in the measurements used. For example, some investigators (e.g., Rossi et al. 1992) used the bank of the Sylvian fissure to estimate planum temporale, whereas others (e.g., DeLisi et al. 1994) used a measure of length. Such variation in measurements likely accounts for the inconsistent findings (57% of studies with positive findings; Table 1–3). More consistent definitions of planum temporale landmarks and measurements are therefore needed in future studies. We recently reported a 28% volume reduction in gray matter in the left planum temporale in patients with chronic schizophrenia compared with control subjects (Kwon et al. 1999). In that study we also found a reversal of planum temporale asymmetry, which may underlie an impairment in language processing and the symptoms of suspiciousness or persecution that are characteristic of schizophrenia.

Frontal Lobe

The frontal cortex is involved in some of the most complex processing of information and modulates many aspects of human functioning. The prefrontal cortex, rostral to the premotor cortex (Broca's area 46), has been widely implicated in the pathophysiology of schizophrenia. MRI findings regarding this brain region have been inconsistent, however, with findings being positive in 55% of studies (Table 1–3). It is difficult to reconcile such conflicting results, although it is clear that one contributing factor may be the small number of slices used to estimate this large brain region. Only two studies, conducted at our laboratory, have evaluated 1.5-mm-thick slices throughout the prefrontal cortex (Wible et al. 1995, 1997).

There is also some suggestion that the conflicting findings may be due to differences in the patient populations studied. There is, for example, some suggestion that patients with more negative symptoms evince more prefrontal lobe abnormalities while patients with more positive symptoms evince more temporal lobe abnormalities (Shenton et al. 1997), thus highlighting the importance of carefully characterizing patient subgroups.

Parietal and Occipital Lobes

Few studies have evaluated the parietal lobe, despite the fact that functions such as language, eye tracking, and attention, which are known to be disrupted in schizophrenia, may involve abnormalities in the parietal lobe (Shenton et al. 1997; Pearlson et al. 1996). In 50% of the studies, findings were positive (Table 1–3). Such equivocal findings are likely due to the fact that the parietal lobe has not been investigated with the same level of detail as that which has characterized MRI studies of the temporal lobe. This difference in level of detail is also true for the small number of occipital lobe studies, which were also inconsistent in terms of findings of abnormalities (Table 1–3).

Other Sites

The category labeled "Other sites" in Table 1–3 includes MRI studies of the basal ganglia, thalamus, corpus callosum, cerebellum, and CSP. The basal ganglia are of particular interest to schizophrenia researchers because the basal ganglia receive dopamine input, and neuroleptics (the mainstay of schizophrenia treatment) block dopamine receptors. In addition, these brain structures, which include the caudate, putamen, and globus pallidus, play important roles in cognitive, sensory, and motor processing (Hokama et al. 1995). Of the 17 MRI studies of these brain structures, 11 found abnormalities and 6 did not (positive findings in 65% of studies).

The most frequently reported abnormality is increased basal ganglia volume in subjects receiving chronic neuroleptic treatment. Chakos and coworkers (1994, 1995) observed a correlation in patients with first-episode schizophrenia between neuroleptic medication and an increase in basal ganglia volume at follow-up. Keshavan and co-workers (1994, 1995) made a similar observation, thus indicating that increased basal ganglia volume may be a function of neuroleptic medication administration. Chakos and co-workers (1995), in fact, further noted that the increase in volume was dose related.

Fewer studies of the thalamus have been conducted, but two-thirds of these studies found abnormalities in schizophrenia (Table 1–3). This structure has reciprocal connections with many brain regions, including prefrontal cortex and limbic structures, and has figured prominently in Andreasen's "cognitive dysmetria" theory regarding schizophrenia (Andreasen 1997). Portas and co-workers (1998), who found no volume differences, did report correlations between thalamic and prefrontal white matter volumes in patients with schizophrenia, a correlation not observed in the control sample. These findings, taken together, suggest that thalamic nuclei, with important connections to limbic and prefrontal cortical regions, should be studied further using higher spatial resolution imaging techniques that optimize the delineation of specific nuclei.

The corpus callosum, the largest white matter tract in the brain, connects the right and left hemispheres. The development of this midline structure is intimately linked to the formation of the CSP, and thus abnormalities in both may reflect dysgenesis during gestation. There is also a reported association between corpus callosum dysgenesis and schizophrenia. Further, given the corpus callosum's role in connecting the two hemispheres, it is reasonable to speculate that if information flow between the hemispheres is disrupted, defective interhemispheric communication might result (see, for example, Gruzelier 1987). Such defective interhemispheric communication might also be manifested as information processing deficits, which are so frequently observed in schizophrenia (see, for instance, Gruzelier 1987).

Approximately 61% of the MRI studies of the corpus callosum found abnormalities in schizophrenia (Table 1–3). Most of these studies, however, used one midsagittal slice to define the area of the corpus callosum. Such an approach is problematic because there is the possibility of errors due to brain alignment, slice thickness, and choice of slice. These methodological problems also make it difficult to compare findings across studies. Gender also needs to be taken into account, because there is evidence to suggest sexual dimorphism in both the shape and size of the corpus callosum (see, for example, DeQuardo et al. 1996). Studies that analyze shape may help to clarify further the presence and role of corpus callosum abnormalities in schizophrenia.

Recent studies suggest that, in addition to having a role in motor function, the cerebellum may play a part in higher cognitive functions (see, for example, Schmahmann 1996; Wassink et al. 1999). As shown in Table 1–3, findings of MRI studies of the cerebellum in schizophrenia have been largely negative.

These studies, however, have generally included only a single midsagittal slice of the vermian area rather than volume measures. Moreover, separation of gray matter and white matter in the cerebellum and in the vermis was not performed in these studies but might be useful to clarify further the role of the cerebellum in the pathophysiology of schizophrenia.

The CSP is the space between the two leaflets of the septum pellucidum, a midline membrane separating the lateral ventricles. In normal development, 85% of individuals show a fusing of these two leaflets within the first 6 months of life (Kwon et al. 1998; Nopoulos et al. 1996, 1997). Fusion of the leaflets may also be associated with the growth of the hippocampus and corpus callosum, at either end of this membrane, and thus incomplete fusion of the septum pellucidum may reflect possible neurodevelopmental abnormalities of these two brain structures. Evidence in support of this speculation comes from Nopoulos and co-workers (1996), who reported a correlation between a large CSP (i.e., a CSP visible on more than four 1.5-mm-thick slices) and temporal lobe volume reduction. Similarly, Kwon et al. (1998) reported a correlation between a large CSP and hippocampal volume reduction in patients with chronic schizophrenia. Additionally, Fukuzako and co-workers (1996), though they found no differences in the CSP between patients with schizophrenia and control subjects, did report a correlation between CSP abnormalities and poorer treatment response and outcome. Thus, although few MRI studies of the CSP have been conducted, findings have been largely positive (positive findings in 90% of studies). These findings are thus robust, and they further suggest a neurodevelopmental abnormality in at least a subgroup of patients with schizophrenia. These MRI findings, indicating a neurodevelopmental abnormality, are also consonant with postmortem findings in schizophrenia (see, for example, Akbarian et al. 1993a, 1993b; Benes 1989; Jakob and Beckmann 1986) and with MRI findings of temporal lobe sulco-gyral pattern abnormalities (see Kikinis et al. 1994).

■ CONCLUSIONS AND FUTURE STUDIES

The search for brain abnormalities in schizophrenia has a long history. However, because brain differences between patients with schizophrenia and control subjects are small (on the order of 10%–20%), detection of brain abnormalities was not possible until improvements in imaging technology had been made. Progress in this area was thus slow, largely because of the lack of tools and secondarily because of less scientific rigor in methodology and a lack of standardized diagnoses. Progress was so slow, in fact, that as late as 1972, Plum urged researchers contemplating careers investigating brain abnormalities in schizophrenia to avoid that "graveyard of neuropathologists." Now, nearly three decades later, because it is possible to discern brain abnormalities in schizophrenia, this field has become one of the most exciting areas of research, and investigators are at the threshold of major discoveries that are likely to have important treatment implications.

Summary of Findings

MRI studies have evolved from studies using 1-cm-thick slices that did not include the entire brain to studies using 1.5-mm-thick slices that include the entire brain. However, even with advances in technology, there is still the difficult task of detecting small morphometric abnormalities against a background of enormous individual and methodological variation. In fact, many of the MRI studies reviewed used different magnetic field strengths, different pulse sequences, or different slice thicknesses, and some studies included gaps between slices whereas others did not. Additionally, there were differences in the selection of both patient and control populations. Nevertheless, there is a remarkable convergence of evidence to suggest that brain abnormalities are not only present but also do not seem to affect all brain regions equally.

More specifically, we conclude that brain abnormalities in patients with schizophrenia are localized rather than diffuse. The most robust findings are lateral ventricular enlargement and temporal lobe abnormalities, the latter including reduced volume in the medial temporal lobe (amygdala-hippocampal complex and parahippocampal gyrus) and reduced neocortical STG. These temporal lobe abnormalities were frequently associated with positive symptoms such as delusions, hallucinations, and functional impairments in language including formal thought disorder and impairments of verbal memory and other associative links in memory. In contrast, frontal lobe volume reductions were more frequently associated with negative symptoms. These latter findings suggest that there may be interesting clinicopathological correlates in schizophrenia that can be better characterized and delineated if careful attention is paid to defining subtypes of schizophrenia. Such subtyping would include categorizing patients not just by diagnostic subtype but also by whether they experience auditory hallucinations, whether they evince formal thought disorder, and so on. Studying such circumscribed disturbances might lead to stronger clinicopathological correlations, as suggested by previous findings (see, for example, Barta et al. 1990; Shenton et al. 1992).

Findings regarding frontal, parietal, and occipital lobes were far less consistent than temporal lobe findings. However, few of these studies examined parcellated regions as carefully as have MRI studies of the temporal lobe. Careful parcellation of frontal, parietal, and occipital lobes is needed because small differences may be missed when only crude measures are used.

Basal ganglia abnormalities appear to be associated with neuroleptic dosage. Few studies have evaluated the thalamus. Moreover, no studies have parcellated individual nuclei of the thalamus; such parcellation is not possible using current MRI technology. The thalamus has, nonetheless, been recognized by many investigators as likely to be implicated in schizophrenia. Andreasen (1997), for example, developed a "cognitive dysmetria" theory of schizophrenia that involves cortico-thalamic circuitry abnormalities. With respect to the corpus callosum, findings were variable, and methodological differences likely account for the inconsistent findings reported. New studies evaluating shape, however, are promising. And with regard to the cerebellum, MRI studies have been sparse, most likely because cognitive functions have only recently been attributed to the cerebellum. Further, separating gray and white matter in this region is technically difficult. Additionally, more careful studies of the cerebellum are needed that go beyond an assessment of one slice. Finally, MRI findings regarding the CSP and sulco-gyral pattern abnormalities are important because they support a neurodevelopmental origin in at least a subgroup of patients with schizophrenia. These findings also suggest the importance of carefully delineating meaningful subgroups of patients to explore more profitably the possibility that different patterns of brain abnormalities might be associated with different, and perhaps specific, subgroups of patients with schizophrenia.

Thus, we conclude that brain abnormalities are evident in schizophrenia and that the most robust MRI findings are lateral ventricular enlargement, medial and neocortical temporal lobe abnormalities, and CSP abnormalities. The evidence is thus in support of more localized changes. However, we are aware that the question of whether schizophrenia is characterized by diffuse, widespread changes or localized abnormalities is one that has generated considerable debate in the field (see, for example, Zipursky et al. 1992). We think this debate is largely one of semantics (see reviews by McCarley et al. 1999; Shenton et al. 1997). For example, if *widespread* or *diffuse* is used to mean there are changes in several brain regions, then the data support this conclusion. If, however, equal severity across all brain regions is meant, then the data do not support this conclusion. And, indeed, a review of MRI studies produces little evidence for diffuse, widespread gray matter volume reduction in schizophrenia. Instead, what one finds is that some regions, such as the temporal lobe, are more profoundly affected than are other brain regions, such as the occipital and frontal lobes.

Pearlson and co-workers (Pearlson et al. 1996; Schlaepfer et al. 1994) also suggest that localized, and not diffuse, brain abnormalities are evident in schizophrenia. These investigators further posit that these localized brain regions are interconnected and reflect abnormalities in heteromodal cortex, which includes dorsolateral prefrontal cortex, inferior parietal lobule, and superior temporal gyrus. This interesting speculation needs to be addressed in future studies. Our laboratory has focused on the temporal lobe, and we are working on a model that would account for the interconnected temporal lobe volume reductions, formal thought disorder, and auditory hallucinations. This model includes a "first hit," which is the vulnerability or genetic predisposition to schizophrenia and which may involve a specific dysregulation of neurotransmission regulated by excitatory amino acid receptors identified by *N*-methyl-D-aspartate (NMDA). Such a dysregulation might disrupt the formation of NMDA neural pathways. The "second hit" occurs at the time of onset of the illness and is caused by a neurotoxic mechanism related to NMDA receptor abnormalities (Grunze et al. 1996; McCarley et al. 1996). Other models of schizophrenia that attempt to account for the findings in schizophrenia have also been proposed (see, for example, Andreasen 1997; Benes 1996; Cohen and Servan-Schreiber 1992; Feinberg 1982; Matthysse et al. 1986).

Unresolved Questions

Are Some Brain Abnormalities Specific to Schizophrenia?

The issue of whether some brain abnormalities are specific to schizophrenia rather than nonspecific concomitants of psychoses is beginning to be addressed (see our question list in Table 1–1). This question is important, although it is not the focus of this chapter. Pearlson and co-workers (1997) reviewed both structural and functional findings in schizophrenia versus affective disorder. At present, findings suggest that mood-disordered patients have amygdala-hippocampal abnormalities (see, for example, Swayze et al. 1992). Additionally, Lim and co-workers (1999) reported diffuse gray matter volume reductions in patients with bipolar disorder that were intermediate between reductions in schizophrenic patients and those in control subjects, with these reductions being similar to patients with schizophrenia. At our laboratory, Hirayasu et al. (1998) found a similar left less than right asymmetry abnormality in medial temporal lobe structures between patients with first-episode bipolar disorder and patients with first-episode schizophrenia. However, STG volume reduction was specific to schizophrenia. The issue, however, of whether some brain abnormalities are specific to schizophrenia and others are concomitants of psychoses, or are specific to affective disorder, has not been adequately addressed, and further studies are needed.

Is Schizophrenia a Neurodevelopmental or a Progressive Disorder?

There is growing evidence to suggest that a subgroup of patients with schizophrenia have brain abnormalities that are neurodevelopmental in origin. The general approach taken is to assume that if certain brain abnormalities could have occurred only during neurodevelopment, then an abnormal finding at a later stage of development confirms a neurodevelopmental origin at that abnormality. For example, the sulco-gyral pattern, as noted previously, is largely formed during the third trimester. Another example would be the increased incidence of CSP, because CSP may result from the aberrant formation of the corpus callosum and hippocampus.

The fact that some structural changes occur in utero, however, does not explain why the symptoms of schizophrenia are not observed until early adulthood or later. Moreover, it is still not established that neurodevelopmental abnormalities, in and of themselves, lead to schizophrenia. Further, it is possible that brain abnormalities that occur late in development are directly related to neurodevelopmental abnormalities, which simply unfold over the course of development. Just as plausibly, some neurodevelopmental abnormalities may be neuroanatomically and functionally linked to brain regions that, though not impaired early in the course of the illness, do show impairments later that are secondary to the initial developmental insult to the brain.

Given this complexity, we find it curious that the issue has been reduced in the literature to the following question: Is schizophrenia a static, neurodevelopmental brain disorder or is it a progressive neurodegenerative brain disorder akin to a neuroencephalopathy? We believe it is more likely that, in some patients, an initial insult to the brain occurs during prenatal or perinatal development. This insult is then followed by a second insult that is either related to the first but occurs later in development around the time of illness onset or else is secondary and independent of the first insult but is an insult that would not result in schizophrenia if the brain had not already been compromised by the first insult. This speculation is similar to Meehl's (1962) hypothesis that a "schizogene" is responsible for producing a "schizotaxic brain," leading to the development of a "schizotypic personality," but that other factors such as an adverse learning or social environment or other genetic influences are necessary for the final outcome of schizophrenia. This speculation is also similar to a "two-hit" model of schizophrenia described elsewhere (McCarley et al. 1996), in which the "first hit" is presumed to be the initial insult and involves errors or defects in neural guiding mechanisms of excitatory amino acid transmission that lead to later use-dependent cellular damage or destruction (the "second hit").

We are thus left with more questions than answers concerning the role of neurodevelopmental abnormalities in schizophrenia. Longitudinal studies[6] are needed to determine the extent to which brain abnormalities change over time. Such studies should also address the question of whether some brain regions become abnormal after the onset of illness. Additionally, the question of whether some brain abnormalities are secondary to more primary brain abnormalities could be better addressed using a longitudinal design. Finally, clinico-structural correlations could be tracked longitudinally to determine whether there are clinical features that characterize a specific interconnected neural network that is damaged in schizophrenia or whether clinical features are epiphenomena that wax and wane and are more state dependent.

What Causes Schizophrenia?

There is as yet no known cause of schizophrenia. There are a host of clinical symptoms that can be used for reliably diagnosing the disorder, but there are as yet no genes or neuropathological lesions that can be identified as the cause of schizophrenia. The investigation of brain abnormalities is a promising area of research with some consistent findings. The cause of these abnormalities, however, is not known, and future work is needed to link the constellation of brain abnormalities discerned in schizophrenia to hard data involving cortical maldevelopment, faulty genes, and so on.

Future Studies

Morphometric MRI studies of schizophrenia clearly document brain abnormalities. These abnormalities are more subtle than in other neuropathological disorders, but there are now tools to detect such subtle deviations. We predict that progress in this area will proceed at a rapid rate, particularly as we begin to combine morphometric analyses with functional brain imaging analyses to

---

[6]Several longitudinal studies have been conducted to address some of these issues (see, for example, DeLisi et al. 1992, 1995, 1997; McCarley et al. 1996; Nair et al. 1997). Our point here is to emphasize the need for many more studies. For a recent review of progressive changes in schizophrenia, see also Anderson et al. (1998b).

understand better the relationship between brain function and structure and the ways in which this relationship goes awry in schizophrenia. Future studies will also likely progress at a faster pace as more automated-segmentation tools are developed for identifying individual brain structures. Such an advance would also help researchers to create a normative database for different brain regions so that normative standards can be developed and pathological brains compared. Finally, the study of well-defined and well-characterized patient groups will be important in reducing unknown variation due to population differences across studies. Moreover, a careful delineation of patient groups will hopefully lead to the discovery of important clinicopathological correlations that might in turn lead to the development of more medications targeted at specific regions of brain dysfunction.

■ SUMMARY

We end this chapter with the observation that, after a long hiatus spanning most of this century, the study of brain abnormalities in schizophrenia has been taken up again. This return is the result of major advances in the ability to observe and measure in vivo brain structure and function, which will likely revolutionize what is now known about brain structure and function in both psychiatrically healthy individuals and patients with schizophrenia.

■ REFERENCES

Akbarian S, Bunney WE Jr, Potkin SG, et al: Altered distribution of nicotinamide-adenine dinucleotide phosphate-diaphorase cells in frontal lobe of schizophrenics implies disturbances of cortical development. Arch Gen Psychiatry 50:169–177, 1993a

Akbarian S, Vinuela A, Kim JJ, et al: Distorted distribution of nicotinamide-adenine dinucleotide phosphate-diaphorase neurons in temporal lobe of schizophrenics implies anomalous cortical development. Arch Gen Psychiatry 50:178–187, 1993b

Alzheimer A: Beitrage zur pathologischen Anatomie der Hirnrinde und zur anatomischen Grundlage einiger Psychosen. Monatsschrift fur Psychiatrie und Neurologie 2:82–120, 1897

Anderson JE, Umans CM, Halle M, et al: Anatomy browser: Java-based interactive teaching tool for learning human neuroanatomy. RSNA Electronic Journal 2:50–97, 1998a (serial online) (http://ej.rsna.org/ej2/0050-97.fin/index.html)

Anderson JE, O'Donnell BF, McCarley RW, et al: Progressive changes in schizophrenia: do they exist and what do they mean? Restorative Neurology and Neuroscience 12:1–10, 1998b

Andreasen NC: Linking mind and brain in the study of mental illnesses: a project for a scientific psychopathology. Science 275:1586–1593, 1997

Andreasen NC, Nasrallah HA, Dunn V, et al: Structural abnormalities in the frontal system in schizophrenia: a magnetic resonance imaging study. Arch Gen Psychiatry 43:136–144, 1986

Andreasen NC, Ehrhardt JC, Swayze VW II, et al: Magnetic resonance imaging of the brain in schizophrenia: the pathophysiologic significance of structural abnormalities. Arch Gen Psychiatry 47:35–44, 1990

Andreasen NC, Flashman L, Flaum M, et al: Regional brain abnormalities in schizophrenia measured with magnetic resonance imaging. JAMA 272:1763–1769, 1994a

Andreasen NC, Arndt S, Swayze VW II, et al: Thalamic abnormalities in schizophrenia visualized through magnetic resonance image averaging. Science 266:294–298, 1994b

Arndt S, Andreasen NC, Flaum M, et al: Longitudinal study of symptom dimensions in schizophrenia: prediction and patterns of change. Arch Gen Psychiatry 52:353–360, 1995

Barr WB, Ashtari M, Bilder RM, et al: Brain morphometric comparison of first episode schizophrenia and temporal lobe epilepsy. Br J Psychiatry 170:515–519, 1997

Barta PE, Pearlson GD, Powers RE, et al: Auditory hallucinations and smaller superior temporal gyral volume in schizophrenia. Am J Psychiatry 147:1457–1462, 1990

Barta PE, Pearlson GD, Brill LB, et al: Planum temporale asymmetry reversal in schizophrenia: replication and relationship to gray matter abnormalities. Am J Psychiatry 154:661–667, 1997a

Barta PE, Powers RE, Aylward EH, et al: Quantitative MRI volume changes in late onset schizophrenia and Alzheimer's disease compared to normal controls. Psychiatry Res 68:65–75, 1997b

Becker T, Elmer K, Mechela B, et al: MRI findings in the medial temporal lobe structures in schizophrenia. Eur Neuropsychopharmacol 1:83–86, 1990

Becker T, Elmer K, Schneider F, et al: Confirmation of reduced temporal limbic structure volume on magnetic resonance imaging in male patients with schizophrenia. Psychiatry Res 67:135–143, 1996

Benes FM: Myelination of cortical-hippocampal relays during late adolescence. Schizophr Bull 15:585–593, 1989

Benes FM: Is there a neuroanatomic basis for schizophrenia? An old question revisited. The Neuroscientist 1:104–115, 1995

Benes FM: The defects of affect and attention in schizophrenia: a possible neuroanatomical substrate, in Psychopathology: The Evolving Science of Mental Disorders. Edited by Matthysse S, Levy D, Kagan J, et al. New York, Cambridge University Press, 1996, pp 127–151

Bilder RM, Wu H, Bogerts B, et al: Absence of regional hemispheric volume asymmetries in first-episode schizophrenia. Am J Psychiatry 151:1437–1447, 1994

Blackwood DHR, Young AH, McQueen JK, et al: Magnetic resonance imaging in schizophrenia: altered brain morphology associated with P300 abnormalities and eye tracking dysfunction. Biol Psychiatry 30:753–769, 1991

Bleuler E: Dementia Praecox or the Group of Schizophrenias (1911). Translated by Zinkin H. New York, International Universities Press, 1950

Bleuler M: Chronische Schizophrenien. Wiener Zeitschrift Nervenheilkunde und Deren Grenzgebiete 29:177–187, 1971

Bogerts B, Meertz E, Schonfledt-Bausch R, et al: Basal ganglia and limbic system pathology in schizophrenia. Arch Gen Psychiatry 42:784–791, 1985

Bogerts B, Ashtari M, Degreef G, et al: Reduced temporal limbic structure volumes on magnetic resonance images in first episode schizophrenia. Psychiatry Res 35:1–13, 1990

Bogerts B, Lieberman JA, Ashtari M, et al: Hippocampus-amygdala volumes and psychopathology in chronic schizophrenia. Biol Psychiatry 33:236–246, 1993a

Bogerts B, Falkai P, Grave B, et al: The neuropathology of schizophrenia: past and present. J Hirnforsch 34:193–205, 1993b

Bornstein RA, Schwarzkopf SB, Olson SC, et al: Third-ventricle enlargement and neuropsychological deficit in schizophrenia. Biol Psychiatry 31:954–961, 1992

Bradley WG, Adey WR, Hasso AN: Magnetic Resonance Imaging of the Brain, Head, and Neck. Rockville, MD, Aspens Systems, 1985

Breier A, Buchanan RW, Elkashef A, et al: Brain morphology and schizophrenia: a magnetic resonance imaging study of limbic, prefrontal cortex, and caudate structures. Arch Gen Psychiatry 49:921–926, 1992

Brown R, Colter N, Corsellis JAN, et al: Postmortem evidence of structural changes in schizophrenia: differences in brain weight, temporal horn area and parahippocampal gyrus compared with affective disorders. Arch Gen Psychiatry 43:36–42, 1986

Bruton CJ, Crow TJ, Frith CD, et al: Schizophrenia and the brain: a prospective clinico-neuropathological study. Psychol Med 20:285–304, 1990

Buchanan RW, Breier A, Kirkpatrick B, et al: Structural abnormalities in deficit and nondeficit schizophrenia. Am J Psychiatry 150:59–65, 1993

Buchsbaum MS, Someya T, Teng CY, et al: PET and MRI of the thalamus in never-medicated patients with schizophrenia. Am J Psychiatry 153:191–199, 1996

Buchsbaum MS, Yang S, Hazlett E, et al: Ventricular volume and asymmetry in schizotypal personality disorder and schizophrenia assessed with magnetic resonance imaging. Schizophr Res 27:45–53, 1997

Buchsbaum MS, Tang CY, Peled S, et al: MRI white matter diffusion anisotropy and PET metabolic rate in schizophrenia. Neuroreport 9:425–430, 1998

Callaghan PT: Principles of Nuclear Magnetic Resonance Microscopy. New York, Oxford University Press, 1991

Carpenter MB: Core Text of Neuroanatomy, 4th Edition. Baltimore, MD, Williams & Wilkins, 1991

Casanova MF, Zito M, Goldberg T, et al: Shape distortion of the corpus callosum of monozygotic twins discordant for schizophrenia. Schizophr Res 3:155–156, 1990

Chakos MH, Lieberman JA, Bilder RM, et al: Increase in caudate nuclei volumes of first- episode schizophrenic patients taking antipsychotic drugs. Am J Psychiatry 151:1430–1436, 1994

Chakos MH, Lieberman JA, Alvir J, et al: Caudate nuclei volumes in schizophrenic patients treated with typical antipsychotics or clozapine. Lancet 345:456–457, 1995

Chien D, Buxton RB, Kwong KK, et al: MR diffusion imaging of the human brain. J Comput Assist Tomogr 14:514–520, 1990

Chua SE, McKenna PJ: Schizophrenia—a brain disease? A critical review of structural and functional cerebral abnormality in the disorder. Br J Psychiatry 166:563–582, 1995

Ciompi L: Catamnestic long-term study on the course of life and aging of schizophrenics. Schizophr Bull 6:606–618, 1980

Cline HE, Lorensen WE, Ludke S, et al: Two algorithms for the three-dimensional reconstruction of tomograms. Med Phys 13:320–327, 1988

Cline HE, Lorensen WE, Kikinis R, et al: Three-dimensional segmentation of MR images of the head using probability and connectivity. J Comput Assist Tomogr 14:1037–1045, 1990

Coffman JA, Schwarzkopf SB, Olson SC, et al: Midsagittal cerebral anatomy by magnetic resonance imaging: the importance of slice position and thickness. Schizophr Res 2:287–294, 1989

Cohen JD, Servan-Schreiber D: Context, cortex, and dopamine: a connectionist approach to behavior and biology in schizophrenia. Psychol Rev 99:45–77, 1992

Colombo C, Abbruzzese M, Livian S, et al: Memory functions and temporal-limbic morphology in schizophrenia. Psychiatry Res 50:45–56, 1993

Colombo C, Bonfanti A, Scarone S: Anatomical characteristics of the corpus callosum and clinical correlates in schizophrenia. Eur Arch Psychiatry Clin Neurosci 243:244–248, 1994

Colter N, Battal S, Crow TJ, et al: White matter reduction in the parahippocampal gyrus of patients with schizophrenia (letter). Arch Gen Psychiatry 44:1023, 1987

Corey-Bloom J, Jernigan T, Archibald S, et al: Quantitative magnetic resonance imaging of the brain in late-life schizophrenia. Am J Psychiatry 152:447–449, 1995

Corkin S: Lasting consequences of bilateral medial temporal lobectomy: clinical course and experimental findings. Semin Neurol 4:249–259, 1984

Crichton-Browne J: On the weight of the brain and its component parts in the insane. Brain 2:42–67, 1879

Crosby EC, Humphrey T, Lauer EW: Correlative Anatomy of the Nervous System. New York, Macmillan, 1962

Crow TJ: Molecular pathology of schizophrenia: more than one disease process? Br Med J 280:66–68, 1989

Crow TJ: The continuum of psychosis and its genetic origins. The sixty-fifth Maudsley lecture. Br J Psychiatry 156:788–797, 1990a

Crow TJ: Temporal lobe asymmetry as the key to the etiology of schizophrenia. Schizophr Bull 16:433–443, 1990b

Dauphinais ID, DeLisi LE, Crow TJ, et al: Reduction in temporal lobe size in siblings with schizophrenia: a magnetic resonance imaging study. Psychiatry Res 35:137–147, 1990

Degreef G, Bogerts B, Ashtari M, et al: Ventricular system morphology in first episode schizophrenia: a volumetric study of ventricular subdivisions on MRI (abstract). Schizophr Res 3:18, 1990

Degreef G, Lantos G, Bogerts B, et al: Abnormalities of the septum pellucidum on MR scans in first-episode schizophrenic patients. Am J Neuroradiology 13:835–840, 1992a

Degreef G, Bogerts B, Falkai P, et al: Increased prevalence of the cavum septum pellucidum in magnetic resonance scans and postmortem brains of schizophrenic patients. Psychiatry Res 45:1–13, 1992b

Degreef G, Ashtari M, Bogerts B, et al: Volumes of ventricular system subdivisions measured from magnetic resonance images in first-episode schizophrenic patients. Arch Gen Psychiatry 49:531–537, 1992c

DeLisi LE, Dauphinais ID, Gershon ES: Perinatal complications and reduced size of brain limbic structures in familial schizophrenia. Schizophr Bull 14:185–191, 1988

DeLisi LE, Hoff AL, Schwartz JE, et al: Brain morphology in first-episode schizophrenic-like psychotic patients: a quantitative magnetic resonance imaging study. Biol Psychiatry 29:159–175, 1991

DeLisi LE, Strizke P, Riordan H, et al: The timing of brain morphological changes in schizophrenia and their relationship to clinical outcome. Biol Psychiatry 31:241–254, 1992

DeLisi LE, Hoff AL, Kushner M, et al: Increased prevalence of cavum septum pellucidum in schizophrenia. Psychiatry Res 50:193–199, 1993

DeLisi LE, Hoff AL, Neale C, et al: Asymmetries in the superior temporal lobe in male and female first-episode schizophrenic patients: measures of the planum temporale and superior temporal gyrus by MRI. Schizophr Res 12:19–28, 1994

DeLisi LE, Tew W, Xie S, et al: A prospective follow-up study of brain morphology and cognition in first-episode schizophrenic patients: preliminary findings. Biol Psychiatry 38:349–360, 1995

DeLisi LE, Sakuma M, Tew W, et al: Schizophrenia as a chronic active brain process: a study of progressive brain structural change subsequent to the onset of schizophrenia. Psychiatry Res 74:129–140, 1997

DeQuardo JR, Bookstein FL, Green WD, et al: Spatial relationships of neuroanatomic landmarks in schizophrenia. Psychiatry Res 67:81–95, 1996

Di Michele V, Rossi A, Stratta P, et al: Neuropsychological and clinical correlates of temporal lobe anatomy in schizophrenia. Acta Psychiatr Scand 85:484–488, 1992

Doran M, Hajnal JV, Van Bruggen N, et al: Normal and abnormal white matter tracts shown by MR imaging using directional diffusion weighted sequences. J Comput Assist Tomogr 14:865–873, 1990

Douek P, Turner R, Pekar J, et al: MR color mapping of myelin fiber orientation. J Comput Assist Tomogr 15:923–929, 1991

Egan MF, Duncan CC, Suddath RL, et al: Event-related potential abnormalities correlate with structural brain alterations and clinical features in patients with chronic schizophrenia. Schizophr Res 11:259–271, 1994

Elkashef AM, Buchanan RW, Gellad F, et al: Basal ganglia pathology in schizophrenia and tardive dyskinesia: an MRI quantitative study. Am J Psychiatry 151:752–755, 1994

Ernst RR, Bodenhausen G, Wokaun A, et al: Principles of Nuclear Magnetic Resonance in One and Two Dimensions. New York, Oxford University Press, 1987

Falkai P, Bogerts B: Cell loss in the hippocampus of schizophrenics. Eur Arch Psychiatry Neurol Sci 236:154–161, 1986

Falkai P, Bogerts B, Rozumek M: Limbic pathology in schizophrenia: the entorhinal region—a morphometric study. Biol Psychiatry 24:515–521, 1988

Feinberg I: Schizophrenia: caused by a fault in programmed synaptic elimination during adolescence? J Psychiatr Res 17:319–334, 1982

Filipek PA, Kennedy DN, Caviness VS, et al: Magnetic resonance imaging-based brain morphometry: development and application to normal subjects. Ann Neurol 25:61–67, 1988

Flaum M, Swayze VW II, O'Leary OS, et al: Effects of diagnosis and gender on brain morphology in schizophrenia. Am J Psychiatry 152:704–714, 1995

Fukuzako T, Fukuzako H, Kodama S, et al: Cavum septum pellucidum in schizophrenia: a magnetic resonance imaging study. Psychiatry Clin Neurosci 50:125–128, 1996

Galaburda AM: Anatomical asymmetry, in Cerebral Dominance: The Biological Foundations. Edited by Geschwind N, Galaburda AM. Cambridge, MA, Harvard University Press, 1984, pp 11–25

Galaburda AM, Corsiglia J, Rosen GD, et al: Planum temporale asymmetry: reappraisal since Geschwind and Levitsky. Neuropsychologia 25:853–868, 1987

Gannon PJ, Holloway RL, Broadfield DC, et al: Asymmetry of chimpanzee planum temporale: humanlike pattern of Wernicke's brain language area homolog. Science 279:220–222, 1997

Gerig G, Kuoni W, Kikinis R, et al: Medical imaging and computer vision: an integrated approach for diagnosis and planning. 11th Die Deutsche Arbeitgemeinschaft fur mustererkennung (DABM) Symposium on Computer Vision, Hamburg, Federal Republic of Germany, October 2–4, 1989, Fach berichte IF B 219, Springer, Berlin, pp 425–443

Gerig G, Kikinis R, Kübler O: Significant Improvement of MR Image Data Quality Using Anisotropic Diffusion Filtering (Technical report BIWI-TR-124). Zurich, Communication Technology Laboratory Image Science Division ETH, 1990

Geschwind N, Levitsky W: Human brain: left-right asymmetries in the temporal speech region. Science 161:186–187, 1968

Gloor P: The role of the human limbic system in perception, memory and affect: lessons from temporal lobe epilepsy, in The Limbic System: Functional Organization and Clinical Disorders. Edited by Doane BK, Livingston KE, New York, Raven, 1986, pp 159–169

Goldberg TE, Ragland JD, Torrey EF, et al: Neuropsychological assessment of monozygotic twins discordant for schizophrenia. Arch Gen Psychiatry 47:1066–1072, 1990

Grunze HCR, Rainnie DG, Hasselmo ME, et al: NMDA-dependent modulation of CA1 local circuit inhibition. J Neurosci 16:2034–2043, 1996

Gruzelier J: Commentary on neuropsychological and information processing deficits in psychosis and neuropsychological syndrome relationships in schizophrenia, in Cerebral Dynamics, Laterality and Psychopathology. Edited by Takahashi R, Flor-Henry P, Gruzelier J, et al. Amsterdam, Elsevier, 1987, pp 23–52

Gudbjartsson H, Maier SE, Mulkern RV, et al: Line-scan diffusion imaging. Magn Reson Med 36:509–519, 1996

Guenther W, Moser E, Petsch R, et al: Pathological cerebral blood flow and corpus callosum abnormalities in schizophrenia: relations to EEG mapping and PET data. Psychiatry Res 29:453–455, 1989

Gunther W, Petsch R, Steinberg R, et al: Brain dysfunction during motor activation and corpus callosum alterations in schizophrenia measured by cerebral blood flow and magnetic resonance imaging. Biol Psychiatry 29:535–555, 1991

Gur RE, Pearlson GD: Neuroimaging in schizophrenia research. Schizophr Bull 19:337–353, 1993

Gur RE, Mozley D, Shtasel DL, et al: Clinical subtypes of schizophrenia: differences in brain and CSF volume. Am J Psychiatry 151:343–350, 1994

Gur RE, Cowell P, Turetsky BI, et al: A follow-up magnetic resonance imaging study of schizophrenia: relationship of neuroanatomical changes to clinical and neurobehavioral measures. Arch Gen Psychiatry 55:145–152, 1998

Hajek M, Huonker R, Boehle C, et al: Abnormalities of auditory evoked magnetic fields and structural changes in the left hemisphere of male schizophrenics: a magnetoencephalographic-magnetic resonance imaging study. Biol Psychiatry 42:609–616, 1997

Hajnal JV, Doran M, Hall AS, et al: MR imaging of anisotropically restricted diffusion of water in the nervous system: technical, anatomic, and pathologic considerations. J Comput Assist Tomogr 15:1–18, 1991

Harvey I, Ron MA, Du Boulay G, et al: Reduction of cortical volume in schizophrenia on magnetic resonance imaging. Psychol Med 23:591–604, 1993

Haug JO: Pneumoencephalographic studies in mental disease. Acta Psychiatr Scand 38 (suppl 165):1–104, 1962

Hauser P, Dauphinais ID, Berrettini W, et al: Corpus callosum dimensions measured by magnetic resonance imaging in bipolar affective disorder and schizophrenia. Biol Psychiatry 26:659–668, 1989

Heyman I, Murray RM: Schizophrenia and neurodevelopment. J R Coll Physicians Lond 26:143–146, 1992

Hirayasu Y, Shenton ME, Salisbury DF, et al: Lower left temporal lobe MRI volumes in patients with first-episode schizophrenia compared with psychotic patients with first-episode affective disorder and normal subjects. Am J Psychiatry 155:1384–1391, 1998

Hoff AL, Riordan H, O'Donnell D, et al: Anomalous lateral sulcus and cognitive function in first-episode schizophrenia. Schizophr Bull 18:257–272, 1992

Hoff AL, Neal C, Kushner M, et al: Gender differences in corpus callosum size in first-episode schizophrenics. Biol Psychiatry 35:913–919, 1994

Höhne KH, Bomans M, Pommert A, et al: Rendering tomographic volume data: adequacy of methods of different modalities and organs, in Imaging in Medicine (NATO ASI Series, Vol F60 3D). Edited by Höhne KH, Fuchs H, Pizer SM. New York, Springer-Verlag, 1990, pp 197–215

Hokama H, Shenton ME, Nestor PG, et al: Caudate, putamen, and globus pallidus volume in schizophrenia: a quantitative MRI study. Psychiatry Res 61:209–229, 1995

Hornak JP: The basics of MRI. 1996. Available at: http://www.cis.rit.edu/htbooks/mri

Horowitz AL: MRI Physics for Radiologists: A Visual Approach, 2nd Edition. New York, Springer-Verlag, 1991

Huber G, Gross G, Schuttler R, et al: A long-term follow-up study of schizophrenia: psychiatric course of illness and prognosis. Acta Psychiatr Scand 52:49–57, 1975

Huber G, Gross G, Schuttler R, et al: Longitudinal studies of schizophrenic patients. Schizophr Bull 6:592–605, 1980

Iosifescu DV, Shenton ME, Warfield SK, et al: An automated registration algorithm for measuring MRI subcortical brain structures. Neuroimage 6:13–25, 1997

Jacobi W, Winkler H, et al: Encephalographische Studien an cronischen Schizophrenen. Arch Psychiatr Nervenkr 81:299–332, 1927

Jacobsen LK, Giedd JN, Vaituzis AC, et al: Temporal lobe morphology in childhood-onset schizophrenia. Am J Psychiatry 153:355–361, 1996

Jakob H, Beckmann H: Prenatal developmental disturbances in the limbic allocortex in schizophrenics. J Neural Transm 65:303–326, 1986

Jakob H, Beckmann H: Gross and histological criteria for developmental disorders in brains of schizophrenics. J R Soc Med 82:466–469, 1989

Jernigan TL, Zisook S, Heaton RK, et al: Magnetic resonance imaging abnormalities in lenticular nuclei and cerebral cortex in schizophrenia. Arch Gen Psychiatry 48:881–890, 1991

Jeste DV, Lohr JB: Hippocampal pathologic findings in schizophrenia: a morphometric study. Arch Gen Psychiatry 46:1019–1024, 1989

Johnston MH, Holzman PS: Assessing Schizophrenic Thinking. San Francisco, CA, Jossey-Bass, 1979

Johnstone EC, Crow TJ, Frith CD, et al: Cerebral ventricular size and cognitive impairment in chronic schizophrenia. Lancet 2:924–926, 1976

Johnstone EC, Owens DG, Crow TJ, et al: Temporal lobe structure as determined by nuclear magnetic resonance in schizophrenia and bipolar affective disorder. J Neurol Neurosurg Psychiatry 52:736–741, 1989

Jurjus GJ, Nasrallah HA, Olson SC, et al: Cavum septum pellucidum in schizophrenia, affective disorder, and healthy controls: a magnetic resonance imaging study. Psychol Med 23:319–322, 1993

Kahlbaum K: Die Katatonie oder der Spannungsirresein. Berlin, Hirshwald, 1874

Kawasaki Y, Maeda Y, Urata K, et al: A quantitative magnetic resonance imaging study of patients with schizophrenia. Eur Arch Psychiatry Clin Neurosci 242:268–272, 1993

Kelsoe JR, Cadet JL, Pickar D, et al: Quantitative neuroanatomy in schizophrenia: a controlled magnetic resonance imaging study. Arch Gen Psychiatry 45:533–541, 1988

Kendler KS, McGuire M, Gruenberg AM, et al: The Roscommon Family Study, III: schizophrenia-related personality disorders in relatives. Arch Gen Psychiatry 50:781–788, 1993

Keshavan MS, Bagwell WW, Haas GL, et al: Changes in caudate volume with neuroleptic treatment (letter). Lancet 344:1434, 1994

Keshavan MS, Bagwell WW, Haas GL, et al: Does caudate volume increase during follow up in first-episode psychosis (abstract)? Schizophr Res 15:87, 1995

Kety SS: Biochemical theories of schizophrenia. Science 129:1528–1532, 1959

Kikinis R, Shenton ME, Jolesz FA, et al: Routine quantitative MRI-based analysis of brain and fluid spaces. J Magn Reson Imaging 2:619–629, 1992

Kikinis R, Shenton ME, Gerig G, et al: Temporal lobe sulco-gyral pattern anomalies in schizophrenia: an in vivo MR three-dimensional surface rendering study. Neurosci Lett 182:7–12, 1994

Kikinis R, Shenton ME, Iosifescu DV, et al: A digital brain atlas for surgical planning, model driven segmentation, and teaching. IEEE Transactions on Visualization and Computer Graphics 2:232–241, 1996

Kirch DG, Weinberger DR: Anatomical neuropathology in schizophrenia: postmortem findings, in Handbook of Schizophrenia, Vol I: The Neurology of Schizophrenia. Edited by Nasrallah HA, Weinberger DR. New York, Elsevier, 1986, pp 325–348

Kleinschmidt A, Falkai P, Huang Y, et al: In vivo morphometry of planum temporale asymmetry in first-episode schizophrenia. Schizophr Res 12:9–18, 1994

Kovelman JA, Scheibel AB: A neurological correlate of schizophrenia. Biol Psychiatry 191:1601–1621, 1984

Kraepelin E: Dementia Praecox (1919). Translated by Barclay E, Barclay S. New York, Churchill Livingstone, 1971

Kretschmer E: Physique and Character. New York, Harcourt Brace Jovanovich, 1925

Krishnan KRR, MacFall JR: Basic principles of magnetic resonance imaging, in Brain Imaging in Clinical Psychiatry. Edited by Krishnan KRR, MacFall JR. New York, Marcel Dekker, 1997, pp 1–11

Kulynych JJ, Vladar K, Fantie BD, et al: Normal asymmetry of the planum temporale in patients with schizophrenia: three-dimensional cortical morphometry with MRI. Br J Psychiatry 166:742–749, 1995

Kulynych JJ, Vladar K, Jones DW, et al: Superior temporal gyrus volume in schizophrenia: a study using MRI morphometry assisted by surface rendering. Am J Psychiatry 153:50–56, 1996

Kumar A, Welti D, Ernst R: NMR Fourier zeugmatography. Magn Reson Imaging 18: 69–83, 1975

Kwon JS, Shenton ME, Hirayasu Y, et al: MRI study of cavum septi pellucidi in schizophrenia, affective disorder, and schizotypal personality disorder. Am J Psychiatry 155:509–515, 1998

Kwon JS, McCarley RW, Hirayasu Y, et al: Left planum temporale volume reduction in schizophrenia. Arch Gen Psychiatry 56:142–148, 1999

Lauriello J, Hoff A, Wieneke MH, et al: Similar extent of brain dysmorphology in severely ill women and men with schizophrenia. Am J Psychiatry 154:819–825, 1997

Le Bihan D: Diffusion and Perfusion Magnetic Resonance Imaging. New York, Raven, 1995

Le Bihan D, Breton E, Lallemand D, et al: MR imaging of intravoxel incoherent motions: application to diffusion and perfusion in neurologic disorders. Radiology 161: 401–407, 1986

Le Bihan D, Berr I, Gelbert F, et al: MR imaging of intravoxel incoherent motions in ischemic and malformative cerebral diseases (abstract). Radiology 165:303, 1987

Lewine RR, Gulleu LR, Risch SC, et al: Sexual dimorphism, brain morphology, and schizophrenia. Schizophr Bull 16:195–203, 1990

Lim KO, Tew W, Kushner M, et al: Cortical gray matter volume deficit in patients with first-episode schizophrenia. Am J Psychiatry 153:1548–1553, 1996

Lim KO, Rosenbloom MJ, Faustman WO, et al: Cortical gray matter deficit in patients with bipolar disorder. Schizophr Res 40:219–227, 1999

Lorensen WE, Cline HE: Marching cubes: a high resolution 3D surface construction algorithm. Computer Graphics 21:163–169, 1987

MacLean PD: Some psychiatric implications of physiological studies on frontotemporal portion of limbic system (visceral brain). Electroencephalogr Clin Neurophysiol 4: 407–418, 1952

Maier SE, Jolesz FA: Line-scan diffusion imaging with a high performance gradient system. Proceedings of the 6th Annual Meeting of the International Society for Magnetic Resonance in Medicine (ISMRM), Sydney, Australia, April 18–24, p. 1389

Maier SE, Hardy CJ, Jolesz FA: Brain and cerebrospinal fluid motion: real-time quantification with M-mode MR imaging. Radiology 193:477–483, 1994

Maier SE, Gudbjartsson H, Patz S, et al: Line-scan diffusion imaging: characterization in healthy subjects and stroke patients. AJR Am J Roentgenol 171:85–93, 1998

Marsh L, Suddath RL, Higgins N, et al: Medial temporal lobe structures in schizophrenia: relationship of size to duration of illness. Schizophr Res 11:225–238, 1994

Marsh L, Harris D, Lim KO, et al: Structural magnetic resonance imaging abnormalities in men with severe chronic schizophrenia and an early age at clinical onset. Arch Gen Psychiatry 54:1104–1112, 1997

Mathew RJ, Partain CL: Midsagittal sections of the cerebellar vermis and fourth ventricle obtained with magnetic resonance imaging of schizophrenic patients. Am J Psychiatry 142:970–971, 1985

Mathew RJ, Partain CL, Prakash MV, et al: A study of the septum pellucidum and corpus callosum in schizophrenia with MR imaging. Acta Psychiatr Scand 72:414–421, 1985

Matthysse S, Holzman PS, Lange K: The genetic transmission of schizophrenia: application of mendelian latent structure analysis to eye tracking dysfunctions in schizophrenia and affective disorder. J Psychiatr Res 20:57–65, 1986

McCarley RW, Shenton ME, O'Donnell BF, et al: Auditory P300 abnormalities and left posterior superior temporal gyrus volume reduction in schizophrenia. Arch Gen Psychiatry 50:190–197, 1993

McCarley RW, Hsiao JK, Freedman R, et al: Neuroimaging and the cognitive neuroscience of schizophrenia. Schizophr Bull 22:703–725, 1996

McCarley RW, Wible CG, Frumin M, et al: MRI anatomy of schizophrenia. Biol Psychiatry 45:1099–1119, 1999

Meehl PE: Schizotaxia, schizotypy, schizophrenia. Am Psychol 17:827–838, 1962

Menon RR, Barta PE, Aylward EH, et al: Posterior superior temporal gyrus in schizophrenia: grey matter changes and clinical correlates. Schizophr Res 16:127–135, 1995

Milner B: Disorders of learning and memory after temporal lobe lesions in man. Clin Neurosurg 19:421–466, 1972

Mion CC, Andreasen NC, Arndt S, et al: MRI abnormalities in tardive dyskinesia. Psychiatry Res 40:157–166, 1991

Moseley ME, Kucharczyk J, Mintorovitch J, et al: Diffusion-weighted MR imaging of acute stroke: correlation with T2-weighted and magnetic susceptibility-enhanced MR imaging in cats. Am J Neuroradiol 11:423–429, 1990

Murray RM, Lewis SW: Is schizophrenia a neurodevelopmental disorder? BMJ 95:681–682, 1987

Nair TR, Christensen JD, Kingsbury SJ, et al: Progression of cerebroventricular enlargement and the subtyping of schizophrenia. Psychiatry Res 74:141–150, 1997

Nasrallah HA, Schwarzkopf SB, Olson SC, et al: Gender differences in schizophrenia on MRI brain scans. Schizophr Bull 16:205–210, 1990

Nestor PG, Shenton ME, McCarley RW, et al: Neuropsychological correlates of MRI temporal lobe abnormalities in schizophrenia. Am J Psychiatry 150:1849–1855, 1993

Nopoulos P, Torres I, Flaum M, et al: Brain morphology in first-episode schizophrenia. Am J Psychiatry 152:1721–1723, 1995

Nopoulos P, Swayze V, Andreasen NC: Pattern of brain morphology in patients with schizophrenia and large cavum septi pellucidi. J Neuropsychiatry Clin Neurosci 8:147–152, 1996

Nopoulos P, Swayze V, Flaum M, et al: Cavum septi pellucidi in normals and patients with schizophrenia as detected by magnetic resonance imaging. Biol Psychiatry 41:1102–1108, 1997

Ohnuma T, Kimura N, Takahashi T, et al: A magnetic resonance imaging study in first- episode disorganized-type patients with schizophrenia. Psychiatry Clin Neurosci 51:9–15, 1997

Ojemann GA: Cortical organization of language. J Neurosci 11:2281–2287, 1991

Ojemann GA, Creutzfeldt O, Lettich E, et al: Neuronal activity in human lateral temporal cortex related to short-term verbal memory, naming and reading. Brain 111:1383–1403, 1988

Olney JW: Excitatory amino acids and neuropsychiatric disorders. Biol Psychiatry 26:505–525, 1989

Park S, Holzman PS: Schizophrenics show spatial working memory deficits. Arch Gen Psychiatry 49:975–982, 1992

Pearlson GD, Marsh L: MRI in psychiatry, in American Psychiatric Press Review of Psychiatry, Vol 12. Edited by Oldham JM, Riba MB, Tasman A. Washington, DC, American Psychiatric Press, 1993, pp 347–381

Pearlson GD, Petty RG, Ross CA, et al: Schizophrenia: a disease of heteromodal association cortex? Neuropsychopharmacology 14:1–17, 1996

Pearlson GD, Barta PE, Powers RE, et al: Ziskind-Somerfeld Research Award 1996. Medial and superior temporal gyral volumes and cerebral asymmetry in schizophrenia versus bipolar disorder. Biol Psychiatry 41:1–14, 1997

Peled S, Gudbjartsson H, Westin CF, et al: Magnetic resonance imaging shows orientation and asymmetry of white matter fiber tracts. Brain Res 780:27–33, 1998

Penfield W, Perot P: The brain's record of auditory and visual experience: a final summary and discussion. Brain 86:595–696, 1963

Penfield W, Roberts L: Speech and Brain Mechanisms. Princeton, NJ, Princeton University Press, 1959

Petty RG, Barta PE, Pearlson GD, et al: Reversal of asymmetry of the planum temporale in schizophrenia. Am J Psychiatry 152:715–721, 1995

Pfefferbaum A, Lim KO, Rosenbloom M, et al: Brain magnetic resonance imaging: approaches for investigating schizophrenia. Schizophr Bull 16:453–476, 1990

Pinel P: Traité medico philosophique sur l'alienation mentale boulamania. Edited by Caille R. Paris, Ravier, 1801

Plum F: Prospects for research on schizophrenia, 3: neuropsychology. Neuropathological findings. Neurosci Res Program Bull 10:384–388, 1972

Portas CM, Goldstein JM, Shenton ME, et al: Volumetric evaluation of the thalamus in schizophrenic patients using magnetic resonance imaging. Biol Psychiatry 43:629–659, 1998

Radamacher J, Galaburda AM, Kennedy DN, et al: Human cerebral cortex: localization, parcellation, and morphometry with magnetic resonance imaging. J Cogn Neurosci 4:352–374, 1992

Raine A, Harrison GN, Reynolds GP, et al: Structural and functional characteristics of the corpus callosum in schizophrenics. Arch Gen Psychiatry 47:1060–1064, 1990

Raine A, Lencz T, Reynolds GP, et al: An evaluation of structural and functional prefrontal deficits in schizophrenia: MRI and neuropsychological measures. Psychiatry Res 45:123–137, 1992

Rauch SL, Renshaw PF: Clinical neuroimaging in psychiatry. Harv Rev Psychiatry 2:297–312, 1995

Reite M, Sheeder J, Teale P, et al: Magnetic source imaging evidence of sex differences in cerebral lateralization in schizophrenia. Arch Gen Psychiatry 54:433–440, 1997

Rosenthal R: Judgement Studies: Design, Analysis and Meta-analysis. New York, Cambridge University Press, 1987

Rossi A, Stratta P, Gallucci M, et al: Standardized magnetic resonance image intensity study in schizophrenia. Psychiatry Res 25:223–231, 1988

Rossi A, Stratta P, Gallucci M, et al: Quantification of corpus callosum and ventricles in schizophrenia with nuclear magnetic resonance imaging: a pilot study. Am J Psychiatry 146:99–101, 1989a

Rossi A, Stratta P, D'Albenzio L, et al: Reduced temporal lobe area in schizophrenia by magnetic resonance imaging: preliminary evidence. Psychiatry Res 29:261–263, 1989b

Rossi A, Galderisi S, Michele VD, et al: Dementia in schizophrenia: magnetic resonance and clinical correlates. J Nerv Ment Dis 178:521–524, 1990

Rossi A, Stratta P, Michele VD, et al: Temporal lobe structure by magnetic resonance in bipolar affective disorders and schizophrenia. J Affective Dis 21:19–22, 1991

Rossi A, Stratta P, Mattei P, et al: Planum temporale in schizophrenia: a magnetic resonance study. Schizophr Res 7:19–22, 1992

Rossi A, Stratta P, Mancini F, et al: Cerebellar vermal size in schizophrenia: a male effect. Biol Psychiatry 33:354–357, 1993

Rossi A, Stratta P, Mancini F, et al: Magnetic resonance imaging findings of amygdala-anterior hippocampus shrinkage in male patients with schizophrenia. Psychiatry Res 52:43–53, 1994a

Rossi A, Serio A, Stratta P, et al: Planum temporale asymmetry and thought disorder in schizophrenia. Schizophr Res 12:1–7, 1994b

Saykin AJ, Shtasel DL, Gur RE, et al: Neuropsychological deficits in neuroleptic naive patients with first episode schizophrenia. Arch Gen Psychiatry 51:124–131, 1994

Schlaepfer TE, Harris GH, Tien AY, et al: Decreased regional cortical gray matter volume in schizophrenia. Am J Psychiatry 151:842–848, 1994

Schmahmann JD: From movement to thought: anatomic substrates of the cerebellar contribution to cognitive processing. Hum Brain Mapp 4:174–198, 1996

Schwartz JM, Aylward E, Barta PE, et al: Sylvian fissure size in schizophrenia measured with the magnetic resonance imaging rating protocol of the Consortium to Establish a Registry for Alzheimer's Disease. Am J Psychiatry 149:1195–1198, 1992

Schwarzkopf SB, Olson SC, Coffman JA, et al: Third and lateral ventricular volumes in schizophrenia: support for progressive enlargement of both structures. Psychopharmacol Bull 26:385–391, 1990

Scott TF, Price TP, George MS, et al: Cerebral malformations and schizophrenia. J Neuropsychiatry Clin Neurosci 5:287–293, 1993

Seidman LJ: Schizophrenia and brain dysfunction: an integration of recent neurodiagnostic findings. Psychol Bull 94:195–238, 1983

Selemon LD, Rajkowska G, Goldman-Rakic PS: Abnormally high neuronal density in schizophrenic cortex: a morphometric analysis of prefrontal area 9 and occipital area 17. Arch Gen Psychiatry 52:805–818, 1995

Shelton RC, Weinberger DR: X-ray computerized tomography studies in schizophrenia: a review and synthesis, in The Handbook of Schizophrenia, Vol I: The Neurology of Schizophrenia. Edited by Nasrallah HA, Weinberger DR. New York, Elsevier, 1986, pp 207–250

Shenton ME: Temporal lobe structural abnormalities in schizophrenia: a selective review and presentation of new MR findings, in Psychopathology: The Evolving Science of Mental Disorders. Edited by Matthysse S, Levy D, Kagan J, et al. New York, Cambridge University Press, 1996, pp 51–99

Shenton ME, Solovay MR, Holzman P: Comparative studies of thought disorders, II: schizoaffective disorder. Arch Gen Psychiatry 44:21–30, 1987

Shenton ME, Kikinis R, McCarley RW, et al: Application of automated MRI volumetric measurement techniques to the ventricular system in schizophrenics and normal controls. Schizophr Res 5:103–113, 1991

Shenton ME, Kikinis R, Jolesz FA, et al: Abnormalities of the left temporal lobe and thought disorder in schizophrenia: a quantitative magnetic resonance imaging study. N Engl J Med 327:604–612, 1992

Shenton ME, Kikinis R, McCarley RW, et al: Harvard Brain Atlas: A Teaching and Visualization Tool. Proceedings from IEEE Computer Society, IEEE Biomedical Visualization, Atlanta, GA, October 30, 1995, pp 10–17

Shenton ME, Wible CG, McCarley RW: A review of magnetic resonance imaging studies of brain abnormalities in schizophrenia, in Brain Imaging in Clinical Psychiatry. Edited by Rama Krishnan KR, Doraiswamy PM. New York, Marcel Dekker, 1997, pp 297–380

Slichter CP: Principles of Magnetic Resonance, Third Edition. Berlin, Springer-Verlag, 1990

Smith RC, Calderon G, Ravichandran GK, et al: Nuclear magnetic resonance in schizophrenia: a preliminary study. Psychiatry Res 12:137–147, 1984

Southard EE: A study of the dementia praecox group in the light of certain cases showing anomalies or scleroses in particular brain regions. American Journal of Insanity 67:119–176, 1910

Southard EE: On the topographic distribution of cortex lesions and anomalies in dementia praecox with some account of their functional significance. American Journal of Insanity 71:603–671, 1915

Squire LR: Memory and the hippocampus: a synthesis from findings with rats, monkeys, and humans. Psychol Rev 99:195–231, 1992

Squire LR, Zola-Morgan S: The medial temporal lobe memory system. Science 253: 1380–1386, 1991

Stevens JR: An anatomy of schizophrenia? Arch Gen Psychiatry 29:177–189, 1973

Stratta P, Rossi A, Gallucci M, et al: Hemispheric asymmetries and schizophrenia: a preliminary magnetic resonance imaging study. Biol Psychiatry 25:275–284, 1989

Suddath RL, Casanova MF, Goldberg TE, et al: Temporal lobe pathology in schizophrenia: a quantitative magnetic resonance imaging study. Am J Psychiatry 146:464–472, 1989

Suddath RL, Christison GW, Torrey EF, et al: Anatomical abnormalities in the brains of monozygotic twins discordant for schizophrenia. N Engl J Med 322:789–794, 1990

Sullivan EV, Mathalon DH, Lim KO, et al: Patterns of regional cortical dysmorphology distinguishing schizophrenia and chronic alcoholism. Biol Psychiatry 43:118–131, 1998

Swayze VW II, Andreasen NC, Alliger RJ, et al: Subcortical and temporal structures in affective disorder and schizophrenia: a magnetic resonance imaging study. Biol Psychiatry 31:221–240, 1992

Torrey EF, Peterson MR: Schizophrenia and the limbic system. Lancet 2:942–946, 1974

Tsuang MT, Woolson RF, Fleming JA: Long-term outcome of major psychosis: schizophrenic and affective disorders compared with psychiatrically symptom-free surgical conditions. Arch Gen Psychiatry 39:1295–1301, 1979

Tsuang MT, Woolson RF, Winokur G, et al: Stability of psychiatric diagnosis: schizophrenia and affective disorders followed up over a 30- to 40-year period. Arch Gen Psychiatry 38:535–539, 1981

Tune L, Barta P, Wong D, et al: Striatal dopamine D2 receptor quantification and superior temporal gyrus: volume determination in 14 chronic schizophrenic subjects. Psychiatry Res 67:155–158, 1996

Uematsu M, Kaiya H: The morphology of the corpus callosum in schizophrenia: an MRI study. Schizophr Res 1:391–398, 1988

Uematsu M, Kaiya H: Midsagittal cortical pathomorphology of schizophrenia: a magnetic resonance imaging study. Psychiatry Res 30:11–20, 1989

Vita A, Dieci M, Giobbio GM, et al: Language and thought disorder in schizophrenia: brain morphological correlates. Schizophr Res 15:243–251, 1995

Warach S, Chien D, Li W, et al: Fast magnetic resonance diffusion-weighted imaging of acute human stroke. Neurology 42:1717–1723, 1992

Warfield S, Dengler J, Zaers J, et al: Automatic identification of grey matter structures from MRI to improve the segmentation of white matter lesions. Proceedings from the 2nd International Symposium on Medical Robotics and Computer Assisted Surgery (MRCAS), Baltimore, MD, November 4–7, 1995. New York, Wiley, 1995, pp 55–62, 1995

Wassink TH, Andreasen NC, Nopoulos P, et al: Cerebellar morphology as a predictor of symptom and psychosocial outcome in schizophrenia. Biol Psychiatry 45:41–48, 1999

Weinberger DR: Implications of normal brain development for the pathogenesis of schizophrenia. Arch Gen Psychiatry 44:660–669, 1987

Weinberger DR, Torrey EF, Neophytides AN, et al: Lateral cerebral ventricular enlargement in chronic schizophrenia. Arch Gen Psychiatry 36:735–739, 1979

Weinberger DR, Berman KF, Suddath R, et al: Evidence of dysfunction of a prefrontal-limbic network in schizophrenia: a magnetic resonance and regional cerebral blood flow study of discordant monozygotic twins. Am J Psychiatry 149:890–897, 1992

Wells WM III, Grimson WEL, Kikinis R, et al: Adaptive segmentation of MRI data. IEEE Trans Med Imaging 15:429–443, 1996

Wernicke C: Der aphasische Symptomenkomplex. Breslau, Germany, Cohen und Weigart, 1874

Westin CF, Peled S, Gudbjartsson H, et al: Geometrical diffusion measures for MRI from tensor basis analysis. Proceedings of the International Society for Magnetic Resonance in Medicine (ISMRM), Vancouver, BC, Canada, April 12–18, 1997, p. 1742

Whalen PJ, Rauch SL, Etcoff NL, et al: Masked presentations of emotional facial expressions modulate amygdala activity without explicit knowledge. J Neurosci 18:411–418, 1998

Wible CG, Shenton ME, Hokama H, et al: Prefrontal cortex and schizophrenia: a quantitative magnetic resonance imaging study. Arch Gen Psychiatry 52:279–288, 1995

Wible CG, Shenton ME, Fischer IA, et al: Parcellation of the human prefrontal cortex in schizophrenia: a quantitative MRI study. Psychiatry Res 1:29–40, 1997

Witelson SF, Pallie W: Left hemisphere specialization for language in the newborn: neuroanatomical evidence of asymmetry. Brain 96:641–646, 1973

Woodruff PW, Pearlson GD, Geer MJ, et al: A computerized magnetic resonance imaging study of corpus callosum morphology in schizophrenia. Psych Med 23:45–56, 1993

Woodruff PW, Philips ML, Rushe T, et al: Corpus callosum size and inter-hemispheric function in schizophrenia. Schizophr Res 23:189–196, 1997a

Woodruff PW, Wright IC, Shuriquie N, et al: Structural brain abnormalities in male schizophrenics reflect fronto-temporal dissociation. Psych Med 27:1257–1266, 1997b

Woods BT, Yurgelun-Todd D, Goldstein JM, et al: MRI brain abnormalities in chronic schizophrenia: one process or more? Biol Psychiatry 40:585–596, 1996

Wyper DJ, Pickard JD, Matheson M: Accuracy of ventricular volume estimation. J Neurol Neurosurg Psychiatry 42:345–350, 1979

Young SW: Nuclear Magnetic Resonance Imaging: Basic Principles. New York, Raven, 1984

Zipursky RB, Lim KO, Sullivan EV, et al: Widespread cerebral gray matter volume deficits in schizophrenia. Arch Gen Psychiatry 49:195–205, 1992

Zipursky RB, Marsh L, Lim KO, et al: Volumetric MRI assessment of temporal lobe structures in schizophrenia. Biol Psychiatry 35:501–516, 1994

Zipursky RB, Seeman MV, Bury A, et al: Deficits in gray matter volume present in schizophrenia but not bipolar disorder. Schizophr Res 26:85–92, 1997

2

MAPPING COGNITIVE FUNCTION IN PSYCHIATRIC DISORDERS

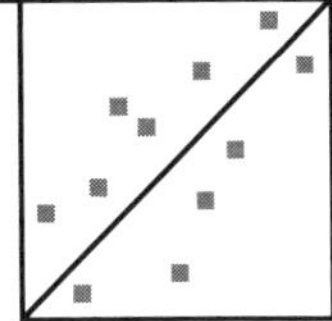

Stephan Heckers, M.D.
Scott L. Rauch, M.D.

Neuroscience research has demonstrated that distributed networks of brain regions govern human behavior (Mesulam 1998). It is now possible to study the neural basis of normal and abnormal behavior in humans using neuroimaging techniques. In this chapter, we review some fundamental principles of imaging cognitive functions in psychiatric disorders. Psychiatrists use neuroimaging technologies primarily to make inferences about psychiatric conditions. Making such inferences requires an understanding of how functional brain images are created, how these images are compared with each other, and what such images indicate about brain function.

■ How Maps Are Created

Basic Principles

Animal preparations allow the direct study of neuronal function (e.g., by recording changes in membrane potential or by sampling proteins and nucleic acids that are amenable to regulation). Human brain function, however, must be assessed indirectly. The study of vascular and metabolic phenomena (e.g., regional cerebral blood flow [rCBF], extraction of oxygen, or metabolism of glucose) is the focus of the most widely used neuroimaging methods in psychiatry: functional magnetic resonance imaging, single photon emission computed tomography, and positron emission tomography. The details of the neuronal-hemodynamic transfer function are still unclear. For the purposes of this chapter, it is sufficient to state that the vascular and metabolic phenomena are indexes of neural activity (Villringer and Dirnagl 1995).

The question of interest in this chapter is, What is the relationship between brain activity and mental state? In most neuroimaging studies involving psychiatric populations, three approaches are used: acquisition of single brain images to study brain activity, acquisition of multiple brain images during the same condition to assess brain activity over time, and acquisition of images during different conditions to assess the recruitment of brain areas.

Study Designs

Single-Image Study: Anatomy of Neural Activity

Single-image studies can be used to assess neural activity at rest or in response to specific stimuli.

Neural activity at rest During studies in which neural activity at rest is being assessed, the subject is not instructed to engage in any activities, except keeping the eyes open or closed. Many functional neuroimaging studies have used resting conditions to compare control subjects with psychiatric patients. Examples of such studies include the decreased anterior-to-posterior rCBF ratio (hypofrontality) in schizophrenia (Ingvar and Franzen 1974) or depression (Ketter et al. 1996) and increased orbitofrontal glucose metabolism in obsessive-compulsive disorder (OCD) (Baxter 1994). Images of brain activity at rest (at times referred to as *random episodic silent thoughts)* may vary considerably (between subjects or even within subjects), because the subject has ample opportunity to engage in various mental activities. It is therefore not surprising that functional imaging studies at rest have often produced inconsistent results.

Despite their inherent limitations, neuroimaging studies at rest can provide information about the relationship between specific mental state abnormalities and distinct patterns of brain activity. For example, decreased prefrontal rCBF at rest was found to correlate with the negative symptoms of schizophrenia (Ebmeier et al. 1993; Liddle et al. 1992; Suzuki et al. 1992; Volkow et al. 1987, 1988; Wiesel et al. 1987; Wolkin et al. 1992) and with the severity of symptoms in major depression (Ketter et al. 1996). Liddle et al. (1992) used factor analysis to demonstrate that three clusters of schizophrenia symptoms (psychomotor poverty, disorganization, and reality distortion) correlate with three distinct rCBF patterns.

Patterns of regional brain activity can also be correlated with behavioral measures or physiological parameters recorded during or independently of the experiment. For example, brain activity can be correlated with psychiatric rating scale scores at the time of the experiment or with variables such as heart rate or blood pressure.

Neural activity during challenge Challenge studies assess the function of a neural network in response to specific stimuli. Challenges can involve exposure to environmental stimuli (symptom provocation; see Chapter 4 of this volume), administration of drugs (see Chapter 9), or engagement in a cognitive task (cognitive activation). Use of such studies is a powerful method for reducing the variance introduced by random neural activity at rest (Gur et al. 1992).

Studies involving low-level-baseline conditions attempt to capture brain activity during a standardized condition that is associated with minimal cognitive, emotional, or sensorimotor demands. For example, a subject might be instructed to fixate on a crosshair in the center of the visual field. Low-level-baseline conditions are often preferred over rest as baseline conditions in studies of multiple conditions (discussed later in this chapter).

Cognitive activation conditions are defined by the performance of a behavioral task during image acquisition. The classic example is the study of rCBF or glucose metabolism during task performance. For example, prefrontal cortex activity is studied during the performance of the Wisconsin Card Sorting Test or the Tower of London, two tests known to involve the frontal cortex. Maps of regional brain activity can then be compared with a baseline condition of the same subject (see the next section) or with maps of other subjects.

Multiple-Image Study During One Condition: Neural Activity Over Time

The multiple-image study involves acquisition of multiple images of the same brain under comparable conditions (i.e., without experimental modulation of brain function). Such studies are often used in clinical neuroimaging but are also used in neuroimaging research. For example, the course of a disease can be followed over time. Patients with Alzheimer's disease, for instance, show progressive degenerative changes in the temporal and parietal cortices that can be documented with studies of glucose metabolism. Treatment effects can also be studied in individual patients. Cognitive-behavioral therapy in OCD, for example, leads to normalization of the increased frontostriatal glucose metabolism (Schwartz et al. 1996).

Multiple-Image Study During Multiple Conditions: Recruitment of Brain Circuits

Images acquired during at least two conditions can provide information about the modulation of brain activity during engagement in a specific behavior. This approach allows the researcher to design experiments to study the contribution of brain function to specific behaviors. The multiple-image, multiple-condition design is therefore more powerful for drawing inferences about brain-behavior relationships than is the collection of images during one condition and the post hoc correlation with behavioral parameters. There are at least three types of the multiple-image, multiple-condition design: the categorical design, the parametric design, and the factorial design.

Categorical design In the categorical design, brain activity during two conditions is compared by subtraction. Two conditions form a contrast (activation condition minus control condition) that is thought to reflect the neural activity characteristic of the activation condition. In a "loose" contrast, the activation condition is compared with rest or a low-level-baseline condition (e.g., involving fixation on a crosshair), whereas in a "tight" contrast, the activation condition is compared with another activation condition that differs by a single contextual element. This design relies on the concept of pure insertion—that a single component of behavior can be removed without any interactions, permitting study of the difference between the full behavioral set and a subset. There are limitations to this assumption, because brain activity and behavior are characterized by the interaction of their components (Friston et al. 1996).

Parametric design In the parametric design, at least two conditions (typically more than two) are correlated with a behavioral measure. The assumption is that brain activity varies monotonically and systematically (but not necessarily linearly) with the degree of processing in the dedicated network.

Factorial design At least two experimental variables (factors) are modulated in the factorial design. The interaction of the factors is then assessed. For example, a pair of tasks (rest and motor activation) is repeated three times. In this way, the effect of activation (factor 1) and the effect of time (factor 2) can be assessed. Another example is the study of rest-activation pairs before and after administration of a drug. The main effects of activation and drug administration can be assessed, as well as the interaction between drug therapy and task performance.

The multiple-image, multiple-condition design allows various analyses of brain-behavior relationships. First, behavior (e.g., attention or memory) can be studied parametrically, with defined increments in components of the behavior (e.g., working memory load or encoding difficulty). Second, activation conditions can be compared with one another so that features shared across behaviors can be studied (conjunction analysis). Third, conditions can be reduced to single-stimulus presentations to permit study of how the brain processes information and how it learns to process stimuli after repeated presentations (single trial design) (Rosen et al. 1998).

Statistical methods (correlation analysis, analysis of variance) are then used to test the hypothesis that the variance between the multiple images can be attributed, at least to a significant amount, to a behavioral index. The behavioral index may be a stimulus feature (e.g., shape or size), an affective valence (e.g., happy, fearful, and sad), or performance (e.g., accuracy or speed), among others.

The recruitment of brain regions can also be assessed during a defined experience (symptom capture; see Chapter 5). In contrast to cognitive activation studies, in which the investigator defines the presentation of stimuli a priori, the subject's behavior (e.g., a tic) or internal state (e.g., a hallucinatory state) defines the condition in these studies. Images are then sorted to represent brain function during the experience of interest and during rest.

■ Comparison of Images

Single-Image Comparison

Single brain images can be used to diagnose an unequivocal or relative deviation from the norm. Such diagnoses are typically made by skilled radiologists, who can compare the single image with images from an extensive database of images of normal brain structure and function. Therefore, the single-subject, single-image study is in fact a comparison of a single subject with a large control group. In addition to qualitative rating of images, quantitative analysis, without knowledge of diagnosis, is also possible. This study design, despite its simplicity, is the gold standard in clinical neuroradiology; inferences about the subject's state of health are drawn on the basis of a single imaging study. Examples of such tests include positron emission tomography glucose metabolism studies to diagnose Alzheimer's disease or seizure disorder.

Multiple-Image Comparison

When more than one image has been acquired, methods are needed to compare multiple images of the same subject or multiple images of multiple subjects. Various sources of variance could give rise to differences between such images, some of which confound testing of inferences. Two issues are briefly mentioned here. First, movement of the subject's head between or during acquisitions of images leads to misalignment at the images. If a group of subjects shows greater head movement (e.g., due to a movement disorder), the comparison of images with those of a control subject could be confounded by movement artifacts (Callicott et al. 1998). Second, differences in brain anatomy make it difficult to compare homologous brain regions between subjects. If one group of subjects has developed brain atrophy, the comparison of differences in brain activity could be confounded by displacement of brain tissue.

Two approaches have been taken for comparing brain images. In one approach, the region-of-interest analysis defines anatomical regions, using either standard templates or high-resolution structural images of the same subject, to assess brain activity in defined spaces. In the second approach, images are transformed, on a voxel-by-voxel basis, into a standardized three-dimensional space that represents an ideal standard brain, which allows comparison of all brain regions.

Once images have been processed for comparison, the following important question arises: Which parameter indicates brain activity? Should the *amplitude* of the signal in a defined location be compared between subjects, or should the focus be on the *extent* of the activation signal within one anatomical area? How does the *variability* of signal changes within one subject affect the comparison of signal changes across subjects and across groups? Although there exist conventions (Friston et al. 1991, 1994) for comparing data sets between groups of investigators, this fact should not be taken as reassurance that maps accurately represent the function of neural circuits.

Between-Group Comparison

The single-subject study is the traditional approach in clinical neuroimaging for making diagnoses, staging diseases, and assessing treatment effects. Between-group comparisons are used 1) when the signal-to-noise ratio is small, in which case averaging the signal across subjects might reveal effects that were too subtle to detect in individual subjects or that were variable between subjects (e.g., the good activator versus the bad activator in functional neuroimaging studies); and 2) when not all of the patients demonstrate similar brain changes.

Functional neuroimaging studies can provide information about psychiatric disorders (Table 2–1). The classic approach is the comparison of a patient sample drawn from a population of psychiatric patients (e.g., schizophrenic patients) with a control group (psychiatrically healthy subjects or a different psychiatric population). The statistical inference is the effect of diagnosis on the image data set: can the variance between the images be attributed, to a significant degree, to the diagnosis? Other contributors to the variance (e.g., age, sex, drug therapy, or behavioral data) are often not considered and may even cloud the picture (in the case of drug therapy, for example). Between-group comparisons of single images test for a main diagnosis effect, whereas comparisons of different images (i.e., those for assessing recruitment of brain regions) test for diagnosis-by-condition interactions (Table 2–1).

In addition to making a statement about the sample of psychiatric patients who participated in an imaging study, investigators also aim to make inferences about the population of patients from which the study sample was drawn. If this goal is to be achieved, study subjects must be treated as though they were chosen randomly from the total population of patients (Holmes and Friston 1998; Neter et al. 1996; Woods 1996). The appropriate statistical methods (mixed or random effects models) typically require large samples and do not allow the intraindividual variability between scans during one condition to enter the statistical comparison (Holmes and Friston 1998). This fact is especially relevant for functional magnetic resonance imaging studies, in which repeated acquisition of images during the same condition is the rule.

■ What Maps Tell Us About Brain Function

Once neuroimaging data sets have been acquired and analyzed, they must be interpreted. It is again helpful to distinguish between single images and multiple images.

Brain-Behavior Correlation

In the case of single images acquired at rest, abnormalities such as decreased blood flow or decreased glucose metabolism are interpreted as evidence of an abnormality that is observable even without the experimentally induced recruitment of neural networks. For example, cell loss in Alzheimer's disease leads to decreased

TABLE 2–1. Inference testing in functional neuroimaging studies of psychiatric disorders

Condition	Inference	Examples
Single images of control subject and patient: neural activity		
Rest	Diagnosis effect	Decreased anterior-to-posterior rCBF ratio (hypofrontality) in schizophrenia (Ingvar and Franzen 1974)
Activation performance	Diagnosis effect	Decreased frontal rCBF during WCST in schizophrenia (Weinberger et al. 1986)
Symptom provocation structures	Symptom effect	Increased paralimbic activity in anxiety disorders (Rauch et al. 1994)
Rest and schizophrenia with symptoms	Symptom effect	Schizophrenia subtypes differentiated by rCBF at rest (Liddle et al. 1992)
Multiple images of control subject and patient: recruitment of neural circuits		
Cognitive activation	Diagnosis-by-condition interaction	Decreased recruitment of prefrontal areas during WCST in schizophrenia (Weinberger et al. 1986) Decreased recruitment of hippocampus during word retrieval in schizophrenia (Heckers et al. 1998) Decreased basal ganglia activity during implicit learning in obsessive-compulsive disorder (Rauch et al. 1997)

Note. rCBF = regional cerebral blood flow; WCST = Wisconsin Card Sorting Test.

glucose metabolism in temporoparietal regions. Other examples include increased orbitofrontal glucose metabolism in OCD and left temporal hyperactivity in schizophrenia (Friston et al. 1992; Liddle et al. 1992).

If multiple images are obtained during engagement in a specific behavior (cognitive activation, symptom provocation), at least two types of brain-behavior relationships may be found:

1. *Regional brain activity correlates positively with a behavioral index.* Such a relationship might reflect the resource allocation within a neural network

in the service of a specific behavior. For example, the degree of medial temporal lobe activation correlates positively with the accuracy of word retrieval (Nyberg et al. 1996). Another example is the linear relationship between prefrontal cortex activity and working memory load in a graded, parametric study (Braver et al. 1997).

2. *The behavioral response is improved but the level of brain activity is decreased.* This pattern has been interpreted as the neural correlate of increased efficiency in the processing of a stimulus. For example, the priming of visual recognition after previous presentation of the target stimulus is associated with decreased activation of visual association areas (Schacter and Buckner 1998).

Group-by-Condition Interactions

In studies involving psychiatric patients, the two groups (control subjects and patients) often demonstrate different brain-behavior relationships. Here we briefly describe three patterns of abnormal brain-behavior relationships in psychiatric disorders.

1. *Patients exhibit behavioral deficits as well as decreased regional brain activity.* For example, patients with schizophrenia score poorly on tests of frontal cortex function (e.g., the Wisconsin Card Sorting Test) and show decreased activity (on single images) or failed recruitment (on multiple images) of the frontal cortex (Kotrla and Weinberger 1995). The crucial question then is, Does the decrease in brain activity represent a failed recruitment of the neural circuit, resulting in poorer performance, or is the impaired performance a consequence of poor motivation or cooperation, leading to lack of recruitment? Investigators have addressed this problematic issue by matching the two samples according to levels of performance. If the decreased regional brain activity is still present after matching for performance, the neural deficits are then often interpreted as primary and the behavioral deficit as secondary.
2. *Patients exhibit behavioral deficits and increased regional brain activity.* This pattern is often interpreted as an inefficient recruitment of brain areas in the effort to complete the task. For example, patients with schizophrenia score poorly on tests of working memory but show greater increases in prefrontal cortex activity (Manoach et al. 1999).
3. *Patients show no behavioral deficits but show decreased regional brain activity in areas activated by the control group (and increased regional brain activity in other areas).* This pattern is interpreted as a failure to activate

the "normal" neural network, with compensatory recruitment of another network. For example, patients with OCD do not activate a basal ganglia network during implicit sequence learning but instead show recruitment of medial temporal lobe structures, while performing the task normally (Rauch et al. 1997).

■ CONCLUSION

Functional neuroimaging holds great promise for elucidating the neural basis of psychiatric disorders. So far, studies have demonstrated abnormal regional brain activity in several psychiatric disorders, abnormal recruitment of neural networks during task performance in psychiatric patients, and an association between abnormal brain activity patterns and distinct psychiatric signs and symptoms. It is the goal of functional neuroimaging in psychiatry to elucidate the neural basis of psychiatric disorders. Progress in this direction will depend in part on how well the methodological issues outlined in this chapter are addressed.

■ REFERENCES

Baxter LR Jr: Positron emission tomography studies of cerebral glucose metabolism in obsessive compulsive disorder. J Clin Psychiatry 55 (suppl):54–59, 1994

Braver TS, Cohen JD, Nystrom LE, et al: A parametric study of prefrontal cortex involvement in human working memory. Neuroimage 5:49–62, 1997

Callicott JH, Ramsey NF, Tallent K, et al: Functional magnetic resonance imaging brain mapping in psychiatry: methodological issues in a study of working memory in schizophrenia. Neuropsychopharmacology 18:186–196, 1998

Ebmeier KP, Blackwood DH, Murray C, et al: Single-photon emission computed tomography with 99mTc-exametazime in unmedicated schizophrenic patients. Biol Psychiatry 33:487–495, 1993

Friston KJ, Frith CD, Liddle PF, et al: Comparing functional (PET) images: the assessment of significant change. J Cereb Blood Flow Metab 11:690–699, 1991

Friston KJ, Liddle PF, Frith CD, et al: The left medial temporal region and schizophrenia: a PET study. Brain 115:367–382, 1992

Friston KJ, Worsley KJ, Frackowiak RSJ, et al: Assessing the significance of focal activations using their spatial extent. Hum Brain Mapp 1:210–220, 1994

Friston KJ, Price CJ, Fletcher P, et al: The trouble with cognitive subtraction. Neuroimage 4:97–104, 1996

Gur RC, Erwin RJ, Gur RE: Neurobehavioral probes for physiologic neuroimaging studies. Arch Gen Psychiatry 49:409–414, 1992

Heckers S, Rauch SL, Goff D, et al: Impaired recruitment of the hippocampus during conscious recollection in schizophrenia. Nat Neurosci 1:318–323, 1998

Holmes AP, Friston KJ: Generalisability, random effects & population inference (abstract). Neuroimage 7:S754, 1998

Ingvar DH, Franzen G: Abnormalities of cerebral blood flow distribution in patients with chronic schizophrenia. Acta Psychiatr Scand 50:425–462, 1974

Ketter TA, George MS, Kimbrell TA, et al: Functional brain imaging, limbic function, and affective disorders. The Neuroscientist 2:55–65, 1996

Kotrla KJ, Weinberger DR: Brain imaging in schizophrenia. Annu Rev Med 46:113–122, 1995

Liddle PF, Friston KJ, Frith CD, et al: Patterns of cerebral blood flow in schizophrenia. Br J Psychiatry 160:179–186, 1992

Manoach DS, Press DZ, Thangaraj V, et al: Schizophrenic subjects activate dorsolateral prefrontal cortex during a working memory task, as measured by fMRI. Biol Psychiatry 45:1128–1137, 1999

Mesulam M-M: From sensation to cognition. Brain 121:1013–1052, 1998

Neter J, Kutner MH, Nachtsheim CJ, et al: Applied Linear Statistical Models, 4th Edition. Chicago, IL, Irwin, 1996

Nyberg L, McIntosh AR, Houle S, et al: Activation of medial temporal structures during episodic memory retrieval. Nature 380:715–717, 1996

Rauch SL, Jenike MA, Alpert NM, et al: Regional cerebral blood flow measured during symptom provocation in obsessive-compulsive disorder using oxygen 15-labeled carbon dioxide and positron emission tomography. Arch Gen Psychiatry 51:62–70, 1994

Rauch SL, Savage CR, Alpert NM, et al: Probing striatal function in obsessive-compulsive disorder: a PET study of implicit sequence learning. J Neuropsychiatry Clin Neurosci 9:568–573, 1997

Rosen BR, Buckner RL, Dale AM: Event-related functional MRI: past, present, and future. Proc Natl Acad Sci U S A 95:773–780, 1998

Schacter DL, Buckner RL: Priming and the brain. Neuron 20:185–195, 1998

Schwartz JM, Stoessel PW, Baxter LR Jr, et al: Systematic changes in cerebral glucose metabolic rate after successful behavior modification treatment of obsessive-compulsive disorder. Arch Gen Psychiatry 53:109–113, 1996

Suzuki M, Kurachi M, Kawasaki Y, et al: Left hypofrontality correlates with blunted affect in schizophrenia. Jpn J Psychiatry Neurol 46:653–657, 1992

Villringer A, Dirnagl U: Coupling of brain activity and cerebral blood flow: basis of functional neuroimaging. Cerebrovasc Brain Metab Rev 7:240–276, 1995

Volkow ND, Wolf AP, Van Gelder P, et al: Phenomenological correlates of metabolic activity in 18 patients with chronic schizophrenia. Am J Psychiatry 144:151–158, 1987

Volkow ND, Wolf AP, Brodie JD, et al: Brain interactions in chronic schizophrenics under resting and activation conditions. Schizophr Res 1:47–53, 1988

Weinberger DR, Berman KF, Zec RF: Physiologic dysfunction of dorsolateral prefrontal cortex in schizophrenia, I: regional cerebral blood flow evidence. Arch Gen Psychiatry 43:114–124, 1986

Wiesel FA, Wik G, Sjogren I, et al: Regional brain glucose metabolism in drug free schizophrenic patients and clinical correlates. Acta Psychiatr Scand 76:628–641, 1987

Wolkin A, Sanfilipo M, Wolf AP, et al: Negative symptoms and hypofrontality in chronic schizophrenia. Arch Gen Psychiatry 49:959–965, 1992

Woods RP: Modeling for intergroup comparisons of imaging data. Neuroimage 4:S84–S94, 1996

3

USING NEUROIMAGING TO STUDY IMPLICIT INFORMATION PROCESSING

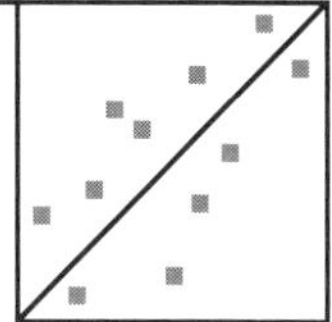

Paul J. Whalen, Ph.D.
Tim Curran, Ph.D.
Scott L. Rauch, M.D.

In this chapter, we focus on a subset of cognitive activation paradigms used to probe information processing that occurs without awareness (i.e., implicit information processing). Such paradigms might be particularly important for studying anxiety disorders, because anxiety disorders have been found to be characterized by an information processing bias that precedes awareness. We present two paradigms that have already been successfully adapted to the neuroimaging environment: an implicit sequence learning task and a passive viewing task that uses backwardly masked face stimuli. These paradigms have been employed to activate the striatum and the amygdala, respectively—two brain regions that are implicated in the pathophysiology of anxiety disorders as well as the processing of information without awareness. Although emerging data suggest that these paradigms will be useful for elucidating the pathophysiology of various neuropsychiatric conditions, in this chapter we present examples related to the study of anxiety disorders.

Learning classified as nonconscious, implicit, or automatic occurs in the absence of awareness or the intention to learn. Although opinion differs concerning the optimal experimental conditions for demonstrating nonconscious processing, there is widespread agreement that perception can occur without benefit of awareness (J. D. Cohen and Schooler 1997; Merikle and Joordens 1997). Numerous cognitive experimental paradigms exist for studying nonconscious processing. Priming studies demonstrate implicit learning through enhanced memory for previously seen but nonrecognized words (A. S. Reber 1989). Serial motor learning tasks demonstrate learning of procedural knowledge through facilitated performance of nonrecognized repeating motor sequences (Nissen and Bullemer 1987). Classical conditioning procedures demonstrate that increased autonomic responses to nonrecognized event contingencies occur without awareness (Clark and Squire 1998; see LeDoux 1996). Finally, backward masking represents a unique strategy for disrupting conscious processing, one that allows investigators to measure autonomic or neuroimaging responses to nonrecognized perceptual stimuli (e.g., backward masking of facial expression [Öhman 1992; Whalen et al. 1998]). All of these experimental approaches have been applied to studies involving psychiatric populations (see, for example, Foa et al. 1997 [priming]; Rauch et al. 1997a [procedural learning]; Pitman et al., in press [classical conditioning]; Öhman 1992 [backward masking]). This body of work has been motivated in part by the following premise: the ability to distinguish between the automatic processing of nonrecognized stimuli and the more elaborative or strategic processing of recognized stimuli will lead to important insights into the pathophysiology, classification, and treatment of psychiatric disorders.

Experimental psychopathologists have invoked a distinction between automatic and elaborative processing in an attempt to test the relevance of this distinction to the study of anxiety (Mathews and MacLeod 1994; McNally 1995). Mathews and MacLeod (1986) demonstrated increased response latencies to neutral stimuli when threat-related words were presented outside awareness in a dichotic listening task. MacLeod and Rutherford (1992) used masked presentations of negative words within a color emotional Stroop paradigm; in subjects with high-trait anxiety who were under stress, the study showed that interference effects occurred, even though the subjects reported not seeing the negative words. Mogg et al. (1993) found that negative words presented outside awareness produced Stroop interference effects in subjects with generalized anxiety disorder, and these investigators showed that anxious, but not depressed, subjects demonstrate these automatic biases in the processing of negative information (Mogg et al. 1995).

Information processing within the automatic channel appears more crude or generalized, in that *all* negative words presented outside awareness produced interference effects in generalized anxiety disorder (Mathews and MacLeod 1994; Mogg et al. 1993). Thus, whereas Stroop words presented overtly produce selective effects in response to content-specific stimuli (McNally et al. 1990), Stroop words presented outside awareness produce interference that is sensitive only to valence (Mathews and MacLeod 1994; McNally 1995). In summary, masking paradigms using word stimuli suggest that subjects with anxiety demonstrate a selective automatic bias and that the automatic (not elaborative) bias may preferentially influence the detection of *general negative* stimuli. This latter point is consistent with Öhman's (1992) demonstration that masked angry faces produce increased skin conductance responses (SCRs) when they predict shock, whereas masked happy faces do not. In contrast, more elaborative (e.g., conscious) processing appears necessary for disorder-specific effects.

Consequently, in the current chapter, we highlight studies that used so-called content-independent stimuli (see McNally 1998). These stimuli have no particular relevance to subjects with anxiety disorders; the studies presented targeted differences in the processing of more generalized information (e.g., word stems, facial expressions, or sequence learning). Thus, it is not the processing of faces or sequences per se that has relevance for anxiety; rather, these stimuli have been shown to activate brain regions implicated in anxiety disorders (i.e., the amygdala and striatum). These studies have provided a foundation for future investigations in psychiatric populations, while yielding basic information about the normal neurobiology of nonconscious processing in humans.

■ Neuroimaging Probe of Nonconscious Processing and the Striatum

Contemporary learning theory acknowledges the existence of different kinds of memory and dissociable neuroanatomic substrates of different learning and memory functions (P. J. Reber and Squire 1994; Squire 1986). *"Implicit" learning and memory* refers to the acquisition and expression of information not accompanied by awareness of its content or influence on behavior (Schacter et al. 1993). *Procedural learning* refers to a subtype of implicit learning, characterized by nonconscious acquisition of skills as a consequence of practice. In contrast, *"explicit"* (or *declarative*) *learning and memory* refers to the acquisition and retrieval of information that is accompanied by awareness of the learned information and its influence on behavior. Explicit memory is believed to be mediated via prefrontal and medial temporal (i.e., the hippocampus and parahippocampal gyrus) structures (Schacter et al. 1996; Squire 1992; Ungerleider 1995). Procedural memory is purportedly mediated via cortico-striato-thalamic circuits. Initially, compelling evidence for the distinct functional neuroanatomy underlying these two types of memory came from both animal studies (see, for example, Packard et al. 1989) and studies of humans with known distributions of brain dysfunction (for instance, see Knopman and Nissen 1991; Willingham and Koroshetz 1993). So-called double dissociation refers to the fact that individuals with medial temporal lesions exhibit impaired explicit memory and preserved procedural memory, whereas individuals with striatal lesions (e.g., early Huntington's disease), exhibit preserved explicit memory, but impaired procedural memory. More recently, functional neuroimaging studies have bolstered the concept that procedural learning is principally mediated by cortico-striato-thalamic circuitry.

Cortico-Striato-Thalamic Circuitry

The striatum is composed of the caudate nucleus, the putamen, and the nucleus accumbens. Historically, the basal ganglia, including the striatum, were thought to play a circumscribed role, limited to the modulation of motor functions. More recently, however, a more complicated scheme has been adopted in which the role of the striatum in cognitive and affective functions is recognized as well. In two landmark articles, Alexander and colleagues (1986, 1990) explicated the organization of multiple, parallel, segregated cortico-striato-thalamic circuits. Although there are several levels of complexity to be considered with regard to the anatomy and function of these circuits, in this chapter we will provide a simplified scheme.

The cortico-striato-thalamic pathway represents a collateral that serves to modulate corticothalamic and thalamocortical transmission at the level of the thalamus. The purported function of the striatum in this context is to process information automatically and without conscious representation. Hence, the healthy striatum, through its influence over thalamic transmission, filters out extraneous input, ensures refined output, and mediates stereotyped, rule-based processes without necessitating the allocation of conscious cortical resources (Graybiel 1995; Houk et al. 1995; Rauch and Savage 1997; Rauch et al. 1995; Wise et al. 1996). In this way, the striatum regulates the content and facilitates the quality of information processing within the explicit (i.e., conscious) domain by fine-tuning input and output. In addition, the striatum enhances the efficiency of the brain by carrying out some nonconscious functions, thereby reducing the computational load on conscious processing systems.

Serial Reaction Time Task

Implicit sequence learning has been widely studied using the serial reaction time (SRT) task of Nissen and Bullemer (1987) (for a review, see Clegg et al. 1998). The SRT task entails serial presentation of visual cues at one of four positions on a viewing screen. The subject is instructed to respond to each cue by pressing one of four buttons on a keypad, on which each button corresponds to one of the possible cue positions. To the subject, the SRT task resembles a simple continuous performance task with attentional, visuospatial, and motor demands. However, unbeknownst to the subject, the cues appear in a pseudorandom order during some series of stimulus presentations, and during other series the cues are presented in a repeating sequence. During blocks of repeating-sequence trials, the subject might become familiar with the sequence and develop a reaction time advantage.

After the performance trials have been completed, debriefing procedures can be used to determine whether subjects were consciously aware that a repeating sequence was present (Rauch et al. 1995; P. J. Reber and Squire 1994; Reed and Johnson 1994). For example, subjects might be tested to determine whether they are able to consciously recall elements of the sequence (Rauch et al. 1995; P. J. Reber and Squire 1994). Hence, when subjects develop a reaction time advantage but are unable to perform better than chance on the recall task, it can be inferred that learning occurred and that this learning was implicit rather than explicit (Rauch et al. 1995; P. J. Reber and Squire 1994). Although many researchers agree that SRT learning can occur without awareness, this claim, like most claims of nonconscious information processing, has been debated (A. Cohen and Curran 1993; Perruchet and Amorrim 1992; Shanks and St. John 1994; Willingham et al. 1993).

Implicit Processing and the Striatum in Obsessive-Compulsive Disorder

The striatum, as well as the orbitofrontal cortex and anterior cingulate cortex, has been implicated in the pathophysiology of obsessive-compulsive disorder (OCD) (see Rauch and Baxter 1998; Rauch et al. 1998b for a review). Morphometric studies of OCD have repeatedly found volumetric abnormalities involving the striatum (see, for example, Robinson et al. 1995). Neutral-state functional imaging studies of OCD have predominantly indicated hyperactivity within the orbitofrontal cortex and anterior cingulate cortex, whereas pretreatment and posttreatment studies of OCD and symptom provocation studies of OCD have suggested that hyperactivity within the orbitofrontal cortex, anterior cingulate cortex, and striatum is associated with the symptomatic state (for instance, see Baxter et al. 1992; Rauch et al. 1994; Swedo et al. 1992). The observation that lesions involving the striatum, including poststreptococcal autoimmune-mediated degeneration (Swedo et al. 1998), can precipitate the presentation of OCD or Tourette's syndrome lends support to the hypothesis that OCD may result from primary striatal pathology.

Cognitive neuroscience provides a perspective that can enrich our understanding of the link between striatal pathology and the phenomenology of OCD. As noted, implicit learning of procedures, skills, or stereotyped serial operations is purportedly mediated via cortico-striato-thalamic systems (Curran 1995; Mishkin and Petri 1984; Rauch and Jenike 1997). Therefore, if OCD and related disorders are referable to striatal dysfunction, their phenomenology might best be understood as a consequence of implicit processing deficits (Mishkin and Petri 1984). OCD is fundamentally characterized by intrusive events that are accompanied by a drive to engage in repetitive behaviors (Miguel et al. 1995; Rauch et al. 1998b). Our working model of OCD proposes that the intrusive events may be conceptualized as a consequence of dysfunctional nonconscious information processing systems. In this way, information that is normally filtered or "put to rest" outside consciousness instead intrudes into the conscious domain. The neurophysiological correlate of this construct is deficient recruitment of the striatum, leading to inadequate "gating" at the level of the thalamus. It has also been hypothesized that this failure in nonconscious information processing leads to aberrant limbic activity (experienced as anxiety or urges) and that repetitive behaviors represent compensatory phenomena that are reinforced by virtue of their efficacy in reducing this limbic hyperactivity, through improved thalamic gating (see, for example, Rauch et al. 1998b; Rauch and Jenike 1997).

In fact, it is plausible that the intrusive events that are the hallmark of OCD represent failures in filtering at the level of the thalamus, attributable to deficient modulation via the cortico-striato-thalamic collateral. To put it another way, information that is normally processed efficiently via cortico-striato-thalamic systems, outside the conscious domain, instead finds access to explicit processing systems because of striatal dysfunction. Until recently, it has not been possible to test this model of OCD empirically. However, the advent of contemporary neuroimaging techniques has made it feasible to investigate the roles of the striatum and thalamus in nonconscious information processing during sequential repetitive behaviors in OCD.

Use of the SRT Task for Studying Obsessive-Compulsive Disorder

Given that neuroimaging and neuropsychological studies suggest that cortico-striato-thalamic systems are critically involved in implicit sequence learning (for reviews, see Curran 1995, 1997), the SRT task appeared to be well suited as a candidate probe for studying the pathophysiology of OCD. In our laboratory, an initial positron emission tomography (PET)–SRT study involving healthy subjects showed activation within the cortex, right striatum, and thalamus for the sequence versus random contrast, in the context of implicit learning (Rauch et al. 1995). An analogous functional magnetic resonance imaging (fMRI) study replicated right striatal recruitment and showed that striatal activity was positively correlated with learning-related reaction time improvements across healthy subjects (Rauch et al. 1997b). Neuroimaging results from other laboratories have generally confirmed the importance of the striatum for implicit sequence learning (Berns et al. 1997; Doyon et al. 1996; Grafton et al. 1995; Hazeltine et al. 1997; Pascual-Leone et al. 1996). Subsequently, using fMRI, we also examined the time course of learning-related brain activity during the SRT task. We found evidence suggesting that the thalamus is *deactivated* during early stages of implicit sequence learning (Rauch et al. 1998). These data indicate that the fMRI-SRT task may be an excellent probe not only of striatal recruitment but also of thalamic gating.

After validating the PET-SRT probe in an initial cohort of healthy subjects, we conducted a study involving subjects with OCD and matched healthy control subjects (Rauch et al. 1997a). The OCD subjects showed normal implicit sequence learning by behavioral measures. However, PET did not show normal right striatal recruitment in the OCD patients, who instead exhibited medial temporal (i.e., hippocampal or parahippocampal) activation, not seen in the healthy comparison group. Given the well-known relationship between medial temporal lobe mechanisms and explicit learning and memory (Aggleton and Brown, in press; Squire 1992), these results suggest that OCD patients may need to tap into conscious information processing systems (e.g., the medial temporal lobe) in situations that normally would be handled by implicit processing systems (e.g., the striatum). Additional preliminary data obtained with the use of the fMRI-SRT probe at our laboratory corroborate our PET findings in OCD.

Applications of the SRT Task: Further Design Considerations

There are numerous factors to be considered in applying the SRT paradigm to studies involving psychiatric populations. First, it is essential that the timing parameters allow for the occurrence of learning, without subjects developing explicit knowledge about the sequence (i.e., "explicit contamination"). Because the learning effects are delicate, minor changes in the interstimulus interval (ISI), sequence structure, and ratio or timing of sequence versus random epochs can eliminate the implicit learning effect or result in explicit contamination. As with any cognitive activation paradigm that is to be studied in conjunction with imaging, it is wise to conduct off-line testing to refine the paradigm before commencing the imaging experiments.

Further, the interpretation of between-group differences in brain activation is complicated by between-group differences in task performance (see Chapter 2 of this volume). Although subtle between-group differences in learning can be accommodated within models of pathophysiology, a gross inability to perform the task by one group would make the probe unsatisfactory. Hence, it is critical to establish that the timing parameters used to validate the probe in healthy subjects do not render the task too challenging for the patient group. For instance, patients with movement disorders or slowed cognition may require longer ISIs.

Another limitation of the SRT task is that this paradigm is not well suited for repeat testing (e.g., pretreatment and posttreatment studies), because prior exposure to a sequence alters learning effects and increases the possibility of explicit contamination. Moreover, subjects cannot be retested once debriefing has occurred (using a conscious recall task to assess explicit knowledge), because the subjects have been made aware that a hidden sequence is present.

Several modified versions of the SRT task have been developed in an effort to augment the implicit learning effect while protecting against explicit contamination. For instance, a simultaneous explicit task can be added to occupy subjects' resources, thereby reducing the risk of explicit contamination (see, for example, Grafton et al. 1995). Similarly, with the use of multiple different sequences, and periodic changing of the sequence to be learned, additional runs can be performed with minimized risk of explicit contamination (for instance, see Rauch et al. 1998).

Adaptation of the SRT Task for Event-Related Experiments

Event-related paradigms are valuable for use in conjunction with techniques that provide superior temporal resolution, such as use of event-related potentials, magnetoencephalography, or event-related fMRI (Buckner 1998). Although many cognitive tasks can be easily modified for use in an event-related paradigm, the SRT task poses a special challenge in this regard because a single stimulus does not a sequence make. We recently developed a new sequence-learning paradigm intended for single-trial, event-related fMRI analyses. Thus far, neuroimaging studies of implicit sequence learning have used paradigms similar to those used in previous behavioral studies, in which stimuli are presented continuously, once every 1–2 seconds. PET studies have used separate blocks of random or sequence stimuli (A. Cohen et al. 1990; Curran and Keele 1993; Rauch et al. 1995). fMRI studies have used intermixed blocks that cycle through random and sequence epochs (Curran 1995; Rauch et al. 1997b; Stadler 1993).

Development of the single-trial SRT paradigm was guided by an understanding of the information that is learned in the SRT task. It is generally believed that subjects learn only chunks of lengthy sequences and that performance improvements result when later elements of the chunk can be predicted from earlier elements (Cleeremans and McClelland 1991; Curran 1997; Stadler 1995). For example, in the case of the sequence 1–2–1–4–2–3–4–1–3–2–4–3 (numbers refer to stimulus or response locations), subjects appear to learn small chunks (e.g., 2–3–4–1) that allow particularly fast reaction times to the latter elements of the chunk (Curran 1997). In other words, subjects learn that 2–3–4 predicts location 1, so subjects are faster to respond when that stimulus appears in location 1. In our neuroimaging studies using the SRT task, we designed conditions so that subjects had to learn chunks of at least three elements for performance to differ between sequence and random conditions. We achieved this result by designing the sequence so that each location followed each of the other locations equally often (Reed and Johnson 1994). Because each element was equally likely to follow each of the other elements, pair-wise associations were not predictive. Subjects had to learn at least second-order associations whereby each element could be uniquely predicted from the previous two locations (e.g., 1–2 predicted 1, 4–2 predicted 3, and 3–2 predicted 4). We believe it is important to use a task that taps learning of at least second-order sequences if striatal function is to be assessed, because the striatum is especially implicated in planning and learning multimovement sequences (Willingham 1998).

Because of the aforementioned constraints on timing and the nature of sequence learning, we developed a single-trial SRT task in which each trial consisted of three stimuli arranged in a triplet. Triplets could be either predictable or unpredictable. For predictable triplets, the location of the third stimulus (S3) could always be predicted from the locations of the first (S1) and second (S2) stimuli. For example, if the location of S1 is location 3 and that of S2 is location 1, then the location of S3 is location 4. For unpredictable triplets, the location of S3 could not be predicted from the locations of S1 and S2 because each S1-S2 pair was followed by three different S3s within the run (e.g., 4–2–1, 4–2–3, and 4–2–4).

The overall paradigm entailed three runs, with 36 of these triplets per run; each triplet or trial was separated by a pause of approximately 5 seconds. Stimulus positions were completely counterbalanced (each stimulus appeared with equal frequency at the locations of S1, S2, and S3); each unpredictable triplet appeared once, and each predictable triplet appeared three times. Initially, pilot testing revealed high levels of explicit contamination. Therefore, we transformed the single-trial SRT task into a dual-task paradigm to minimize explicit learning. Specifically, in addition to performing the basic SRT task, subjects were required to maintain a series of seven letters in working memory during each block of trials. Research with the SRT task suggests that working memory loads have only a small effect on implicit sequence learning (Stadler 1995) and reduce explicit learning. This refined version of the single-trial SRT paradigm has now been piloted off-line in our laboratory, and results appear to support a significant implicit learning effect in the context of a dual-task format.

The single-trial SRT paradigm promises to provide a method for investigating implicit learning–related striatal responses at superior temporal resolution. Moreover, a dual-task version of the SRT paradigm will enable investigators to further explore the relationship between implicit and explicit processing in OCD. We predict that if, as we have hypothesized, patients with OCD compensate for striatal dysfunction by using frontotemporal systems during SRT learning, a simultaneous working memory load would disproportionately interfere with their performance, because unlike healthy control subjects, patients with OCD lack intact dissociable systems with which to support parallel processing of this type. Experiments are ongoing in our laboratory to test this hypothesis.

Summary

SRT paradigms 1) have been studied using functional imaging and have been shown to reliably produce detectable right striatal activation and thalamic deactivation in healthy subjects, 2) provide a framework for examining the hypothesis that patients with OCD exhibit abnormal nonconscious information processing, and 3) appear to yield replicable patterns of abnormal brain activity in OCD. Moreover, further modifications of this paradigm can enable investigators to study the finer temporal aspects of implicit sequence learning in the brain, the parallel processing deficiency hypothesis of OCD, and a range of other disorders in which basal ganglia dysfunction is implicated.

■ NEUROIMAGING PROBE OF NONCONSCIOUS PROCESSING AND THE AMYGDALA

The amygdala, a brain structure located within the medial temporal lobe, has been implicated in the response to biologically relevant stimuli such as aversive events, appetitive reward, and stimuli that predict these events (Aggleton 1992). Most of what is known about the amygdala concerns its role in the acquisition and expression of conditioned fear responses. During pavlovian conditioning, an initially neutral stimulus, such as a tone, comes to predict the occurrence of an aversive event, such as a mild electric current. With sufficient experience, the tone becomes a conditioned stimulus, leading to amygdala activation and many of the same autonomic and somatomotor responses that originally followed the shock itself. Furthermore, lesions of the amygdala attenuate fear conditioning in animals (Kapp et al. 1979). Electrical stimulation of neurons in this region produces the same learned responses observed in fear conditioning (e.g., heart rate and respiration changes). Recordings of activity in amygdala neurons reveal learned increases in firing rate to aversively conditioned stimuli (Davis 1992; Kapp et al. 1992; LeDoux 1996). Finally, complementary research has demonstrated that the biologically relevant predictive stimuli about which the amygdala learns need not produce intense fear (see Whalen 1998 for further discussion).

The Amygdala and Anxiety

The amygdala's primary role in learning about stimuli that predict aversive events makes the structure a prime candidate for initiating activation in efferent systems that support anxiety (Davis 1998; Whalen 1998). Subjects with anxiety disorders demonstrate amygdala activation in association with symptoms (see, for example, Rauch et al. 1996; Shin et al. 1997). In part on the basis of animal studies demonstrating a direct, short-latency pathway from the thalamus to the amygdala (LeDoux et al. 1985), LeDoux (1996) proposed that the amygdala might survey emotionally valenced stimuli without awareness. Thus, the hypothesis that anxiety is associated with an automatic information processing bias for negative information immediately implicates the amygdala. As LeDoux (1996) pointed out, such a system makes false alarms possible, even probable, but also makes for an organism that will scarcely be caught off guard. Further, anxiety disorders may be the price paid by some individuals for an automated vigilance system that bolsters evolutionary longevity of the human species.

The fMRI probe described later in this chapter uses masked stimulus presentations of facial expressions in an attempt to elucidate the amygdala's role in the clinical phenomena observed across the anxiety disorders (e.g., hypervigilance, failure to habituate, and exaggerated startle). The continued study of automaticity might be particularly relevant to anxiety, given that symptoms such as obsessions and panic attacks appear to be involuntary and spontaneous.

Practical Issues Regarding Probe Development

Aversive classical conditioning procedures have increased our understanding of biologically relevant learning as well as normal and pathological fear. Indeed, such paradigms have already been used in nonimaging studies of anxiety disorders (for instance, see Öhman 1992; Pitman et al., in press). Classical conditioning used in conjunction with scanning should prove useful for assessing the amygdala's involvement in anxiety. However, the brain imaging environment is novel. Even healthy subjects may decide that they cannot tolerate the confined space of the magnet bore. Thus, this environment alone may present a daunting obstacle for some patients with anxiety disorders. Consequently, for our initial neuroimaging studies, we sought a paradigm that would reliably activate the amygdala but that would be more innocuous than shock presentations. Neuropsychological evidence pointed to the use of facial expressions.

Patients with lesions of the amygdala have been studied extensively and offer another source of information concerning the role of the amygdala. These patients consistently demonstrate deficits in the processing of facial expression (Adolphs et al. 1995; Calder et al. 1996). Specifically, it appears that fearful facial expressions present the greatest problem for these patients in terms of identification and interpretation of intensity (Adolphs et al. 1995, 1999; Calder et al. 1996). In two initial neuroimaging studies in which healthy subjects viewed pictures of fearful, happy, or neutral facial expressions, amygdala activity was greatest during viewing of pictures of fearful facial expressions (Breiter et al. 1996; Morris et al. 1996). In addition to the amygdala, other brain areas also showed greater activation in response to pictures of fearful faces. Thus, these initial studies did not resolve the respective roles of these various brain regions, nor did they address the automaticity of the amygdala response.

Neuroimaging and Backward Masking of Facial Expression

Backward masking involves the presentation of two stimuli, with presentation of the second stimulus following the first so quickly that the observer reports seeing only the second stimulus. It is the immediate presentation of the second stimulus (coincident with the offset of the first) that does the trick. If a stimulus—for instance, a picture of a fearful face—is presented for 33 milliseconds (ms), subjects will unanimously report its presence. But if the fearful face stimulus is presented for 33 ms and is immediately followed by a picture of a face with a neutral expression, subjects will report seeing only the second, neutral face. This maneuver is called backward masking. The appearance of the second face (the mask stimulus) apparently interrupts ongoing processing of the first (the target stimulus) before the latter stimulus has a chance to activate brain systems that give rise to awareness (Rolls and Tovee 1994). The amount of time between the onset of the target stimulus and the onset of the mask is referred to as the *stimulus onset asynchrony* (SOA), which appears to be the critical parameter that determines whether subjects will report seeing the target facial expression (Esteves and Öhman 1993).

Pioneering Work of Öhman and Colleagues

Arne Öhman of the Karolinska Institute in Stockholm realized the relevance of such a paradigm to the study of psychiatric disorders. Öhman and his colleagues (Öhman 1992) have used the backward masking of facial expressions combined with pavlovian fear conditioning to demonstrate automatic biologically relevant learning processes in healthy subjects and associated dysfunction in patients with anxiety disorders. Although Öhman recently collaborated on a functional neuroimaging study using backward masking (Morris et al. 1998), the bulk of what is known about masking aversively conditioned stimuli was established by measuring changes in skin conductance response (SCR).

Öhman's basic strategy has been to condition the presentation of a facial expression (e.g., an angry face) to predict the occurrence of an aversive shock presentation in human subjects. To determine whether negative expressions are better suited or "prepared" to predict such an event, Öhman counterbalanced the use of angry (i.e., negative) and happy (i.e., positive) faces as predictive stimuli. In one strategy, these facial expressions are presented overtly (i.e., nonmasked) during conditioning and then testing is conducted to determine whether the facial expression that predicts the aversive event evokes larger SCRs during masked presentations. Thus, after a subject has learned that a stimulus predicts an aversive event, can SCRs demonstrate that this learned stimulus is *detected* when later presented below the subject's level of awareness? In a second strategy, these phases are reversed, with backward masking used during conditioning to assess whether subsequent overt presentations produce greater SCRs to the face that had predicted the aversive event during masked presentations. Thus, can these subjects *learn* this predictive relationship when these stimulus contingencies are presented below the level of awareness?

Öhman's programmatic research using fear conditioning procedures, backward masking of facial expression, and the measurement of SCRs can be summarized (and possibly oversimplified) as follows: Greater SCRs to aversively conditioned facial expressions are recorded when these expressions are presented backwardly masked, after overt conditioning. Thus, this automatic system is capable of demonstrating that it previously learned about stimuli currently being presented below the level of awareness. Greater SCRs to facial expressions presented overtly, after masked conditioning, are also recorded. Thus, this same system is capable of demonstrating that it can learn predictive relationships among biologically relevant stimuli presented below the level of awareness. Öhman was also able to draw some preliminary conclusions concerning how readily this system associates negative versus positive facial expressions with an aversive outcome. After overt conditioning, angry faces support learning more quickly than do happy faces (i.e., subjects take longer to demonstrate conditioned SCRs to aversively conditioned happy faces). During masked presentations after overt conditioning, only the angry faces produce greater SCRs. Similarly, when angry and happy faces are presented backwardly masked during conditioning, only angry faces later produce increased SCRs during overt presentations. It appears that this automatic system is better prepared to associate negative information in the environment with negative outcomes. Öhman and colleagues (Öhman 1992; Öhman and Soares 1994) successfully applied these principles and paradigms to the study of anxiety disorders.

Initial Neuroimaging Study of the Amygdala's Response to Masked Stimuli

The work of Öhman and colleagues suggested a paradigm that might prove useful in isolating amygdala response to fearful face stimuli, in the absence of awareness. In a study involving 10 healthy, male control subjects, we presented masked fearful and masked happy facial expressions (Ekman and Friesen 1976) while acquiring functional magnetic resonance images (Whalen et al. 1998).

The masked fearful and masked happy stimuli are shown in Figure 3–1, A. Each photograph represents a single frame on a film. Because VHS videotape moves at a rate of 30 frames per second, the first fearful or happy target face was visible for 33 ms. This stimulus was immediately followed by five frames of another individual's neutral mask face, visible for 167 ms. Shown in Figure 3–1, B, is how these stimuli were presented to subjects during scanning. Each epoch was 28 seconds long. The masked stimuli were presented every 500 ms (i.e., two masked stimuli were presented per second). Thus, all

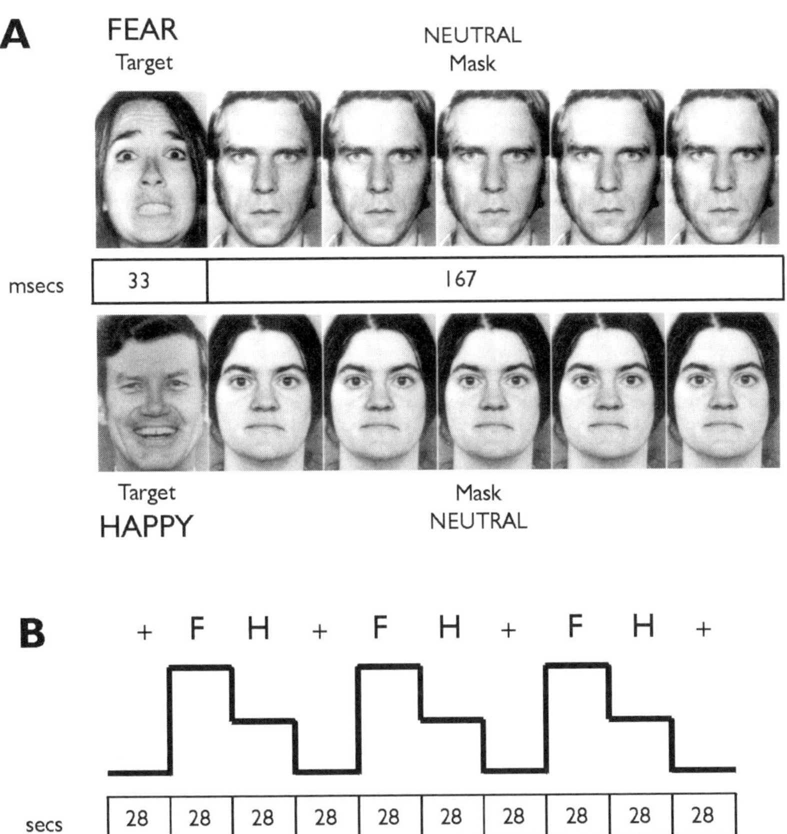

FIGURE 3–1. Design of a masked faces study.
(A) Each masked stimulus consisted of a 33-millisecond (ms) presentation of a fearful or happy expression (target) immediately followed by a 167-ms presentation of a neutral expression (mask). Stimuli were taken from *Pictures of Facial Affect* (Ekman and Friesen 1976). We used fearful, happy, and neutral facial expressions of the same eight individuals (both men and women). The fearful and happy target faces of each person were masked by each of the seven other individuals' neutral expressions, resulting in 56 masked fearful and 56 masked happy stimuli. Masked stimuli were presented twice per second in a pseudorandom order constrained by the requirement that the same identity could occur only twice in a row (as either the target or mask). *(B)* Subjects were presented, in alternating 28-second epochs, with masked fearful face targets (F) masked happy face targets (H), or a single cross that served as a low-level fixation condition (+). Ten epochs made up a run of 4 minutes and 40 seconds. Each subject viewed two runs. The order of epochs was counterbalanced within and across subjects; half of the subjects viewed masked fearful followed by masked happy targets during the first run (+, F, H, +, F, H, +, F, H, +), and the other half viewed masked happy followed by masked fearful targets during the first run (+, H, F, +, H, F, +, H, F, +). The order of fearful and happy target epochs was then reversed for the second run for all subjects.

stimuli were presented in a pseudorandom order within each epoch. Each subject completed two scanning runs; the order of stimulus presentations was fully counterbalanced within and between subjects.

Depicted in Figures 3–2 and 3–3 are fMRI signal changes in the amygdala in response to masked fearful faces versus masked happy faces for the eight subjects who demonstrated no explicit knowledge that these stimuli had been presented. Significantly greater fMRI signal intensity was observed in the amygdala in response to masked fearful faces compared with masked happy faces. Although numerous brain regions make activity-based distinctions between fearful and neutral faces (Breiter et al. 1996) and between fearful and happy faces (Morris et al. 1996), the amygdala appears critical to an early, automatic discrimination between threat- and non-threat-related facial expressions.

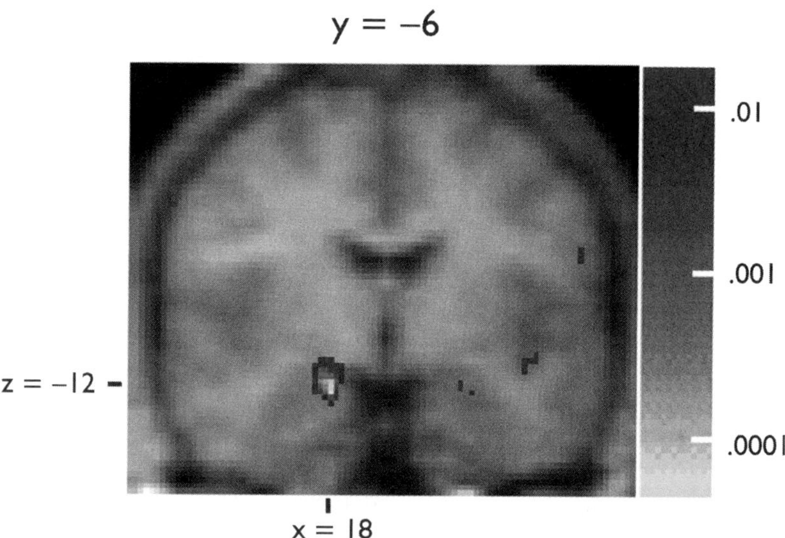

FIGURE 3–2. Amygdala activation to masked fearful faces versus masked happy faces. A coronal slice 6 mm posterior to the anterior commissure depicting average amygdala activation for eight subjects who reported not having seen the fearful or happy target faces. The figure is displayed according to radiological convention (i.e., left=right; right=left; top=superior; bottom=inferior). The colorized statistical map is superimposed over the averaged high-resolution structural data for these eight subjects. Both functional and structural data were placed in a normalized space according to the coordinate system of Talairach and Tournoux (1988).

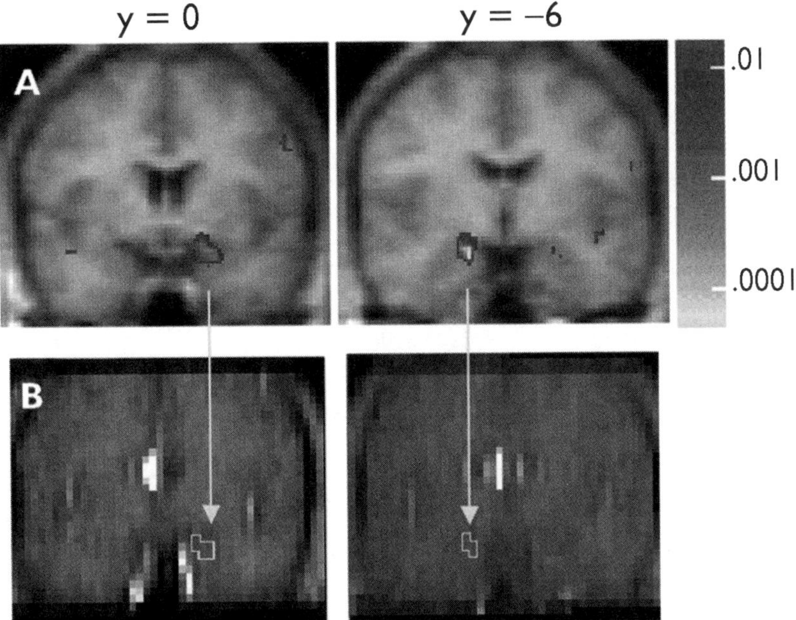

FIGURE 3–3. Activation in the amygdaloid region.
(A) Activation throughout the amygdaloid region was observed at y=0 in addition to y=–6 (depicted in Figure 3–2). Image parameters are as in Figure 3–2. *(B)* Coronal display of analogous averaged magnetic resonance angiograms for these eight subjects was also placed into normalized Talairach space. Thus, the observed composite functional magnetic resonance imaging activation (outlined in yellow) overlaid gray matter and not the location of large arteries (white voxels) medial to the temporal lobe. Veins in this region are known to lie within close proximity to these arteries. The software for placing angiograms in Talairach space was provided by Aiping Jiang and Sean McInerney of Massachusetts General Hospital, Boston, MA.

Selection of the Stimulus Onset Asynchrony

We used a backward masking procedure previously demonstrated to interrupt processing of emotionally expressive faces (Esteves and Öhman 1993; Rolls and Tovee 1994). Face stimuli consisted of PICT files that were assembled frame by frame into a film using Adobe Premiere software. Digital PICT information was then transferred to videotape synchronized with the headsweeps of the videocassette recorder so that stimuli would not be distorted. A videocassette recorder was used to play the tape, and the output was projected (using a Sharp XG-2000U liquid crystal display) onto a screen within the imaging chamber visible on a 1.5-by-3.5-inch mirror approximately 6.5 inches from the subject's face. We chose to use tape for stimulus presentation because tape permitted consistent timing of the 33-ms target stimuli, without the memory constraints of computer presentation.

Esteves and Öhman (1993) demonstrated that if the SOA (i.e., the interval between the onset of the target and the mask) is sufficiently brief (less than 40 ms), human subjects are not aware (as shown by the results of objective forced-choice tasks and by subjective report) of the emotionally expressive target face. Because stimulus contrast and intensity can differ across laboratories, the SOA described here requires pilot testing to confirm adequate masking effects.

Selection of the Interstimulus Interval

The temporal spacing of masked stimuli is critically related to how subjects' awareness of stimuli is assessed (see "Selection of a Measure of Awareness"). This ISI between each masked stimulus should not be confused with the interval between presentation of the target stimulus and presentation of the mask stimulus [i.e., the SOA]. Ideally, the ISI would be long enough for subjects to produce some response that allowed for the determination of their awareness of the target stimulus (e.g., 2 seconds). The ISI used for our initial study (500 ms) did not allow time for such a response as subjects passively viewed masked stimuli. Because our study was the first exploration of fMRI response in the amygdala to masked stimuli, we sought to maximize the number of presented masked stimuli so that the likelihood of detecting amygdala activation would be maximized. This strategy limited our ability to assess subjects' awareness objectively but nonetheless produced a powerful probe of amygdala function; it was appreciated that parameters such as the ISI could later be modified for the purpose of objectively assessing subjects' awareness.

Selection of Baseline Conditions: When Happy May Be Neutral

It will be critical to understand the response of the amygdala to fearful and happy faces relative to its response to neutral faces. This condition is easily implemented during overt stimulus presentations. But implementation of this condition during masked presentations is complicated by the fact that neutral faces also serve as masks in all conditions. Although it seems reasonable simply to add a condition in which neutral faces are masked by neutral faces, there are problems with that design. Any differences observed between masked fearful or happy faces compared with masked neutral faces may be due not to expression but rather to the fact that the subject has seen neutral faces four times as often as either fearful or happy faces. A reasonable solution to this problem would be to have the target faces differ in identity as a group from those of the mask faces. Thus, neutral target faces would be seen just as often as fearful and happy targets. But the assumption behind this solution is that the amygdala responds on the basis of identity in the masked condition. If the amygdala does so respond, this design will suffice. But if the amygdala does not, then the structure will still have been presented with neutral faces four times as often as it has been presented with happy or fearful faces. It has not yet been established that the amygdala responds on the basis of identity per se, especially under masked conditions, and therefore such a baseline condition remains questionable.

In pavlovian conditioning, a stimulus that predicts an aversive event (CS+) is traditionally compared with a stimulus (presented at baseline) that predicts the absence of this event (CS–). Thus, fearful and happy faces might serve as analogous naturalistic stimuli. Like the CS– condition, the happy face baseline condition is, by design, not a neutral condition but a nonthreat condition. The happy face sets a nonthreat baseline against which to contrast the amygdala response to the stimulus that predicts an increased probability of threat. Implicit in this conceptualization is the notion that subjects have had reinforced experience with these stimuli in their lifetimes (probably intermittent experience), and thus these contingencies were learned naturalistically before the subjects entered the study.

Our study design also included epochs of equal duration during which a fixation crosshair was presented on an otherwise blank screen (see Figure 3–1). This fixation stimulus was placed at a level on the screen where the bridge of the nose would appear in face presentations. This additional baseline condition provided a reference from which to assess the direction of fMRI signal changes in the amygdala during presentation of masked fearful and happy faces.

Selection of the Mask Stimulus: Where in the Brain Does Masking of Facial Expression Occur?

The visual pathway for processing of facial stimuli is known to include primary visual cortex followed by processing throughout the ventral pathway involving numerous association cortices, including fusiform gyrus, inferior temporal cortex (IT) and the superior temporal sulcus (STS). Studies in monkeys suggest that neurons responsive to faces and facial expression reside within the STS (Hasselmo et al. 1989; Rolls and Tovee 1994). For the sake of discussion, it will be assumed that activation in the STS for a requisite length of time produces activation within additional brain circuits that give rise to awareness of facial expression.

Backward masking might be achieved in the following fashion: The fearful target face arrives at the STS. If activation were allowed to continue, it would spread through the neural network that supports awareness and the subject would report seeing the face. Instead, however, a masked face arrives at the STS, interrupting or inhibiting activation associated with the target. Recordings from neurons in the STS in monkeys suggest that neurons activated by the neutral masked face inhibit activation in neurons activated by the fearful target face. Rolls and Tovee (1994) presented data suggesting that a process of lateral inhibition is at work. We find this hypothesis intriguing because 1) Öhman and colleagues (Öhman 1992) have consistently used pictures of expressions of different individuals as the target and the mask and 2) we have noticed in our own work that masking is more efficient if the mask and target are pictures of the faces of different individuals (P.J. Whalen, unpublished data, 1998). To elaborate, if the target and mask are pictures of the same individual, subjects report experiencing the tandem stimuli in terms of motion within the face. But if the neutral mask is a picture of a different individual, masking is more efficient. A picture of one individual might activate a given constellation of neurons within the STS, and a picture of another individual might activate different but adjacent neurons within the STS. Thus, activation of neurons in the STS in response to one identity inhibits ongoing activation in response to another identity in adjacent STS neurons through lateral inhibition as hypothesized by Rolls and Tovee (1994). Consequently, to support effective masking, a mask stimulus must be selected that is both sufficiently similar to and sufficiently different from the target. In the case of face stimuli, use of a mask matched to the target in terms of size and contrast, but differing from the target with respect to identity and/or facial expression, seems to minimize development of awareness.

Selection of a Measure of Awareness

Our initial neuroimaging study using masked stimuli (Whalen et al. 1998) was designed as a study of the automaticity of the amygdala with implications for the study of nonconscious processing. This emphasis is evident in two key facets of our study design. First, to maximize the probability of activating the amygdala, we used a relatively short ISI. Second, subjects were unaware of our experimental hypotheses and design and therefore had no reason to suspect that faces with emotional expressions were being masked by neutral faces. In this way, amygdala activation would suggest that the amygdala constantly monitors the environment for predictive stimuli of biological relevance. Because we chose to maximize stimulus presentations and not to inform subjects that masked fearful and happy facial expressions were being presented, we used subjective recall to assess subjects' awareness immediately after image acquisition. Subjective reports of not having seen the target facial expressions correlated with relatively isolated amygdala activation in this study. In contrast, in previous studies using nonmasked (i.e., overt) presentations of fearful facial expressions, unanimous subjective reporting of these expressions occurred, and activation of numerous brain regions in addition to the amygdala was noted (Breiter et al. 1996; Morris et al. 1996). It would be premature to assume that this distinction in fMRI response defines nonconscious processing. However, the observed response dissociation does provide a neuroimaging-based distinction between automatic and more elaborative processing of facial expression. Thus, if isolation of amygdala activity is the goal, then masked presentations and subjective report following stimulus presentations satifies this criterion.

A more rigorous measure of nonconscious processing is an objective forced-choice measure used during stimulus presentations (see Greenwald et al. 1996). This measure requires that subjects be informed of the presence of the target facial expressions before the experiment begins. After presentation of each masked stimulus, subjects report whether the neutral mask face was preceded by a fearful or happy face (for example). If subjects perform at chance levels, then objective evidence exists that they are unaware of the presence of the target stimuli. Use of this more rigorous measure of awareness will allow investigators to design studies directly addressing the role of the amygdala in nonconscious compared with conscious processing. The backward masking study of Morris and colleagues (1998) approached this goal; those researchers assessed awareness during stimulus presentations. Future studies might add to these data by using forced-choice options to direct subjects' responses. Psychiatric neuroimaging studies will continue to address these issues in healthy subjects while determining the usefulness of current subjectively and objectively defined implicit processing probes for studies involving groups of psychiatric patients.

■ Conclusions and Future Directions

Interplay Between Conscious and Nonconscious Information Processing

From an evolutionary perspective, it may be most germane to note that nonconscious information processing is carried out particularly efficiently at the cost of some flexibility, whereas conscious processing is more flexible (and hence more complex), but at the cost of some efficiency. As McNally (1995) pointed out, cognitive psychology's study of basic functional processes such as nonconscious processing, perception without awareness, or automaticity should not be confused with Freud's theory of an unconscious mind complete with wishes, desires, and feelings. Cognitive psychology generally conceptualizes nonconscious processes as being less complex than those portrayed in psychodynamic theory (Greenwald 1992; Loftus and Klinger 1992).

Neuroimaging offers psychiatry a new level of organization from which to address models of conscious and nonconscious information processing. Delineation of brain systems responsible for supporting awareness in healthy subjects will undoubtedly have implications regarding neural dysfunction that contributes to psychiatric illness in a top-down fashion. Likewise, identification of dysfunction in nonconscious systems that have early perceptual access to sensory stimuli might elucidate "bottom-up" contributions to psychiatric illness. Though activity within collective neuronal networks apparently gives rise to awareness of one's perceptual experiences, clearly the brain must do most of its processing below the level of awareness (Crick and Koch 1998). Even humans are simply not aware of most of the information that their brains are processing; if they were, life would be chaos. By using paradigms intended to isolate nonconscious processing, neuroimaging can also serve to localize the brain regions involved in these processes. Finally, it may be that the interplay between conscious and nonconscious information processing systems represents a critical substrate for psychiatric disease.

Summary

In this chapter, we provided two examples to illustrate how probes of immplicit information processing can be developed. Classic implicit information processing paradigms, drawn from the psychology and cognitive neuroscience literature, were modified for use in conjunction with functional neuroimaging. In both cases, these probes were first validated by studying healthy subjects to establish normal behavioral responses and brain activiation profiles. Now that this has been accomplished, these probes are ready to be used to assess implicit information processing abilities and the functional integrity of relevant brain systems in psychiatric populations.

We propose that by using probes of nonconscious as well as conscious information processing, investigators will be able to determine the top-down influence of cortical territories on the amygdala (Morris et al. 1998; Whalen et al. 1998). Likewise, through use of implicit and explicit learning paradigms, the interplay between cortico-striato-thalamic and frontotemporal systems can be systematically assessed (Rauch et al. 1997a). Investigators can then begin to use these probes to study other psychiatric conditions, to identify predictors of treatment response, and to explore the neural substrates of the extinction process in humans, which purportedly underlies behavioral therapies.

■ References

Adolphs R, Tranel D, Damasio H, et al: Fear and the human amygdala. J Neurosci 15:5879–5891, 1995

Adolphs R, Russell JA, Tranel D: A role for the human amygdala in recognizing emotional arousal from unpleasant stimuli. Psychological Science 10:167–171, 1999

Aggleton JP (ed): The Amygdala: Neurobiological Aspects of Emotion, Memory, and Mental Dysfunction. New York, Wiley-Liss, 1992

Aggleton JP, Brown MW: Episodic memory, amnesia, and the hippocampal-anterior thalamic axis. Behav Brain Sci (in press)

Alexander GE, DeLong MR, Strick PL: Parallel organization of functionally segregated circuits linking basal ganglia and cortex. Annu Rev Neurosci 9:357–381, 1986

Alexander GE, Crutcher MD, DeLong MR: Basal ganglia-thalamocortical circuits: parallel substrates for motor, oculomotor, "prefrontal" and "limbic" functions. Prog Brain Res 85:119–146, 1990

Baxter LR Jr, Schwartz JM, Bergman KS, et al: Caudate glucose metabolic rate changes with both drug and behavior therapy for obsessive-compulsive disorder. Arch Gen Psychiatry 49:681–689, 1992

Berns GS, Cohen JD, Mintun MA: Brain regions responsive to novelty in the absence of awareness. Science 276:1272–1275, 1997

Breiter HC, Etcoff NL, Whalen PJ, et al: Response and habituation of the human amygdala during visual processing of facial expression. Neuron 17:875–887, 1996

Buckner RL: Event-related fMRI and the hemodynamic response. Hum Brain Mapp 6:373–377, 1998

Calder AJ, Young AW, Rowland D, et al: Facial emotion recognition after bilateral amygdala damage: differentially severe impairment of fear. Cognitive Neuropsychology 13:699–745, 1996

Clark RE, Squire L: Classical conditioning and brain systems: the role of awareness. Science 280:77–81, 1998

Cleeremans A, McClelland JL: Learning the structure of event sequences. J Exp Psychol Gen 120:235–253, 1991

Clegg BA, DiGirolamo GJ, Keele SW: Sequence learning. Trends in Cognitive Sciences 2:275–281, 1998

Cohen A, Curran T: On tasks, knowledge, correlations, and dissociations: comment on Perruchet and Amorim. J Exp Psychol Learn Mem Cogn 19:1431–1437, 1993

Cohen A, Ivry RI, Keele SW: Attention and structure in sequence learning. J Exp Psychol Learn Mem Cogn 16:17–30, 1990

Cohen JD, Schooler JW (eds): Scientific Approaches to the Study of Consciousness. Mahwah, NJ, Erlbaum, 1997

Crick F, Koch C: Consciousness and neuroscience. Cereb Cortex 8:97–107, 1998

Curran T: On the neural mechanisms of sequence learning. Psyche 2, 1995 (serial online) (http://psyche.cs.monash.edu.au/volume2-1/psyche-95-2-12-sequence-1-curran.html)

Curran T: Implicit sequence learning from a cognitive neuroscience perspective: what, how, and where? in Handbook of Implicit Learning. Edited by Stadler MA, Frensch PA. Thousand Oaks, CA, Sage, 1997, pp 365–400

Curran T, Keele SW: Attentional and nonattentional forms of sequence learning. J Exp Psychol Learn Mem Cogn 19:189–202, 1993

Davis M: The role of the amygdala in conditioned fear, in The Amygdala: Neurobiological Aspects of Emotion, Memory and Mental Dysfunction. Edited by Aggleton JP. New York, Wiley, 1992, pp 255–306

Davis M: Are different parts of the extended amygdala involved in fear vs. anxiety? Biol Psychiatry 44:1239–1247, 1998

Doyon J, Owen AM, Petrides M, et al: Functional anatomy of visuomotor skill learning in human subjects examined with positron emission tomography. Eur J Neurosci 8:637–648, 1996

Ekman P, Friesen WV: Pictures of Facial Affect. Palo Alto, CA, Consulting Psychologists Press, 1976

Esteves F, Öhman A: Masking the face: recognition of emotional facial expressions as a function of the parameters of backward masking. Scand J Psychol 34:1–18, 1993

Foa E, Amir N, Gershuny B: Implicit and explicit memory in obsessive-compulsive disorder. J Anxiety Disord 2:119–129, 1997

Grafton ST, Hazeltine E, Ivry R: Functional mapping of sequence learning in normal humans. J Cogn Neurosci 7:497–510, 1995

Graybiel AM: Building action repertoires: memory and learning functions of the basal ganglia. Curr Opin Neurobiol 5:733–741, 1995

Greenwald AG: New look 3: unconscious cognition reclaimed. Am Psychol 47:766–779, 1992

Greenwald AG, Draine SC, Abrams RL: Three cognitive markers of unconscious semantic activation. Science 273:1699–1702, 1996

Hasselmo ME, Rolls ET, Baylis GC: The role of expression and identity in the face-selective responses of neurons in the temporal visual cortex of the monkey. Behav Brain Res 32:203–218, 1989

Hazeltine E, Grafton ST, Ivry R: Attention and stimulus characteristics determine the locus of motor-sequence encoding: a PET study. Brain 120:123–140, 1997

Houk JC, Davis JL, Beiser DG (eds): Models of Information Processing in the Basal Ganglia. Cambridge, MA, MIT Press, 1995

Kapp BS, Frysinger RC, Gallagher M, et al: Amygdala central nucleus lesions: effects on heart rate conditioning in the rabbit. Physiol Behav 23:1109–1117, 1979

Kapp BS, Whalen PJ, Supple WF, et al: Amygdaloid contributions to conditioned arousal and sensory information processing, in The Amygdala: Neurobiological Aspects of Emotion, Memory and Mental Dysfunction. Edited by Aggleton JP. New York, Wiley, 1992, pp 229–254

Knopman D, Nissen MJ: Procedural learning is impaired in Huntington's disease: evidence from the serial reaction time task. Neuropsychologia 29:245–254, 1991

LeDoux JE: The Emotional Brain. New York, Simon & Schuster, 1996

LeDoux JE, Ruggiero DA, Reis DJ: Projections to the subcortical forebrain from anatomically defined regions of the medial geniculate body in the rat. J Comp Neurol 242:182–213, 1985

Loftus EF, Klinger MR: Is the unconscious smart or dumb? Am Psychol 47:761–765, 1992

MacLeod C, Rutherford EM: Anxiety and the selective processing of emotional information: mediating roles of awareness, trait and state variables, and personal relevance of stimulus materials. Behav Res Ther 30:479–491, 1992

Mathews A, MacLeod C: Discrimination of threat cues without awareness in anxiety states. J Abnorm Psychol 95:131–138, 1986

Mathews A, MacLeod C: Cognitive approaches to emotion and emotional disorders. Annu Rev Psychol 45:25–50, 1994

McNally RJ: Automaticity and the anxiety disorders. Behav Res Ther 33:747–754, 1995

McNally RJ: Information-processing abnormalities in anxiety disorders: implications for cognitive neuroscience. Cognition and Emotion 12:479–495, 1998

McNally RJ, Kaspi SP, Riemann BC, et al: Selective processing of threat cues in posttraumatic stress disorder. J Abnorm Psychol 99:407–412, 1990

Merikle PM, Joordens S: Parallels between perception without attention and perception without awareness. Conscious Cogn 6:219–236, 1997

Miguel EC, Coffey BJ, Baer L, et al: Phenomenology of intentional repetitive behaviors in obsessive-compulsive disorder and Tourette's syndrome. J Clin Psychiatry 56: 246–255, 1995

Mishkin N, Petri HL: Memory and habits: some implications for the analysis of learning and retention, in Neuropsychology of Memory. Edited by Squire LR, Butters N. New York, Guilford, 1984, pp 287–296

Mogg K, Bradley BP, Williams R, et al: Subliminal processing of emotional information in anxiety and depression. J Abnorm Psychol 102:304–311, 1993

Mogg K, Bradley BP, Williams R: Attentional bias in anxiety and depression: the role of awareness. Br J Clin Psychol 34:17–36, 1995

Morris JS, Frith CD, Perrett DI, et al: A differential neural response in the human amygdala to fearful and happy facial expressions. Nature 383:812–815, 1996

Morris JS, Öhman A, Dolan RJ: Conscious and unconscious emotional learning in the human amygdala. Nature 393:467–470, 1998

Nissen MJ, Bullemer P: Attentional requirements of learning: evidence from performance measures. Cogn Psychol 19:1–32, 1987

Öhman A: Fear and anxiety as emotional phenomena: clinical phenomenology, evolutionary perspectives, and information-processing mechanisms, in Handbook of Emotions. Edited by Lewis M, Haviland JM. New York, Guilford, 1992, pp 511–536

Öhman A, Soares JJF: "Unconscious anxiety": phobic responses to masked stimuli. J Abnorm Psychol 103:231–240, 1994

Packard MG, Hirsch R, White NM: Differential effects of fornix and caudate nucleus lesions on two radial arm maze tasks: evidence for multiple memory systems. J Neurosci 9:1465–1472, 1989

Pascual-Leone A, Wassermann E, Grafman J, et al: The role of dorsolateral prefrontal cortex in implicit procedural learning. Exp Brain Res 107:479–485, 1996

Perruchet P, Amorim M: Conscious knowledge and changes in performance in sequence learning: evidence against dissociation. J Exp Psychol Learn Mem Cogn 18:785–800, 1992

Pitman R, Shalev AY, Orr SP: Posttraumatic stress disorder: emotion, conditioning and memory, in The Cognitive Neurosciences, 2nd Edition. Edited by Gazzaniga MS. Cambridge, MA, MIT Press (in press)

Rauch SL, Baxter LR Jr: Neuroimaging of OCD and related disorders, in Obsessive-Compulsive Disorders: Practical Management. Edited by Jenike MA, Baer L, Minichiello WE. Boston, MA, Mosby, 1998, pp 289–317

Rauch SL, Jenike MA: Neural mechanisms of obsessive-compulsive disorder. Current Review of Mood and Anxiety Disorders 1:84–94, 1997

Rauch SL, Savage CR: Neuroimaging and neuropsychology of the striatum, in Neuropsychiatry of the Basal Ganglia. Psychiatr Clin North Am 20:741–768, 1997

Rauch SL, Jenike MA, Alpert NM, et al: Regional cerebral blood flow measured during symptom provocation in obsessive-compulsive disorder using ^{15}O-labeled CO_2 and positron emission tomography. Arch Gen Psychiatry 51:62–70, 1994

Rauch SL, Savage CR, Brown HD, et al: A PET investigation of implicit and explicit sequence learning. Hum Brain Mapp 3:271–286, 1995

Rauch SL, van der Kolk BA, Fisler RE, et al: A symptom provocation study of posttraumatic stress disorder using positron emission tomography and script-driven imagery. Arch Gen Psychiatry 53:380–387, 1996

Rauch SL, Savage CR, Alpert NM, et al: Probing striatal function in obsessive-compulsive disorder: a PET study of implicit sequence learning. J Neuropsychiatry Clin Neurosci 9:568–573, 1997a

Rauch SL, Whalen PJ, Savage CR, et al: Striatal recruitment during an implicit sequence learning task as measured by functional magnetic resonance imaging. Hum Brain Mapp 5:124–132, 1997b

Rauch SL, Whalen PJ, Curran T, et al: Thalamic deactivation during early implicit sequence learning: a functional MRI study. Neuroreport 9:865–870, 1998a

Rauch SL, Whalen PJ, Curran T, et al: Thalamic deactivation during early implicit sequence learning: a functional MRI study. Neuroreport 9:865–870, 1998a

Rauch SL, Whalen PJ, Dougherty DD, et al: Neurobiological models of obssessive compulsive disorders, in Obssessive-Compulsive Disorders: Practical Management. Edited by Jenike MA, Baer L, Minichiello WE. Boston, MA, Mosby, 1998b, pp 222–252

Reber PJ, Squire LR: Parallel brain systems for learning with and without awareness. Learn Mem 1:217–229, 1994

Reed J, Johnson P: Assessing implicit learning with indirect tests: determining what is learned about sequence structure. J Exp Psychol Learn Mem Cogn 20:585–594, 1994

Robinson D, Wu H, Munne RA, et al: Reduced caudate nucleus volume in obsessive-compulsive disorder. Arch Gen Psychiatry 52:393–398, 1995

Rolls ET, Tovee MJ: Processing speed in the cerebral cortex and the neurophysiology of visual masking. Proc R Soc Lond B Biol Sci 257:9–15, 1994

Schacter DL, Chiu CP, Ochsner KN: Implicit memory: a selective review. Annu Rev Neurosci 16:159–182, 1993

Schacter DL, Alpert NM, Savage CR, et al: Conscious recollection and the human hippocampal formation: evidence from positron emission tomography. Proc Natl Acad Sci U S A 93:321–325, 1996

Shanks DR, St. John MF: Characteristics of dissociable human learning systems. Behav Brain Sci 17:367–447, 1994

Shin LM, Kosslyn SM, McNally RJ, et al: Visual imagery and perception in posttraumatic stress disorder. Arch Gen Psychiatry 54:233–241, 1997

Squire LR: Mechanisms of memory. Science 232:1612–1619, 1986

Squire LR: Memory and the hippocampus: a synthesis from findings with rats, monkeys, and humans. Psychol Rev 99:195–231, 1992

Stadler MA: Implicit serial learning: questions inspired by Hebb (1961). Mem Cognit 21:819–827, 1993

Stadler MA: Role of attention in implicit learning. J Exp Psychol Learn Mem Cogn 21:674–685, 1995

Swedo SE, Pietrini P, Leonard HL, et al: Cerebral glucose metabolism in childhood-onset obsessive-compulsive disorder: revisualization during pharmacotherapy. Arch Gen Psychiatry 49:690–694, 1992

Swedo SE, Leonard HL, Garvey M, et al: Pediatric autoimmune neuropsychiatric disorders associated with streptococcal infections: clinical description of the first 50 cases. Am J Psychiatry 155:264–271, 1998

Talairach J, Tournoux P: Co-planar Stereotaxic Atlas of the Human Brain. New York, Thieme, 1988

Ungerleider LG: Functional brain imaging studies of cortical mechanisms for memory. Science 270:769–775, 1995

Whalen PJ: Fear, vigilance, and ambiguity: initial neuroimaging studies of the human amygdala. Current Directions in Psychological Science 7:177–188, 1998

Whalen PJ, Rauch SL, Etcoff NL, et al: Masked presentations of emotional facial expressions modulate amygdala activity without explicit knowledge. J Neurosci 18:411–418, 1998

Willingham DB: COBALT: a neuropsychological theory of motor skill learning. Psychol Rev 105:558–584, 1998

Willingham DB, Koroshetz WJ: Evidence for dissociable motor skills in Huntington's disease patients. Psychobiology 21:173–182, 1993

Willingham DB, Greenley DB, Bardone AM: Dissociation in a serial response time task using a recognition measure: comment on Perruchet and Amorim (1992). J Exp Psychol Learn Mem Cogn 19:1424–1430, 1993

Wise SP, Murray EA, Gerfen CR: The frontal cortex-basal ganglia system in primates. Crit Rev Neurobiol 10:317–356, 1996

4

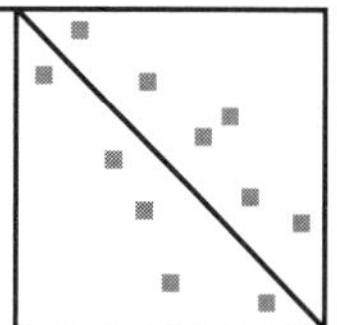

SYMPTOM PROVOCATION STUDIES

The Example of Anxiety Disorders

Lisa M. Shin, Ph.D.
Scott L. Rauch, M.D.
Roger K. Pitman, M.D.

In the field of psychiatric neuroimaging, several paradigms have been implemented to study brain activity in patients with psychiatric disorders. One such paradigm is symptom provocation, which is used to determine the brain systems that mediate symptomatic states. In separate conditions within a symptom provocation study, individuals with a psychiatric disorder undergo neuroimaging during exposure to both neutral and symptom-provoking stimuli; subsequently, blood flow in these two conditions is compared, and brain areas that are differentially active during the symptomatic state are delineated.

The use of symptom provocation paradigms in conjunction with functional neuroimaging can help elucidate the pathophysiology of specific disorders. In addition, symptom provocation can be implemented before and after treatment, to determine how the mediating neuroanatomy might change after treatment and whether the pretreatment brain activity predicts response to treatment (see Chapter 7 in this volume).

In this chapter, we describe the basic elements of the symptom provocation paradigm, review the literature regarding symptom provocation in patients with anxiety disorders and emotional state induction in healthy individuals, and discuss some special considerations and limitations of symptom provocation studies.

■ ELEMENTS OF A SYMPTOM PROVOCATION STUDY

Study Groups

Because some disorders are not easily studied within the context of a symptom provocation paradigm, the selection of a proper study group is important. Anxiety disorders, such as posttraumatic stress disorder (PTSD), obsessive-compulsive disorder (OCD), and specific phobia, are the most amenable to study because their respective symptomatic states occur fairly reliably in the presence of specific stimuli. For example, the symptomatic state of specific phobia occurs reliably in response to a feared stimulus, such as a snake or a spider.

As in most neuroimaging studies, the study group is selected using strict inclusion and exclusion criteria. Typically excluded from symptom provocation studies are patients with histories of head injury or severe medical conditions, patients taking medications with psychotropic or cardiovascular effects, and patients with significant comorbid psychiatric conditions, such as current alcohol dependence or psychotic disorders.

Often in symptom provocation studies, researchers include both a patient group and a comparison group, which typically comprises healthy individuals without the disorder of interest. For example, in a symptom provocation study focusing on combat veterans with PTSD, researchers might also include a group of combat veterans without PTSD (Bremner et al. 1999a; Shin et al. 1997). Such a comparison group would then be matched with the patient group for variables such as age, education, sex, and handedness. In some circumstances, subjects in the comparison group may be matched with the patient group for the presence of other psychiatric disorders. For example, depression is exceedingly common in combat veterans with PTSD, and it is often difficult to locate PTSD patients without comorbid depression. If a researcher decides to include a certain number of PTSD patients with comorbid depression, he or she might consider also including the same number of comparison subjects with depression.

Stimuli

Symptomatic states are typically provoked through exposure to disorder-relevant stimuli, which can vary both in content and in mode of presentation. *Content* refers to what the stimulus depicts (e.g, a snake), and *mode of presentation* refers to how the stimulus is shown to subjects (e.g., in the form of a real snake, a picture of a snake, or a mental image of a snake). Researchers can adjust both the content and mode of stimulus presentation to ensure that the stimulus is optimally provocative yet tolerable to subjects. In addition to provocative stimuli, neutral control stimuli are shown to subjects in a separate condition; these neutral control stimuli should be matched with the provocative stimuli for basic visual characteristics (such as approximate size, color, movement, or detail) and duration of presentation. The following is a description of different modes of presentation used in symptom provocation studies.

In Vivo Exposure

In vivo exposure involves exposing subjects to the actual feared stimulus, as well as a neutral stimulus, during scanning. For example, in a study of specific phobia, the provocative stimulus might be an actual spider placed in a container next to the subject (Rauch et al. 1995); in a study of OCD, the provocative stimulus might be a "dirty" glove placed on the subject's hand (Breiter et al. 1996; Rauch et al. 1994). Occasionally, researchers ask subjects (before scanning) to construct hierarchical lists of symptom-provoking items, ranging from least to most provocative. These hierarchies can then be presented to subjects in different scanning conditions to determine the neural correlates of various symptomatic levels (McGuire et al. 1994). One limitation of in vivo exposure is that this mode of stimulus presentation cannot easily be used to study some anxiety disorders, such as PTSD and panic disorder, because in vivo provocative stimuli are either not available (e.g., past traumatic events cannot be re-created in the laboratory) or not reliable (e.g., specific stimuli may not always trigger a panic attack in panic disorder).

Exposure Using Audiovisual Material

When using an in vivo stimulus is not possible or practical, researchers may elect to present provocative and neutral stimuli using still photographs, videotape, or audiotape. For example, symptom provocation studies of combat-related PTSD have included still photographs and videotapes of combat-related scenes, as well as audiotapes of combat-related sounds (Bremner et al. 1999a; Liberzon et al. 1999; Shin et al. 1997). In addition, audiovisual stimuli have been used extensively in studies of emotional state induction in healthy individuals. For example, emotional film clips have been used to study normal states of happiness, sadness, fear, and disgust (Lane et al. 1997b; Paradiso et al. 1997; Reiman et al. 1997). In most cases, the audiovisual stimuli presented to subjects are standardized, not personalized; in other words, all subjects are exposed to the same stimuli, and those stimuli are not based on any one subject's personal experience.

Script-Driven Imagery

In script-driven imagery, a paradigm that was first developed by Lang and colleagues (Lang 1985; Lang et al. 1983), audiotaped descriptions (i.e., scripts) of personal events guide subjects through the recollection and imagery of those events for the purpose of inducing the desired emotional state. Scripts are constructed in the following manner: First, subjects provide detailed, written descriptions of both emotionally provocative and neutral personal events. These descriptions are then modified (through adjustment of length, tense, voice, and person) according to established procedures and are audiotaped for later playback during scanning. This basic paradigm was adapted by Pitman and colleagues (1987, 1990) for the study of psychophysiologic responses in PTSD and was later used in neuroimaging studies of PTSD (Rauch et al. 1996; Shin et al. 1999) and normal emotional state induction (Dougherty et al. 1999; Lane et al. 1997b; Rauch et al. 1999; Reiman et al. 1997; Shin et al. 2000). Because all scripts are personalized, subjects in any given study will generate and be exposed to different scripts. Script-driven imagery is especially useful when stimuli cannot be presented in vivo or be re-created using audiovisual materials.

Pharmacologic Challenge

Often the stimuli that researchers use to provoke anxiety symptoms are not, and cannot be, audiovisual or imagery based. In pharmacologic challenge studies, specific substances (e.g., carbon dioxide, sodium lactate, or yohimbine) are used to induce symptomatic states in patients with disorders such as panic disorder or PTSD. For example, yohimbine has been used in pharmacologic challenge studies of PTSD because it increases noradrenergic activity and has been shown to induce panic, reexperiencing, and numbing symptoms in veterans with PTSD (Bremner et al. 1997; Southwick et al. 1993). Pharmacologic challenge neuroimaging studies can be particularly informative, because they provide data not only about regional brain activation but also about the possible role of specific neurotransmitter systems in the disorder of interest. Pharmacologic challenge studies can also be conducted in healthy individuals to determine the neural correlates of normal responses to those challenges (Benkelfat et al. 1995; Ketter et al. 1996; Servan-Schreiber et al. 1998).

Procedures

Neuroimaging

Symptom provocation paradigms can be used in conjunction with positron emission tomography (PET), functional magnetic resonance imaging (fMRI), or single photon emission computed tomography (SPECT). However, most symptom provocation studies in the literature have used PET and [^{15}O]water or carbon dioxide. PET and ^{15}O are particularly well suited for use in symptom provocation paradigms because 1) the short half-life of ^{15}O allows researchers to perform multiple scans in a single subject in a single session; 2) blood flow can be measured in discrete periods of approximately 1 minute, with ample debriefing time between scans; 3) subjects are not enclosed in a small space; and 4) anterior paralimbic regions of the brain (e.g., orbitofrontal cortex) can be visualized easily. In addition, because the offset of a symptomatic state is gradual, symptom provocation is not easily achieved using fMRI paradigms that require rapidly alternating conditions (i.e., block on–block off or single-trial paradigms).

Selection of Study Conditions

In symptom provocation studies, brain activity is measured in at least two conditions: provoked and neutral. Occasionally, other conditions may be added. For example, some studies have included neutral teeth-clenching conditions, to control for possible spontaneous jaw muscle contraction in the provoked condition (Rauch et al. 1996; Shin et al. 1999). Some researchers have chosen to use two different types of provoked conditions (e.g., in vivo exposure and imaginal flooding [Zohar et al. 1989]). As noted earlier, other researchers have presented subjects with a hierarchical range of provocative stimuli in separate conditions (McGuire et al. 1994).

Documentation of Symptomatic or Emotional Change

Typically, symptom severity is assessed immediately after every scan during which exposure to a neutral or provocative stimulus occurs. Symptoms can be assessed using analog scales (e.g., Likert-type scales) or standard inventories (e.g., the State-Trait Anxiety Inventory, State Form [Spielberger et al. 1983]). In either case, the provoked condition should be associated with a greater number and/or greater severity of symptoms than the neutral condition. In studies of emotional states in healthy individuals, analog or standard scales may be used to assess the intensity of the emotional state of interest.

Measurement of Psychophysiologic Response

Because subjective reports of symptoms are vulnerable to bias, more objective measures of symptomatic states are desirable (e.g., psychophysiologic measures, such as heart rate, skin conductance, and muscle tension [Lang 1985; Pitman et al. 1987]). For example, a vast amount of research has indicated that individuals with PTSD have larger psychophysiologic responses to trauma-related stimuli than to neutral stimuli and that these responses to trauma-related stimuli are greater in subjects with PTSD than in comparison subjects without PTSD (see, for instance, Blanchard et al. 1986; Pitman et al. 1987, 1990; Rauch et al. 1996; Shin et al. 1999).

Monitoring of Behavioral Changes

In some disorders, the symptomatic state may be associated with observable behavioral changes that should be monitored and documented in symptom provocation studies. For example, when experiencing trauma-related script-driven imagery, individuals with PTSD may display behavior suggestive of a flashback. Patients with panic disorder might be monitored for other directly observable behaviors, such as hyperventilation or shaking.

Data Analysis

Contrasts Between Conditions

Brain activity in the provoked condition can be compared with that of the neutral condition by means of a direct statistical contrast, revealing regions that are more (or less) active in the provoked condition. In symptom provocation studies, two general approaches to data analysis have been taken: a region of interest–based approach and a voxel-wise, statistical parametric mapping approach. The former approach involves targeting one or more specific brain regions of interest and analyzing data only in those regions; this approach can be quite conservative and hypothesis driven but is also vulnerable to type II errors. The latter approach involves conducting voxel-by-voxel comparisons between the provoked and neutral conditions throughout the whole brain; when combined with a priori hypotheses and appropriately conservative significance thresholds (to reduce the risk of type I errors), this method may be more powerful than the region of interest–based approach.

Correlational Analyses

In addition to performing contrasts between conditions, some researchers compute correlations between brain activity and symptom ratings. These correlations reveal whether activity in certain regions of the brain is significantly related to symptomatic changes. For example, McGuire et al. (1994) measured blood flow during exposure to increasingly provocative stimuli and conducted correlational analyses between blood flow and symptom ratings across different conditions. Furthermore, correlational analyses may be useful in pretreatment-posttreatment neuroimaging studies, in that such analyses may help researchers determine whether pretreatment blood flow in specific regions of the brain is correlated with degree of treatment response. Correlational analyses also have been conducted in studies of emotional state induction in healthy individuals. For example, Cahill et al. (1996) reported a significant positive correlation between glucose metabolic rate in the amygdaloid complex and the number of emotionally arousing film clips that subjects subsequently remembered.

■ Symptom Provocation Studies of Anxiety Disorders

The elements of symptom provocation studies are illustrated further in the following review of relevant research on PTSD, OCD, specific phobia, and panic disorder. To demonstrate that similar designs can be implemented to study emotional state induction in healthy individuals, we review that literature as well. PET has been used most often in studies of symptom provocation, and, unless otherwise stated, the studies reviewed here used PET to examine regional cerebral blood flow (rCBF).

Posttraumatic Stress Disorder

Rauch et al. (1996) used script-driven imagery to examine rCBF patterns in eight individuals with PTSD. In separate conditions, subjects were prompted by audiotaped scripts to recall and imagine neutral and traumatic autobiographical events. In a teeth-clenching control condition, subjects recalled and imagined a neutral event while clenching their teeth. Heart rate and subjective ratings of anxiety, fear, sadness, disgust, anger, and guilt were higher in the traumatic condition than in the neutral condition. Significant rCBF increases occurred in the traumatic condition, compared with the control condition, in right medial orbitofrontal cortex, right insular cortex, right anterior temporal pole, anterior cingulate gyrus, right amygdala, right medial temporal cortex, right secondary visual cortex, and bilateral sensorimotor cortex. In addition, rCBF decreases were found in left middle temporal cortex and left inferior frontal gyrus (Broca's area).

Shin and colleagues (1999) examined rCBF in 16 female survivors of childhood sexual abuse: 8 with PTSD and 8 without PTSD. During separate scans, subjects imagined neutral and traumatic autobiographical events. A teeth-clenching neutral condition was also used in the study. The PTSD group had greater heart rate responses to traumatic imagery than did the comparison group. In the traumatic condition, relative to the control conditions, both groups exhibited rCBF increases in orbitofrontal cortex and anterior temporal poles; however, these increases were significantly greater in the PTSD group than in the comparison group. Furthermore, only the PTSD group exhibited rCBF decreases in left inferior frontal gyrus (Broca's area), and only the comparison group exhibited rCBF increases in anterior cingulate gyrus.

Using similar methods, Bremner et al. (1999b) also studied women with histories of childhood sexual abuse. In this study, 10 women with PTSD and 12 women without PTSD underwent PET while listening to scripts describing neutral and traumatic events. The traumatic versus neutral comparison revealed that relative to the control group, the PTSD group exhibited greater rCBF decreases in subcallosal gyrus (Brodmann's area 25), a failure to activate anterior cingulate gyrus, and greater rCBF increases in posterior cingulate cortex and anterolateral prefrontal cortex.

Shin et al. (1997) studied patterns of rCBF associated with exposure to neutral, negative, and combat-related pictures in seven combat veterans with PTSD and seven combat veterans without PTSD. In separate conditions, subjects either viewed or generated visual mental images of these three types of pictures. In the PTSD group, rCBF increases occurred in right amygdala and ventral anterior cingulate gyrus in the combat imagery conditions. In addition, the PTSD group exhibited rCBF decreases in left inferior frontal gyrus (Broca's area).

Using a different paradigm, Bremner et al. (1999a) studied 20 Vietnam combat veterans: 10 with PTSD and 10 without PTSD. While undergoing PET, subjects were presented with combat-related and neutral slides and sounds. In the combat versus neutral comparison, the PTSD group was found to exhibit rCBF decreases in medial prefrontal cortex (subcallosal gyrus) and anterior cingulate cortex. According to a group-by-condition interaction, areas with decreased rCBF in subjects with PTSD and increased rCBF in control subjects were medial prefrontal cortex (subcallosal gyrus), middle temporal gyrus, and thalamus. Areas with increased rCBF in PTSD subjects and decreased rCBF in control subjects were inferior parietal lobule, lingual gyrus, cerebellum-pons-parahippus, midcingulate gyrus, and motor cortex.

Liberzon et al. (1999) used SPECT and technetium Tc 99m hexamethylpropylene-amine oxime to study rCBF in 14 Vietnam veterans with PTSD, 11 combat veteran control subjects, and 14 healthy nonveteran subjects. In separate scanning sessions, subjects were presented with combat sounds and white noise. In the combat sounds versus white noise comparison, all three groups were found to show activation in anterior cingulate/medial prefrontal gyrus medial prefrontal gyrus, but only the PTSD group exhibited activation in the left amygdaloid region.

Bremner et al. (1997) examined the effect of yohimbine challenge on glucose metabolic rates in 10 combat veterans with PTSD and 10 nonveteran subjects without PTSD. Administration of yohimbine, which activates noradrenergic neurons by blocking α_2-adrenergic receptors, has been shown to induce panic, reexperiencing, and numbing symptoms in veterans with PTSD (Southwick et al. 1993). Only the PTSD group reported increased anxiety and panic symptoms after yohimbine administration. Furthermore, in the yohimbine condition, relative to the placebo condition, brain glucose metabolism decreased in a wide variety of cortical areas in the PTSD group but not in the comparison group.

In summary, symptom provocation studies of PTSD have revealed activation of the amygdala and anterior paralimbic regions of the brain (e.g., orbitofrontal cortex, anterior temporal poles, and anterior insular cortex) and deactivation of Broca's area during the symptomatic state in PTSD. Activation of the amygdala is consistent with the role that this structure appears to play in fear conditioning and the processing of stimuli with affective significance (LeDoux 1992). PTSD may be differentiated from other anxiety disorders by the presence of activation of the amygdala during symptom provocation; however, only two studies have found such amygdala activation in PTSD. Thus, further research is required before conclusions about the role of the amygdala in PTSD can be drawn. Activation in visual cortex may reflect reexperiencing phenomena in the form of imagery. Deactivation in Broca's area is consistent with clinical observations that patients with PTSD often have difficulty constructing narrative accounts of traumatic events (see, for example, van der Kolk and Fisler 1995).

Five of the completed studies described here actually used comparison groups of trauma-exposed individuals without PTSD, and findings of these studies suggest some differences in brain activation between individuals with and those without PTSD. Specifically, individuals with PTSD appeared to have greater activation in some regions of the brain (e.g., orbitofrontal cortex and anterior temporal poles) but less activation in certain portions of medial frontal cortex, including anterior cingulate gyrus. This finding is interesting given that medial prefrontal cortex is thought to be involved in the extinction of conditioned fear responses (Morgan et al. 1993) and may perform a compensatory role in the regulation of emotion (Mayberg 1997). Medial prefrontal cortex may function abnormally in PTSD.

Obsessive-Compulsive Disorder

Using the ^{133}Xe inhalation technique, Zohar et al. (1989) measured rCBF in 10 patients with OCD and washing compulsions. Subjects participated in three conditions: relaxation, imaginal flooding, and in vivo exposure. Heart rate and blood pressure were higher and the severity of OCD symptoms was greater in the in vivo exposure and imaginal flooding conditions than in the relaxation condition. rCBF in temporal cortex was higher in the imaginal flooding condition than in the relaxation condition. rCBF in many cortical areas was reduced in the in vivo exposure condition, relative to the relaxation and imaginal flooding conditions.

Rauch et al. (1994) measured rCBF in eight patients with OCD during symptomatic and neutral states. In separate conditions, subjects were presented with individually tailored provocative stimuli (e.g., a "contaminated" glove) and neutral control stimuli (e.g., a clean glove). Subjective ratings of anxiety and OCD symptoms were higher during the provoked condition than during the neutral condition. The provoked versus neutral comparison revealed rCBF increases in right caudate nucleus, left anterior cingulate gyrus and bilateral orbitofrontal cortex. rCBF in left anterior orbitofrontal cortex during the provoked condition was positively correlated with OCD symptom severity.

Breiter et al. (1996) used fMRI to study 10 patients with OCD and 5 healthy control subjects. Subjects were presented with provocative and neutral stimuli in different scanning conditions. The OCD patients reported significant increases in obsessions, compulsions, and anxiety in the provoked condition relative to the neutral condition, and the control subjects reported smaller, but significant, increases. In the provoked versus neutral comparison, at least 70% of OCD patients were found to show activation in bilateral anterior and posterior medial orbital gyri; bilateral superior, middle, and inferior frontal gyri; bilateral anterior cingulate gyrus; bilateral temporal cortex; right caudate; left lenticulate; left insular cortex; and bilateral amygdala. None of the control subjects exhibited activations in any brain region.

McGuire and colleagues (1994) studied four OCD patients with contamination fears and hand-washing rituals. In 12 separate conditions, subjects were exposed to different "contaminants" that provoked a range of urges to ritualize. OCD symptom intensity was positively correlated with rCBF in right inferior frontal gyrus, right caudate, right putamen, right thalamus, left hippocampus, left posterior cingulate gyrus, and left cuneus.

Cottraux and colleagues (1996) examined rCBF during mental imagery of neutral and obsession-related events in 10 patients with OCD and 10 matched control subjects. Both groups exhibited increased rCBF in middle and inferior orbitofrontal gyri during obsessional imagery relative to neutral imagery.

In summary, the existing literature suggests that the symptomatic state of OCD is accompanied by activation of anterior paralimbic structures, caudate, and thalamus. At least one study has demonstrated a direct relationship between rCBF in orbitofrontal cortex and OCD symptom severity.

Specific Phobias

Mountz et al. (1989) studied seven subjects with small-animal phobia during both rest and confrontation with phobic stimuli. Self-reported anxiety and psychophysiologic responses were higher in the fear condition than in the rest condition. However, rCBF differences between the conditions disappeared after carbon dioxide partial pressure (P_{CO_2}) was corrected.

Wik et al. (1993) measured rCBF in six female subjects with snake phobia. In separate conditions, subjects viewed videotapes depicting snakes, other generally aversive scenes, and neutral scenes. Heart rate and anxiety ratings were higher in the snake condition than in the neutral condition. In the snake condition, relative to the neutral condition, rCBF increases occurred in secondary visual cortex; rCBF decreases were observed in hippocampus, prefrontal cortex, orbitofrontal cortex, temporopolar cortex, and posterior cingulate cortex. Fredrikson et al. (1993) also found rCBF increases in secondary visual cortex during symptom provocation in individuals with snake phobia. Fredrikson and colleagues (1995) reported similar results in a study of spider phobia.

Rauch et al. (1995) measured rCBF during symptom provocation in seven individuals with simple phobia. In separate conditions, subjects were presented with provocative stimuli (e.g., a spider in a container) and neutral stimuli (e.g., an empty container) and then were scanned with their eyes closed. Heart rate, respiration rate, and ratings of subjective anxiety were higher in the provoked condition than in the neutral condition. In the provoked versus neutral comparison, rCBF was found to be increased in left somatosensory cortex, the left thalamus, and the following paralimbic regions: right anterior cingulate gyrus, left insular cortex, left posterior orbitofrontal cortex, and right anterior temporal pole.

The results summarized here suggest that paralimbic structures mediate symptoms of simple phobia. The discrepancy between the findings of Rauch et al. (1995) and those of Wik et al. (1993) and Fredrikson et al. (1993, 1995) may be due to differences in mode of stimulus presentation (in vivo vs. videotape) or scanning procedure (eyes closed vs. eyes opened).

Panic Disorder

Reiman et al. (1989) studied rCBF changes during lactate infusions in 17 patients with panic disorder and 15 healthy control subjects. In the 8 patients who had a lactate-induced panic attack, rCBF increases occurred in bilateral temporopolar cortex, bilateral claustrum-insula-putamen, bilateral superior colliculi, and anterior cerebellar vermis. These increases were not observed in the healthy control subjects or in patients who did not experience a panic attack. However, according to Drevets et al. (1992) and Benkelfat et al. (1995), temporopolar blood flow increases in the panicking patients may have been extracranial artifacts of muscular origin.

Woods et al. (1988) used SPECT to study the effects of yohimbine (vs. saline placebo) on rCBF in six patients with panic disorder and six healthy control subjects. In patients with panic disorder, anxiety levels increased and frontal blood flow decreased in the yohimbine condition, relative to the saline placebo condition.

Three Anxiety Disorders

To elucidate further the mediating neuroanatomy of pathological anxiety, Rauch et al. (1997) combined the results of their previous symptom provocation studies of three different anxiety disorders: OCD (Rauch et al. 1994), simple phobia (Rauch et al. 1995), and PTSD (Rauch et al. 1996). In the provoked versus control comparison, Rauch et al. (1997) found rCBF increases in right inferior frontal cortex, right posterior medial orbitofrontal cortex, bilateral insular cortex, bilateral lenticular nuclei, and bilateral brain stem. In addition, rCBF in left brain stem was positively correlated with subjective anxiety ratings.

■ EMOTIONAL STATE INDUCTION

In this section, we review the literature regarding emotional state induction in healthy individuals because the general methods used in such studies are similar to those used in symptom provocation studies of anxiety disorders and because the results of these studies can inform our theories regarding the normal function of certain brain systems and how those systems may function abnormally in anxiety disorders. Findings from negative emotional conditions within each of the following studies are highlighted because they are the most relevant to the research on anxiety disorders.

State Induction and Emotional Stimuli

The following studies involved inducing an emotional state using imagery or audiovisual emotional stimuli or both.

Pardo et al. (1993) studied rCBF associated with mild sadness in seven healthy individuals. In the sad condition, subjects imagined situations that would make them sad. In the resting condition, subjects lay quietly with their eyes closed. In the sad versus rest contrast, rCBF increases were found in superior frontal gyrus, inferior frontal gyrus, and orbitofrontal cortex.

Baker et al. (1997) studied nine healthy male subjects after induction of a depressed, elated, or neutral mood state. Subjects also performed verbal fluency and word repetition tasks during scanning. Compared with the neutral mood state, the depressed state was associated with rCBF increases in inferior frontal or orbitofrontal cortex, middle frontal gyrus, premotor cortex, supplementary motor area, and posterior cingulate gyrus. rCBF decreases occurred in medial frontal cortex, middle frontal gyrus, and caudate nucleus.

Dougherty et al. (1999) included eight healthy men in a script-driven imagery study of anger. During the anger condition, subjects recalled and imagined personal events involving a maximal amount of anger; in the neutral condition, subjects recalled and imagined emotionally neutral events. The anger versus neutral comparison revealed rCBF increases in the orbitofrontal cortex, anterior cingulate gyrus, and anterior temporal poles. These subjects were also studied in a condition involving guilt-related script driven imagery (Shin et al. 2000); the guilt versus neutral comparison revealed activation in anterior cingulate gyrus, anterior temporal poles, and anterior insular cortex/inferior frontal gyrus.

George et al. (1995) studied the neural correlates of transient sadness and happiness in 11 healthy women. In separate scanning conditions, subjects recalled neutral, sad, and happy events, viewed affect-appropriate faces, and attempted to experience the emotion corresponding to each facial expression. In the sad condition, relative to the neutral condition, rCBF increases occurred in right medial frontal gyrus, left cingulate gyrus, right putamen, caudate, left cingulate/orbitofrontal cortex, and left thalamus. The happy versus neutral contrast revealed no significant rCBF increases. Data from 10 of the female subjects were reanalyzed after 10 healthy men were added to the subject pool (George et al. 1996). In the sad versus neutral comparison, both men and women exhibited blood flow increases in left insular cortex, and only the female subjects showed additional blood flow increases in anterior cingulate gyrus.

Using a similar paradigm, Kimbrell et al. (1999) studied anxiety, anger, and neutral states in 16 healthy adults. Relative to the neutral condition, the anxiety condition was associated with rCBF increases in left anterior cingulate gyrus and left temporal pole and rCBF decreases in right medial and middle frontal gyri. The anger versus neutral comparison revealed rCBF increases in bilateral temporal poles, medial frontal gyrus, and thalamus.

Lane and colleagues (1997b) examined rCBF during induced states of happiness, sadness, and disgust in 12 healthy female subjects. In separate scans, each of these emotions was induced using a film clip (film condition) and script-driven recall (recall condition). Subjects also participated in neutral conditions consisting of neutral film clips and script-driven recall. When the film and recall conditions were combined, all three emotional states were associated with rCBF increases in thalamus, medial prefrontal cortex, and anterior temporal cortex; the sadness condition was associated with additional rCBF increases in the cerebellum, midbrain, caudate, and putamen. Within the recall condition only, rCBF increases during sadness occurred in insular cortex. Within the film condition only, rCBF increases during sadness occurred in bilateral amygdala, and increases during happiness occurred in left amygdala/nucleus accumbens.

Schneider et al. (1995) examined patterns of rCBF during states of happiness and sadness in 16 healthy volunteers. Subjects viewed slides of happy and sad facial expressions and were asked to feel the emotions displayed by the faces. Neutral comparison tasks consisted of a resting baseline task and a gender judgment task (in which subjects attempted to determine whether faces shown were women's or men's faces). The sad condition was associated with relative rCBF increases in left amygdala and caudate nucleus and decreases in right amygdala and mamillary body. The happy condition was associated with rCBF increases in mamillary body, marginal increases in the posterior cingulate gyrus, and decreases in caudate nucleus. Using the same basic paradigm, but with fMRI, Schneider et al. (1997) found increased activation of left amygdala during both sad and happy conditions.

Fischer et al. (1996) studied brain activation in six bank officials while they viewed security camera videotape of a robbery that they had experienced previously. The control condition involved viewing a neutral videotape. Heart rate, skin conductance fluctuations, and ratings of distress were higher in the robbery condition than in the neutral condition. Relative to the neutral condition, the robbery condition was associated with rCBF increases in orbitofrontal cortex, visual cortex, and posterior cingulate gyrus; rCBF decreases occurred in Broca's area, left angular gyrus, operculum, and secondary somatosensory cortex.

Lane et al. (1997c) presented sets of neutral, pleasant, and unpleasant pictures to 12 healthy women. Skin conductance magnitude was larger in the unpleasant and pleasant conditions than in the neutral condition. In the unpleasant condition, compared with the neutral condition, rCBF increases occurred in left amygdala, midbrain, thalamus, hypothalamus, prefrontal cortex, hippocampus, parahippocampal gyrus, occipitotemporal cortex, and cerebellum. In the pleasant condition, compared with the neutral condition, rCBF increases occurred in midbrain, thalamus, hypothalamus, prefrontal cortex, and caudate.

Lane et al. (1997a) also presented 10 healthy male subjects with neutral, pleasant, and unpleasant pictures. However, this study was unique in that there were no comparisons between conditions involving different types of emotional stimuli (e.g., unpleasant vs. neutral); rather, comparisons were between two different conditions in which subjects' attentional focus with regard to the pictures was varied. In the internal focus condition, subjects indicated whether the picture evoked a neutral, pleasant, or unpleasant feeling. In the external focus condition, subjects indicated whether the scene was indoors, outdoors, or either. The internal focus versus external focus comparison revealed rCBF increases in medial frontal gyrus/anterior cingulate gyrus, ventral anterior cingulate gyrus, right temporal pole, and frontal operculum or insula. The external focus versus internal focus comparison demonstrated rCBF increases in the bilateral parieto-occipital cortex.

Paradiso et al. (1997) studied rCBF in eight healthy elderly subjects while the subjects viewed soundless film clips rated as evoking happiness, disgust, fear/disgust, or no prominent emotion. In the happy versus neutral comparison, rCBF decreases were found in several paralimbic regions, including anterior cingulate gyrus, orbitofrontal cortex, and medial frontal cortex. The disgust versus neutral comparison revealed bilateral thalamic activation, and the fear/disgust versus neutral comparison revealed activation in the orbitofrontal cortex, among other areas.

Cahill et al. (1996) used PET and [^{18}F]fluorodeoxyglucose to measure cerebral glucose metabolic rate in the amygdaloid complex in eight healthy male subjects who viewed emotionally arousing and emotionally neutral film clips. Subjects rated the emotional intensity of each film clip immediately after viewing the clip. Approximately 3 weeks later, subjects were asked to recall as many film clips as possible. Subjects recalled more emotionally arousing clips than neutral clips. Although glucose metabolism in the amygdaloid complex did not differ between the emotionally arousing and neutral conditions, glucose metabolism in the right amygdaloid complex during the emotionally arousing condition was positively correlated with the number of emotionally arousing clips later recalled. Glucose metabolism in the right amygdaloid complex during the neutral condition was not associated with the number of neutral clips recalled. Hamann et al. (1999) conducted a similar type of study using negative and positive emotional pictures and found a positive correlation between rCBF in the amygdala during exposure to those pictures and recognition accuracy scores.

In summary, neuroimaging studies involving healthy individuals demonstrate that negative emotional states may be mediated by anterior paralimbic regions of the brain. Furthermore, the patterns of brain activation in different types of negative states (e.g., anger vs. sadness) do not appear to differ greatly, although more research on this issue is necessary before conclusions can be drawn. Amygdala activation is reported in studies that involve presentation of audiovisual emotional stimuli.

Pharmacologic Challenge

Benkelfat et al. (1995) examined rCBF changes associated with administration of cholecystokinin tetrapeptide (CCK-4) versus saline in eight healthy individuals. Blood flow was also measured during an anticipatory anxiety condition, in which subjects expected to receive CCK-4 but actually received saline. CCK-4 administration was associated with increased heart rate and panic symptoms. In the anticipatory anxiety versus saline comparison, rCBF increases occurred in left orbitofrontal cortex and cerebellar vermis. In the CCK-4 versus anticipatory anxiety comparison, blood flow increases occurred in right cerebellar vermis, left anterior cingulate gyrus, bilateral claustrum-insula-amygdala, and bilateral temporal poles. However, further analyses suggested that the apparent temporal pole activations were attributable to extracranial artifacts of jaw muscle contraction and that the bilateral activations in the claustrum-insula-amygdala may have reflected blood volume changes in insular arteries.

Ketter et al. (1996) studied the effects of procaine on rCBF in 32 individuals without histories of psychiatric disorders. In the procaine condition, relative to the saline condition, rCBF increases occurred in the amygdala and anterior paralimbic structures, including anterior cingulate gyrus, insular cortex, and orbitofrontal cortex. Subjects who reported fear exhibited greater blood flow increases in left amygdala than did subjects who reported euphoria. In addition, blood flow in left amygdala was positively correlated with fear intensity and negatively correlated with euphoria intensity.

In a similar experiment, Servan-Schreiber et al. (1998) examined patterns of brain activation associated with procaine administration in 10 healthy individuals. Subjects were given injections of either procaine or saline placebo without being informed which substance was being administered. In the procaine condition, relative to the placebo condition, subjects reported greater levels of euphoria, anxiety, depression, fear, derealization, and somatic sensations; four subjects experienced a panic attack during the procaine condition. Heart rate did not differ significantly between conditions. In the procaine condition, relative to the placebo condition, rCBF increases occurred in limbic and paralimbic regions, including anterior cingulate gyrus, insular cortex, and bilateral amygdala-parahippocampal regions. rCBF in left amygdala was positively correlated with anxiety ratings. Subjects who had low anxiety scores (and did not panic) during the procaine condition had greater rCBF increases in the tip of anterior cingulate gyrus and in left inferior frontal cortex than did subjects who did have a panic attack.

In summary, the results of pharmacologic challenge studies are similar to those of other emotional state induction studies in healthy individuals. Interestingly, both of the procaine studies just described found positive correlations between amygdala activation and ratings of fear or anxiety.

■ Summary, Considerations, and Limitations

The results of the symptom provocation studies described in this chapter suggest that anterior paralimbic regions (i.e., orbitofrontal cortex, anterior cingulate gyrus, anterior temporal poles, and anterior insular cortex) mediate symptomatic states in PTSD, OCD, phobias, and panic disorder. In addition, some of these paralimbic structures appear to mediate negative emotional states in psychiatrically healthy individuals. Symptom provocation studies also suggest that the caudate nucleus may play a special role in OCD, whereas the amygdala and anterior cingulate gyrus may play a special role in PTSD. Like other types of studies, symptom provocation studies are not without special considerations and limitations, as presented in the following.

Matching of Conditions

In symptom provocation studies, the neutral condition should be adequately matched to the provoked condition. For example, in a study of phobia, an eyes-closed resting baseline condition would not be adequately matched to a provoked condition that involved viewing film clips of spiders. Although this example is an exaggerated one, the message is clear: inadequate matching of conditions complicates interpretation of blood flow differences between conditions. Such inadequate matching is therefore a limitation of many studies in the literature. However, stringent matching of conditions is not always possible when stimuli are complex, as in the case of script-driven imagery. Furthermore, exactly which variables are the most important to match is often unclear.

Order of Conditions

In most symptom provocation studies, researchers must determine the presentation order of their conditions. It is always most scientifically rigorous to counterbalance the order of conditions, so that half the subjects received the provoked condition first and half receive the neutral condition first. Without counterbalancing, the type of condition and its position in the scanning order are confounded. However, counterbalancing is not always practical. In studies of some disorders, such as OCD and panic disorder, the provoked conditions are often placed last in the scanning order to prevent residual anxiety in the provoked condition from carrying over into the subsequent neutral condition. The decision regarding whether to counterbalance the order of conditions depends on the disorder studied, the severity of the symptomatic state, and the degree to which patients can quickly return to baseline after symptom provocation.

Manipulation Checks

In some studies of symptom provocation and normal emotion, subjects are essentially asked to enter some type of emotional state. Unfortunately, emotional states are subjective and researchers must often rely on self-reports to verify that the desired emotional state was achieved. Although subjective reports of emotional states are necessary, they may not be sufficient to establish that subjects are performing the task as instructed. Because of the limitations associated with subjective reports, some researchers have relied on more objective measures, such as psychophysiologic responses and behavioral responses in a cognitive task. Not all the published symptom provocation studies included psychophysiologic measures, but those that did typically found greater psychophysiologic responses in provoked conditions, compared with neutral conditions, in patients with anxiety disorders. Thus, at least for patients with anxiety disorders, psychophysiologic measures may be helpful in checking provocation manipulation.

In some studies of normal emotional state induction, subjects perform emotion-irrelevant cognitive tasks (such as a gender judgment task), which typically yield behavioral data (i.e., response times and error rates) that can be examined to ensure that subjects are actually attending to the stimuli. This approach may make good experimental sense, especially if the cognitive task is the same in both the emotional and neutral conditions. However, one could argue that the addition of such a cognitive task might actually distract subjects and thus minimize the emotional response that the stimuli were intended to evoke. Lane et al. (1997a) found different patterns of brain activation when subjects focused on nonemotional versus emotional aspects of a set of pictures. Thus, the addition of a cognitive task may be viewed as an asset or a limitation, depending on the research question posed.

Personalized Versus Standardized Stimuli

Researchers have used both personalized and standardized stimuli in symptom provocation studies. Personalized stimuli are tailored to individual subjects' concerns and thus differ among subjects in a given study; for example, imagery scripts are personalized stimuli because they are based on descriptions of subjects' autobiographical events. Standardized stimuli typically consist of well-validated audiovisual material that is presented systematically to all subjects in a study (e.g., aversive pictures from the International Affective Picture System developed by Lang and colleagues [1988]).

Personalized stimuli are almost certainly more emotionally provocative than are standardized stimuli; however, the use of personalized stimuli can lead to increased variability of data because different subjects are exposed to different stimuli, and because personalized stimuli in different conditions cannot always be well matched. Thus, although the use of personalized stimuli may increase the emotional effect, such use may also increase variability and decrease experimental control. The choice of personalized versus standardized stimuli depends on the precise experimental question that is posed and the researchers' tolerance for variability and threats to experimental control.

Mode of Stimulus Presentation

The results of symptom provocation and normal emotional state induction studies are not always consistent with each other. Possible reasons for this discrepancy include differences in subject samples, tasks, data acquisition, and data analysis. Some researchers have proposed that differences in mode of stimulus presentation also may account for some of the discrepancies in the literature (Reiman et al. 1997; Whalen 1998). For example, some symptom provocation and normal emotional state induction studies have used external stimuli (e.g., pictures presented on a video monitor), whereas others have used internal stimuli (e.g., recollection and imagery of past events).

In the only PET study to directly examine rCBF responses to external and internal emotional stimuli, 12 healthy female subjects were scanned while they viewed emotional film clips (film condition) and recalled emotional autobiographical events (recall condition) (Reiman et al. 1997). (The data set and design were identical to those of Lane et al. [1997b].) Although subjective ratings of emotion were significantly higher in the recall than in the film condition, several brain regions were more active in the film condition than in the recall condition: anterior temporal cortex (including the amygdala and hippocampal formation), occipito-temporo-parietal cortex, hypothalamus, and lateral cerebellum. No brain regions had greater activation in the recall condition than in the film condition. These findings suggest that in healthy individuals, some regions of the brain (such as the amygdala) may respond more strongly to external stimuli than to internal stimuli. The amygdala may be involved in monitoring the external environment for possible threat, even in the absence of an emotional response (Whalen 1998); thus, it might not be surprising that greater amygdala activation was found in the film condition despite the fact that this condition was less emotion-provoking than the recall condition.

■ CONCLUSION

When used in conjunction with current neuroimaging techniques and appropriate methods, the symptom provocation paradigm can be a powerful means of determining the regions of the brain that mediate symptomatic states in patients with anxiety disorders. Using this approach, researchers have found that symptomatic states of PTSD, OCD, phobia, and panic disorder are accompanied by activation of anterior paralimbic regions of the brain and that the activation of some structures (such as caudate nucleus and amygdala/

anterior cingulate gyrus) may be specific to particular disorders (such as OCD and PTSD, respectively). Normal emotional state induction studies, which are analogous to symptom provocation studies, have also demonstrated anterior paralimbic activation in negative emotional states.

Identifying the mediating functional neuroanatomy of symptomatic states in psychiatric disorders is particularly important because psychiatric disorders are defined by their symptoms. In the future, symptom provocation studies will continue to highlight specific brain systems that function abnormally in anxiety disorders, and these systems may be further examined with other neuroimaging paradigms, such as the cognitive activation paradigm (see Chapter 2 in this volume). The ultimate goal of psychiatric neuroimaging research is to identify the underlying pathophysiology of psychiatric disorders, and this goal can be approached with the use of symptom provocation studies, along with cognitive activation, receptor characterization, and spectroscopy studies.

■ References

Baker SC, Frith CD, Dolan RJ: The interaction between mood and cognitive function studied with PET. Psychol Med 27:565–578, 1997

Benkelfat C, Bradwejn J, Meyer E, et al: Functional neuroanatomy of CCK_4-induced anxiety in normal healthy volunteers. Am J Psychiatry 152:1180–1184, 1995

Blanchard EB, Kolb LC, Gerardi RJ, et al: Cardiac response to relevant stimuli as an adjunctive tool for diagnosing post-traumatic stress disorder in Vietnam veterans. Behavioral Therapy 17:592–606, 1986

Breiter HC, Rauch SL, Kwong KK, et al: Functional magnetic resonance imaging of symptom provocation in obsessive compulsive disorder. Arch Gen Psychiatry 53: 595–606, 1996

Bremner JD, Innis RB, Ng CK, et al: Positron emission tomography measurement of cerebral metabolic correlates of yohimbine administration in combat-related post-traumatic stress disorder. Arch Gen Psychiatry 54:246–254, 1997

Bremner JD, Staib L, Kaloupek D, et al: Neural correlates of exposure to traumatic pictures and sound in Vietnam combat veterans with and without posttraumatic stress disorder: a positron emission tomography study. Biol Psychiatry 45:806–816, 1999a

Bremner JD, Narayan M, Staib LH, et al: Neural correlates of memories of childhood sexual abuse in women with and without posttraumatic stress disorder. Am J Psychiatry 156:1787–1795, 1999b

Cahill L, Haier RJ, Fallon J, et al: Amygdala activity at encoding correlated with long-term, free recall of emotional information. Proc Natl Acad Sci U S A 93:8016–8021, 1996

Cottraux J, Gérard D, Cinotti L, et al: A controlled positron emission tomography study of obsessive and neutral auditory stimulation in obsessive-compulsive disorder with checking rituals. Psychiatry Res 60:101–112, 1996

Dougherty DD, Shin LM, Alpert NM, et al: Anger in healthy men: a PET study using script-driven imagery. Biol Psychiatry 46:466–472, 1999

Drevets WC, Videen TO, MacLeod AK, et al: PET images of blood flow changes during anxiety: correction (letter). Science 256:1696, 1992

Fischer H, Wik G, Fredrikson M: Functional neuroanatomy of robbery re-experience: affective memories studied with PET. Neuroreport 7:2081–2086, 1996

Fredrikson M, Wik G, Greitz T, et al: Regional cerebral blood flow during experimental fear. Psychophysiology 30:126–130, 1993

Fredrikson M, Wik G, Annas P, et al: Functional neuroanatomy of visually elicited simple phobic fear: additional data and theoretical analysis. Psychophysiology 32: 43–48, 1995

George MS, Ketter TA, Parekh PI, et al: Brain activity during transient sadness and happiness in healthy women. Am J Psychiatry 152:341–351, 1995

George MS, Ketter TA, Parekh PI, et al: Gender differences in regional cerebral blood flow during transient self-induced sadness or happiness. Biol Psychiatry 40:859–871, 1996

Hamann SB, Ely TD, Grafton ST, et al: Amygdala activity related to enhanced memory for pleasant and aversive stimuli. Nat Neurosci 2:289–293, 1999

Ketter TA, Andreason PJ, George MS, et al: Anterior paralimbic mediation of procaine-induced emotional and psychosensory experiences. Arch Gen Psychiatry 53:59–69, 1996

Kimbrell TA, George MS, Parekh PI, et al: Regional brain activity during transient self-induced anxiety and anger in healthy adults. Biol Psychiatry 46:454–465, 1999

Lane RD, Fink GR, Chau PM-L, et al: Neural activation during selective attention to subjective emotional responses. Neuroreport 8:3969–3972, 1997a

Lane RD, Reiman EM, Ahern GL, et al: Neuroanatomical correlates of happiness, sadness, and disgust. Am J Psychiatry 154:926–933, 1997b

Lane RD, Reiman EM, Bradley MM, et al: Neuroanatomical correlates of pleasant and unpleasant emotion. Neuropsychologia 35:1437–1444, 1997c

Lang PJ: The cognitive psychophysiology of emotion: fear and anxiety, in Anxiety and the Anxiety Disorders. Edited by Tuma AH, Maser J. Hillsdale, NJ, Erlbaum, 1985, pp 131–170

Lang PJ, Levin DN, Miller GA, et al: Fear behavior, fear imagery, and the psychophysiology of emotion: the problem of affective response integration. J Abnorm Psychol 92:276–306, 1983

Lang PJ, Öhman A, Vaitl D: The International Affective Picture System (Photographic Slides). Gainesville, FL, Center for Research in Psychophysiology, University of Florida, 1988

LeDoux JE: Emotion and the amygdala, in The Amygdala: Neurobiological Aspects of Emotion, Memory, and Mental Dysfunction. Edited by Aggleton JP. New York, Wiley-Liss, 1992, pp 339–351

Liberzon I, Taylor SF, Amdur R, et al: Brain activation in PTSD in response to trauma-related stimuli. Biol Psychiatry 45:817–826, 1999

Mayberg HS: Limbic-cortical dysregulation: a proposed model of depression. J Neuropsychiatry Clin Neurosci 9:471–481, 1997

McGuire PK, Bench CJ, Frith CD, et al: Functional anatomy of obsessive-compulsive phenomena. Br J Psychiatry 164:459–468, 1994

Morgan MA, Romanski LM, LeDoux JE: Extinction of emotional learning: contribution of medial prefrontal cortex. Neurosci Lett 163:109–113, 1993

Mountz JM, Modell JG, Wilson MW, et al: Positron emission tomographic evaluation of cerebral blood flow during state anxiety in simple phobia. Arch Gen Psychiatry 46:501–504, 1989

Paradiso S, Robinson RG, Andreasen NC, et al: Emotional activation of limbic circuitry in elderly normal subjects in a PET study. Am J Psychiatry 154:384–389, 1997

Pardo JV, Pardo PJ, Raichle ME: Neural correlates of self-induced dysphoria. Am J Psychiatry 150:713–719, 1993

Pitman RK, Orr SP, Forgue DF, et al: Psychophysiologic assessment of posttraumatic stress disorder imagery in Vietnam combat veterans. Arch Gen Psychiatry 44:970–975, 1987

Pitman RK, Orr SP, Forgue DF, et al: Psychophysiologic responses to combat imagery of Vietnam veterans with posttraumatic stress disorder versus other anxiety disorders. J Abnorm Psychol 99:49–54, 1990

Rauch SL, Jenike MA, Alpert NM, et al: Regional cerebral blood flow measured during symptom provocation in obsessive-compulsive disorder using oxygen 15-labeled carbon dioxide and positron emission tomography. Arch Gen Psychiatry 51:62–70, 1994

Rauch SL, Savage CR, Alpert NM, et al: A positron emission tomographic study of simple phobic symptom provocation. Arch Gen Psychiatry 52:20–28, 1995

Rauch SL, van der Kolk BA, Fisler RE, et al: A symptom provocation study of posttraumatic stress disorder using positron emission tomography and script-driven imagery. Arch Gen Psychiatry 53:380–387, 1996

Rauch SL, Savage CR, Alpert NM, et al: The functional neuroanatomy of anxiety: a study of three disorders using positron emission tomography and symptom provocation. Biol Psychiatry 42:446–452, 1997

Rauch SL, Shin LM, Dougherty DD, et al: Neural activation during sexual and competitive arousal in healthy men. Psychiatry Res 91:1–10, 1999

Reiman EM, Raichle ME, Robins E, et al: Neuroanatomical correlates of a lactate-induced anxiety attack. Arch Gen Psychiatry 46:493–500, 1989

Reiman EM, Lane RD, Ahern GL, et al: Neuroanatomical correlates of externally and internally generated human emotion. Am J Psychiatry 154:918–925, 1997

Schneider F, Gur RE, Mozley LH, et al: Mood effects on limbic blood flow correlate with emotional self-rating: a PET study with oxygen-15 labeled water. Psychiatry Res 61:265–283, 1995

Schneider F, Grodd W, Weiss U, et al: Functional MRI reveals left amygdala activation during emotion. Psychiatry Res 76:75–82, 1997

Servan-Schreiber D, Perlstein WM, Cohen JD, et al: Selective pharmacological activation of limbic structures in human volunteers: a positron emission tomography study. J Neuropsychiatry Clin Neurosci 10:148–159, 1998

Shin LM, Kosslyn SM, McNally RJ, et al: Visual imagery and perception in posttraumatic stress disorder: a positron emission tomographic investigation. Arch Gen Psychiatry 54:233–241, 1997

Shin LM, McNally RJ, Kosslyn SM, et al: Regional cerebral blood flow during script-driven imagery in childhood sexual abuse-related posttraumatic stress disorder: a positron emission tomographic investigation. Am J Psychiatry 156:575–584, 1999

Shin LM, Dougherty DD, Orr SP, et al: Activation of anterior paralimbic structures during guilt-related script-driven imagery. Biol Psychiatry 48:43–50, 2000

Southwick SM, Krystal JH, Morgan A, et al: Abnormal noradrenergic function in posttraumatic stress disorder. Arch Gen Psychiatry 50:266–274, 1993

Spielberger CD, Gorsuch RL, Lushene R, et al: Manual for the State-Trait Anxiety Inventory. Palo Alto, CA, Consulting Psychologists Press, 1983

van der Kolk BA, Fisler R: Dissociation and the fragmentary nature of traumatic memories: overview and exploratory study. J Trauma Stress 8:505–525, 1995

Whalen PJ: Fear, vigilance, and ambiguity: initial neuroimaging studies of the human amygdala. Current Directions in Psychological Science 7:177–188, 1998

Wik G, Fredrikson M, Ericson K, et al: A functional cerebral response to frightening visual stimulation. Psychiatry Res 50:15–24, 1993

Woods SW, Koster K, Krystal JK, et al: Yohimbine alters regional cerebral blood flow in panic disorder (letter). Lancet 2:678, 1988

Zohar J, Insel TR, Berman KF, et al: Anxiety and cerebral blood flow during behavioral challenge. Arch Gen Psychiatry 46:505–510, 1989

5

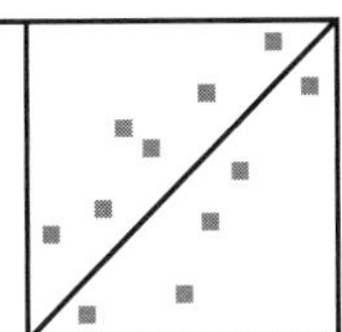

SYMPTOM CAPTURE

A Strategy for Pathophysiologic Investigation in Functional Neuropsychiatric Imaging

Emily Stern, M.D.
David A. Silbersweig, M.D.

■ Rationale for the Symptom-Oriented Approach

Psychiatric disorders are currently defined descriptively (see DSM-IV [American Psychiatric Association 1994]), as combinations of symptoms that tend to occur together. This descriptive approach has provided an agreed-on and empirically based taxonomy that has greatly facilitated research and patient care. Such an approach can also promote research on the etiology of characteristic clinical syndromes. There is, however, significant heterogeneity in the clinical presentation of patients within a given diagnostic category, and many patients do not fit neatly into these classification schemes. To date, there has also been a relative lack of sensitive or specific biological markers that could be closely associated with individual descriptive syndromes.

When attempts are being made to identify the brain circuits underlying psychiatric diseases, use of a symptom-oriented, rather than syndrome-oriented, strategy can be an effective way to increase specificity. Particular psychiatric symptoms, such as delusions, do not necessarily segregate with descriptive diag-

We acknowledge the essential work of our collaborators at the Hammersmith Hospital and the Wellcome Department of Cognitive Neurology in London. We also acknowledge the substantial support of our chairman, Dr. Jack Barchas, and of the DeWitt-Wallace Fund of the New York Community Trust, in establishing the Functional Neuroimaging Laboratory at Cornell, where symptom-oriented studies are ongoing.

nostic categories, and may occur in different syndromes, such as schizophrenia or affective disorders (Kaplan and Sadock 1993). Psychopharmacologic agents that act on specific neurochemical systems, such as neuroleptics, can be used to successfully treat particular symptoms, such as delusions, whether in the setting of schizophrenia or affective disorders (Arana and Hyman 1991). Symptoms, rather than syndromes, can more readily be described as dysfunctions of specific cognitive, perceptual, emotional or behavioral functions. Symptoms can therefore be mapped more readily onto neural substrates. Functional neuroimaging studies have suggested that similar symptoms, such as psychomotor poverty in schizophrenia and psychomotor retardation in depression, are associated with similar profiles of cerebral activity, regardless of different DSM diagnoses (Dolan et al. 1993). Conversely, diverse neurologic lesions (such as strokes, tumors, abscesses) in particular brain regions (such as Wernicke's area) or nodes in circuits (such as primary motor cortex in the neocortical pyramidal motor system) tend to elicit specific neuropsychological or neurological symptoms (such as receptive aphasia or a particular distribution of upper motor neuron paralysis).

All of these observations suggest that a neurology-type distinction between disease etiology and pathophysiological mechanism of symptom formation can be useful in psychiatry. Symptom formation in psychiatric conditions can thus be seen as resulting from disordered functioning in specific neural circuits (or nodes within those circuits) that represent final common pathways of perceptual, cognitive, emotional and behavioral integration (Silbersweig and Stern 1997). These observations also suggest that a focus on symptoms, rather than on descriptive categories, may be particularly conducive to a more neuroscientifically based approach to understanding pathophysiology (Silbersweig and Stern 1997). Such an understanding would, in turn, provide a foundation for more targeted, biologically based diagnostic and therapeutic strategies.

In contrast to the symptom-oriented approach, there is another approach to the study of psychiatric syndromes that is quite reasonable and that is used by many investigators in the field. This approach involves trying to identify a "fundamental" neuropsychological abnormality that is associated with a psychiatric syndrome and that might underlie or tie together many of the symptoms that are expressed (e.g., Goldman-Rakic 1994; Wiser et al. 1998). This is a noble goal, and unifying theories are appealing. Furthermore, this approach has achieved important and promising results. However, such an approach assumes that a pathological system or condition can be most effectively modeled as a disruption of a specific normal function and is highly reliant on the correct choice of neuropsychological function to be probed. It must also address the fact that neuropsychological abnormalities are rarely syndrome specific and are themselves phenotypic expressions or symptoms. Finally, even with significant findings, claims of causality are difficult to substantiate.

We believe that our contrasting approach, by targeting the neuropathophysiology of known, major symptoms, may provide a direct, non–model-dependent route toward the shared goal of understanding the neurobiology of these devastating disorders. In fact, these approaches are not mutually exclusive, and each has strengths and limitations. Advances are most likely to be achieved if the two approaches are used nondogmatically in a complementary fashion.

■ Development of New Functional Neuroimaging Methods

Functional neuroimaging provides a direct, noninvasive means of identifying the brain states associated with normal and abnormal mental states in vivo. Functional neuroimaging is particularly relevant for the study of psychiatric disorders that are not associated with macroscopic lesions of known etiology (although subtle morphometric abnormalities have recently been noted) and for which animal models, blood and cerebrospinal fluid examinations, and postmortem studies have provided helpful, but limited, insights.

Whereas the application of existing methods can be suitable for the investigation of many scientific questions, the development of new methods is essential for the examination of phenomena not previously amenable to study, or the examination of previously studied phenomena with greater sensitivity, specificity, and (spatial and temporal) resolution. Neuropsychiatric functional neuroimaging experiments are highly interdisciplinary, integrating expertise from many fields, including clinical neuropsychiatry, cognitive psychology, behavioral neuroscience, biophysics, mathematics, statistics, and electrical engineering. A detailed understanding of the principles and paradigms within each of these disciplines, as well as the way in which these approaches can be most effectively integrated, is a necessary prerequisite for the development of novel and rigorous methods. This is because, in functional neuroimaging research, the elements of hypothesis, study design, neuropsychological activation paradigm, image acquisition, image processing, and image analysis are highly inter-related. Choices concerning each element inform and constrain choices concerning all the other elements.

Equally essential, if not more so, is the identification of an important medical scientific problem or challenge that drives and shapes the entire process. This first step must be undertaken with great care, as there are an unlimited number of questions one can ask, and as the development of new methods is a risky, time-consuming, and resource intensive way to find answers. New techniques must be carefully conceived, developed, optimized, and then validated before they can be employed to address cognitive neuroscientific or pathophysiologic questions.

■ SYMPTOM-ORIENTED IMAGING APPROACHES

We chose symptom capture as a strategy and goal for this process. The rationale for a symptom-oriented approach to psychiatric research has been described above. There are a number of symptom-oriented functional neuroimaging approaches, among which symptom capture is one possibility.

One such alternate approach is the *top-down approach* (Silbersweig and Stern 1996). This approach is based on theories regarding specific neuropsychological functions that are thought to be impaired, leading to symptom formation. A neuropsychological task probing the implicated neuropsychological function is used as an "activation" task while brain activity is being imaged. A control task that shares sensorimotor or cognitive components other than the implicated neuropsychological function is often used as a comparison imaging condition for analyses that isolate the cognitive component of interest. One can use this top-down study design with patients who are currently experiencing or who have previously experienced the symptom of interest, compared with patient or control subjects. One can then determine whether abnormal performance on this task and/or an abnormal pattern of corresponding brain activity are associated with the presence of, or predisposition toward, the symptom of interest.

With colleagues in London, we have used this approach with high-sensitivity $H_2{}^{15}O$–positron emission tomography (PET) techniques (described later in this chapter) to test hypotheses concerning the role of abnormal inner speech and auditory-verbal imagery in the genesis of hallucinations in schizophrenia (McGuire et al. 1995, 1996). Patients with a predisposition to hallucinate, compared with matched patient controls without a history of hallucinations and healthy control subjects, showed no difference in the activation pattern for inner speech, but showed decreased supplementary motor and left middle temporal gyrus activation associated with auditory-verbal mental imagery. These findings support a frontotemporal deficit in the volitional control and evaluation of auditory-linguistic percepts, rather than a primary inner speech deficit model of symptom formation.

A variant of this approach is illustrated by a functional magnetic resonance imaging (fMRI) study in which schizophrenic patients with and without current hallucinations listened to externally presented speech (Woodruff et al. 1995). This was based on the premise that interference (and hence decreased performance and/or activity) would occur if the endogenous hallucinations and the exogenous task placed demands on similar psychological functions and associated brain regions—in this case, superior temporal gyrus (where the hypothesized effect was noted). These top-down approaches have the benefits of drawing on and evaluating cognitive experimental psychological models and techniques that have been developed over the past half century. Such model dependency can also be a relative limitation, however, because the model may be associated with incorrect assumptions, may not be applicable, or may not be causally related to symptom formation.

Symptom provocation represents another useful and well-developed symptom-oriented functional neuroimaging approach. Here the symptom state of interest is provoked in the scanning environment and imaged, often in comparison with a control state (controlling for sensorimotor aspects of the provocation procedure). Rauch and colleagues (Breiter and Rauch 1996; Rauch et al. 1996, 1997) have performed outstanding studies of this type in patients with anxiety disorders, such as phobias, posttraumatic stress disorder, and obsessive compulsive disorder. The background and details of these studies are discussed by them elsewhere in this volume and will therefore not be detailed here. Strengths of this strategy include the fact that the symptom state is directly observable and under careful experimental control. Relative limitations include the possibilities that a provoked symptom and its brain state may not be identical to a naturally occurring one and that the method of provocation may introduce confounding elements that can not be fully controlled for. Another consideration, and potential concern, is that the provoking stimuli may be different across subjects. One therefore has to choose between using the same stimuli for all subjects, with possible differential efficacy/effect, and using different stimuli optimally tailored to each subject, which introduces another confounding experimental variable.

Symptom capture is a naturalistic, symptom-oriented strategy that avoids some of the limitations of the top-down and provocation approaches. Each of the three approaches, however, has its strengths and provides unique information that is complementary to, and convergent with, the others in working toward the common goal of understanding the pathogenesis of symptoms. The aim of the symptom capture approach is to capture the brain state associated with the symptom state in a direct manner that is not model dependent and not provoked. Instead of probing psychological or neural systems, symptom capture uses methods of study design, image acquisition, and image analysis that are tailored to the target symptom. This requires that exquisite attention be paid to the phenomenology and timing of symptom expression, as well as the mechanisms of brain imaging signal transduction and detection.

If performed successfully, this results in the localization of the pattern of brain activity associated with natural occurrence of major elements of psychopathology. This approach also allows the study of symptoms that otherwise would not be amenable to study with traditional techniques, because they are transient, unpredictable or randomly occurring, involuntary, or even subjective. Furthermore, there is not necessarily a need for "control" conditions, which can greatly influence results and are liable to be based on incorrect assumptions concerning cognitive and neuronal processing (Price and Friston 1997). The relative limitations or constraints of this approach include the facts that only certain well-defined, stereotyped, repetitive types of symptoms are appropriate for such study; that the symptoms must occur discretely with a great enough frequency to be adequately sampled within the study session (and that this may only be seen in a subset of patients with the disorder); and that the timing of the onset and offset of each individual symptom (relative to scanning parameters) must be determined by some observable measure or reliable report. As with any methodologically intensive approach, the limitations of the technology also determine what is possible to achieve, although the pursuit of symptoms may also lead to the development of new methods to transcend apparent limitations, as will presently be discussed.

■ DEVELOPMENT OF PET SYMPTOM CAPTURE TECHNIQUES

PET provides robust indices of neuronal activity throughout the entire brain. [^{18}F]fluorodeoxyglucose (FDG) provides excellent basal measures of brain glucose metabolism which is coupled to neuronal activity over a half-hour integrated period. $H_2{}^{15}O$ is a diffusible tracer that allows the measure of cerebral blood flow (Raichle 1987), which is coupled to neuronal activity. The tracer's brief half life of 2.07 minutes permits multiple scans to be performed during a study session, making it possible to compare and contrast the brain states associated with several different mental states during the session.

In the early 1990s, the norm for $H_2{}^{15}O$ PET studies was to perform group studies using two-dimensional techniques, 30–60 millicuries (mCi) of radiotracer per scan, approximately six scans per study session, and "subtraction" design (Posner et al. 1988), in which were compared two or three different psychological tasks that were repeated continuously during each scan. These methods would not permit symptom capture.

The advent of newer, high-sensitivity three-dimensional (3D) scanning techniques, which produce a four- to sixfold increase in noise equivalent counts (Bailey et al. 1991), a measure of signal-to-noise, allowed increased sampling (with decreased dose of radiotracer per scan) and the ability to obtain statistically significant activation results in single subjects. Such improved sampling would increase the chance of capturing transient symptoms, whereas the analysis of individual results would be helpful when examining heterogeneous psychiatric symptoms.

A new paradigm for $H_2{}^{15}O$ activation studies that consisted of 3D scanning and 12 scans per study session was therefore developed to facilitate symptom capture (Silbersweig et al. 1993) . The following parameters were optimized: the dose of radiotracer (10–15 mCi of $H_2{}^{15}O$ per scan); the mode of delivery of radiotracer (slow bolus resulting in a rapid rise of counts in the head, over approximately 30 seconds); the duration of image acquisition (90 seconds); the coordination of timing between radiotracer delivery, image acquisition, and psychological task performance; and the determination and delineation of the period during which brain/mental activity was sampled during each scan (the 30 seconds of first-pass arterial input of radiotracer into the brain). This slow-bolus technique (Silbersweig et al. 1993) allowed the detection of statistically significant activations with high sensitivity over the entire brain during a highly defined period, in individual subjects. These conditions were necessary prerequisites for capturing symptoms such as hallucinations. Further advances were needed, however.

Because hallucinations are involuntary, transient, randomly occurring events, it is not possible to tell a patient with schizophrenia to hallucinate continuously for 30 seconds during some scans and not to hallucinate at all for 30 seconds during other, control scans. Furthermore, the signal from brief hallucinations, which often last only a few seconds, would be lost in a single measure that integrates all the counts emitted from the radiotracer over 30 seconds. Finally, because it takes many seconds for radiotracer to reach the brain after injection, the scanning protocol could not be triggered by the occurrence of the target events.

One could consider, however, that the integrated measure is composed of a series of dynamic instantaneous measures (Iida et al. 1991). This allows one to deconvolve the integrated measure, make use of information concerning which instants represent radiotracer deposition associated with the target mental events and take into consideration the fact that all time is not the same within the critical 30-second period (because of the continually changing rate of radiotracer deposition). One can then determine the contribution of the target mental events (via vascular change and radiotracer deposition) to voxel signal intensity in the resultant image. This contribution can be represented as a mathematical score for each scan (Figure 5–1). Scans can be performed at

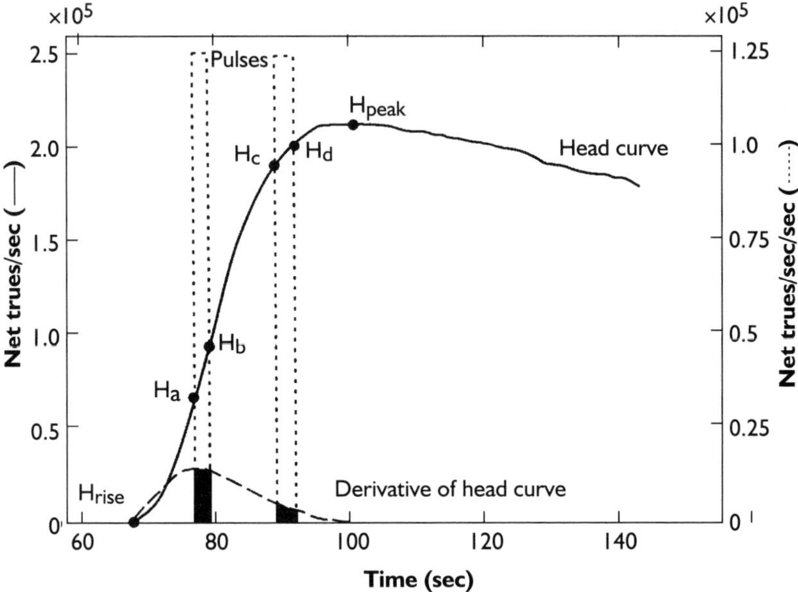

FIGURE 5–1. Calculation of an event-related scan score from the event pulse data (indicating the timing and duration of the target mental events) and the simultaneous whole-brain time activity curve data (indicating the entry of radiotracer to the brain). The score weights for the amount of radiotracer entering the brain during the events, as a proportion of the total amount of radiotracer entering during the scan. This can be expressed by

$$[(H_b - H_a) + (H_d - H_c)]/(H_{peak} - H_{rise})$$

where H_x is the curve value at point x. This can also be represented by the sum of the integrals of the differentiated curve from each pulse start time to each pulse finish time (shaded areas), as a proportion of the total integral of the differentiated curve. Note that the contribution of an event (per unit of time) to the resultant image is greater if the event occurs during a period of greater radiotracer delivery. The relative contribution of the target mental events to each scan varies over the course of a multiscan experiment. A statistical analysis is then performed to identify voxels in the series of images (corresponding to brain regions) in which signal intensity correlates highly with the scan scores. This constitutes a statistical map of the brain regions active during the target mental events.

preset 10-minute (5 half-life) intervals and can therefore capture various amounts of the randomly occurring target events within their 30-second critical periods. The variance in timing, duration, and frequency of target events over the multiple scans within the study session, combined with the dynamic nature of the input function in each scan, result in a spread of scan scores over the study session. A statistical analysis can then be performed for each voxel of the functional image (representing each point in the brain), within the context of statistical parametric mapping (Friston et al. 1995), to identify those brain regions in which voxel intensity is highly correlated with the target event scan score. This analysis produces a map of brain regions active during the target event, regardless of the distribution of the event in time. This method has been designated an *event-related count rate correlational analysis* (Silbersweig et al. 1994).

Before the slow-bolus technique and event-related count rate correlational analysis were used to identify the unknown neural correlates of ephemeral symptoms in neuropsychiatric patients, the techniques were validated by determining their ability to detect brain activations of known localization associated with transient, randomly occurring neuropsychological events in healthy subjects (Silbersweig et al. 1993, 1994).

■ Use of Symptom Capture PET Techniques to Study Hallucinations and Tics

The methods just discussed were used to study the functional neuroanatomy of hallucinations in schizophrenia and tics in Tourette's syndrome—afferent and efferent examples, respectively, of transient, randomly occurring neuropsychiatric symptoms.

Hallucinations are perceptions in the absence of external stimuli. They are present in up to 74% of patients with schizophrenia (Wing et al. 1974). They are most commonly auditory-verbal, usually take the form of voices talking to or about the patient in a derogatory fashion, and are often experienced as real and emotionally relevant (Schneider 1959). These characteristics make this symptom extremely debilitating and at first may seem to defy neurobiologic explanation, yet they may provide clues as to possible neural substrates.

Earlier functional imaging studies suggested a number of frontal, temporal, and striatal brain areas that may be involved in the predisposition to hallucinate (Cleghorn 1991; Cleghorn et al. 1990; DeLisi et al. 1989; McGuire et al. 1993; Suzuki et al. 1993; Volkow et al. 1987). These studies did not, however, have the temporal discrimination necessary to isolate the brain state associated with this symptom. Using the specifically designed methods of PET image acquisition and analysis discussed in the previous section, five schizophrenic patients with classic auditory-verbal hallucinations, and one drug-naive patient with both visual and auditory-linguistic hallucinations were studied (Silbersweig et al. 1995). All the patients had well-documented histories of hallucinosis, were thought by their clinicians to be reliable reporters of their symptoms, and participated in a practice and evaluative session. The patients were asked to report the occurrence of each hallucination during the scanning protocol by pressing a button (linked to a digitalized computer output, time-synched with the scanner clock) that allowed the exact timing of the hallucinations to be noted relative to radiotracer delivery to the brain. The event-related count rate correlational analysis (Silbersweig et al. 1994) was then performed to locate the brain regions in which activity was highly correlated with hallucination occurrence.

In the individual subject with visual and auditory-verbal hallucinations, prominent activity was detected in bilateral (left>right) visual and auditory-linguistic association cortices and in left posterior cingulate, right parahippocampal/mesotemporal, and temporal pole (para)limbic regions, as well as in right striatum. The regions of activation common to the group of five patients with auditory-verbal hallucinations were deep (para)limbic and subcortical structures, including the bilateral hippocampus and parahippocampal gyrus, right anterior cingulate gyrus, bilateral thalamus, and right ventral striatum (although neocortical activations were detected in each individual subject as well) (Figure 5–2).

Similar methodology was used to identify the brain circuits associated with tics in Tourette syndrome (Stern et al. 2000). Tourette syndrome is a striking neuropsychiatric disorder characterized by multiple motor and vocal tics, which may be simple or complex in nature. Although basal ganglia dysfunction had been implicated (Robertson 1989; Singer and Walkup 1991), the neural correlates of tics had not previously been defined, although a number of FDG-PET resting studies have been performed (Braun et al. 1993, 1995; Eidelberg et al. 1997; Stoetter et al. 1992), and an fMRI study of tic suppression has been performed (Peterson et al. 1998).

In the event-related PET study, six right-handed male patients with Tourette syndrome and frequent tics were studied. Tics were monitored with two video cameras (one focused on the face and one on the body) as well as a throat microphone and tape recorder. Information about the exact timing of the tics relative to radiotracer delivery to the brain was used to identify brain regions in which activity was highly correlated with tic occurrence.

The pattern of increased brain activity highly correlated with tics included executive motor cortices (supplementary motor, premotor, anterior cingulate, and dorsolateral prefrontal), primary motor cortices, language cortices (including Broca's area), other paralimbic cortices (posterior cingulate, and insula), and subcortical regions (striatum and midbrain tegmentum).

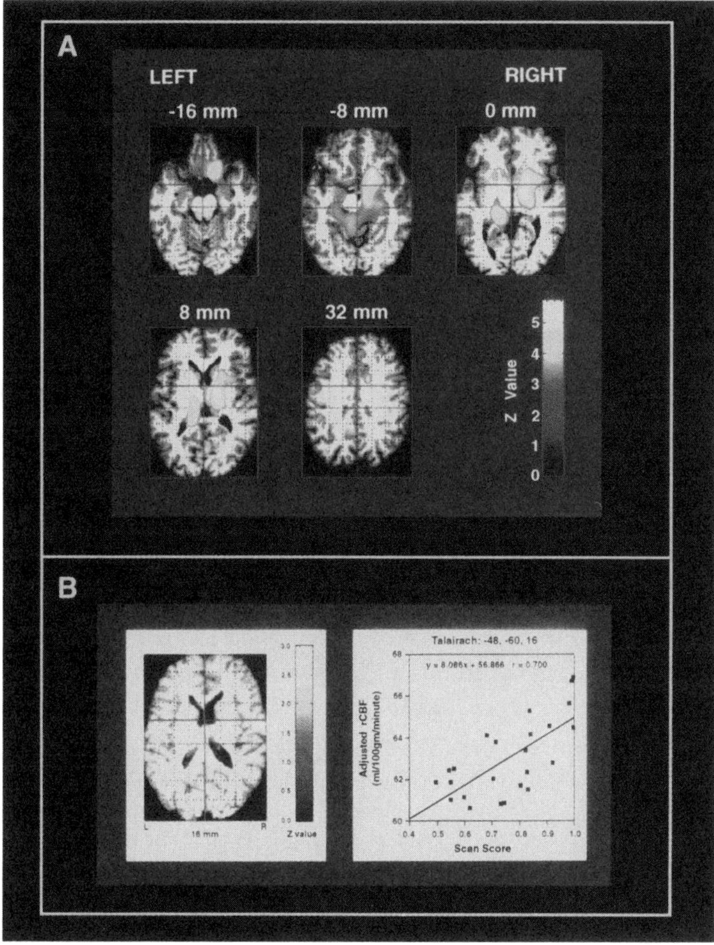

FIGURE 5–2. *(A)* Axial sections demonstrating brain regions with significantly increased activity during auditory-verbal hallucinations in a group of five patients with schizophrenia. Functional positron emission tomography results ($P<0.001$) are displayed in color and are superimposed on a single structural magnetic resonance scan transformed into stereotactic space for anatomical reference. *(B)* Axial section and a regression plot demonstrating left temporoparietal activity (in Brodmann's areas 22 and 39; as reflected by adjusted regional cerebral blood flow [rCBF]) highly correlated with reports of hallucinations (as reflected by event-related scan scores) over 24 scans in an individual patient. Note the presence of neocortical activity in an auditory-linguistic region, complementing the subcortical and limbic activity common to the group.

These symptom capture studies suggest that dysfunction in specific neural circuits is associated with the occurrence major positive neuropsychiatric symptoms. The circuits are distributed and have neocortical, paralimbic, limbic, and subcortical components. The findings also show modality and/or somatotopic specificity that is consistent with the clinical phenomenology of the symptom (Silbersweig and Stern 1997). For example, the perceptual symptom of hallucinations is correlated with activity in afferent postrolandic cortices, whereas the behavioral symptom of tics is correlated with activity predominantly in efferent prerolandic cortices. Moreover, in the bimodal hallucination patient, the presence of both auditory-verbal and visual hallucinations was associated with activity in both auditory-linguistic and visual association cortices. Similarly, vocal and motor tics in the Tourette syndrome patients were associated with activity in Broca's area and motor cortices. An additional possibility (supported by the behavioral neuroanatomic literature and discussed at greater length elsewhere [Silbersweig and Stern 1996, 1997]) is that the emotional/motivational attributes of hallucinations may be associated with the paralimbic and ventral striatal activations, and the urges associated with tics may be associated with the medial prefrontal executive system activations.

These paralimbic, limbic, and subcortical activations are perhaps the most relevant for issues of pathogenesis. Such deeper, phylogenetically older regions are highly interconnected and have convergent and divergent connections to and from widespread areas of cortex (Pandya and Yeterian 1985). The regions thereby constitute a foundation for mnemonic, attentional, emotional, and intentional processing and are necessary for the organism to label and evaluate the relevance of sensory data and to select an appropriate action (Mesulam 1985). Dysfunction in these regions or the interactions (or functional connectivity [Friston and Frith 1995]) among them may therefore contribute to the inappropriate labeling of percepts in hallucinations and the inappropriate initiation of actions in tics. Details of possible contributions to symptom formation of each of the regions detected are discussed more fully elsewhere (Silbersweig and Stern 1996; Stern et al. 2000).

These discussions draw on convergent findings from more basic investigations into behavioral neuroscience and psychiatric pathophysiology. In the case of schizophrenia, these findings include subtle morphometric abnormalities that have recently been described in some of the (para)limbic and subcortical regions we have implicated in symptom formation (Barta et al. 1990), as well as cytoarchitectonic and neurochemical abnormalities in these regions that provide plausible basic mechanisms (including abnormal γ-aminobutyric acid [GABA]–glutamate–dopamine (D_4) connectivity and interactions in interneuron populations) that could underlie symptom formation (Benes et al. 1992; Mrzljak et al. 1996; Olney and Farber 1995). In the case of Tourette syndrome, these findings include work on the executive motor cortico-striato-pallido-thalamo-cortical circuits described by Alexander and DeLong (Alexander et al. 1986, 1990), as well as work on the executive functions of anterior cingulate and supplementary motor cortices (Deiber et al. 1991; Devinsky et al. 1995), the direct and indirect pathways that provide a balance of excitation and inhibition within them (Parent and Hazrati 1995), and the dopaminergic projections from the midbrain tegmentum (a region activated in the study) that are involved in their modulation (Alexander et al. 1986).

■ Conclusions and Future Directions

Symptom capture is a powerful strategy for pathophysiologic investigation in functional neuropsychiatric imaging. Symptom capture can be seen in the context of the symptom-oriented approach to identifying the brain circuits in which abnormal activity is associated with, and contributes to the expression of, major neuropsychiatic disorders. Although non–symptom-oriented approaches certainly represent a major and important line of investigation, symptom-oriented approaches offer a direct route with fewer assumptions. Among the symptom-oriented approaches, symptom capture is the most direct and assumption free. In this regard, it is important to note that symptoms are not necessarily merely "superficial epiphenomena" of a "deeper" underlying process, and that it is not necessarily the case that fewer assumptions means fewer hypotheses. In fact, rigorous functional imaging study designs that are carefully targeted and thought out (combined with whole brain, in addition to or instead of region of interest analyses) can result in data-driven observations that open up new possibilities for future hypotheses and investigations.

Symptom capture is also a powerful strategy for methodologic development in functional neuropsychiatric imaging. This approach provides a compelling rationale for the mobilization of an interdisciplinary team and resources, and provides exciting intellectual challenges linked to a tangible, practically important, and meaningful goal. This can be time consuming and risky, however, as great care must be taken to coordinate and work through the many technical details on many interrelated levels of paradigm development, without guarantee of success.

Examples were provided of methods of high-sensitivity $H_2{}^{15}O$ PET study design, image acquisition, and image analysis, and their application to the problems of hallucinations in schizophrenia and tics in Tourette syndrome. These methods and studies, as with any, have strengths and limitations that must be understood to use or extend them in an appropriate and effective manner. They do not constitute the only or necessarily the best tool with which to explore a given question. Such methods are most effectively used in a convergent fashion with other complementary, symptom or non–symptom-oriented techniques, and are most effectively interpreted in light of basic and clinical behavioral neuroscientific findings from related fields. In fact, once symptom-specific abnormal activity is localized to a particular brain region, information concerning the neurochemistry and neural modulation of that region can help to develop novel, targeted therapeutic interventions.

In addition to extending these paradigms to the study of other neuropsychiatric symptoms, future directions also involve incorporating other technologies, each with its own strengths and limitations that must be considered. One of these is fMRI. This technology offers the possibility of increased spatial and temporal resolution and a greater number of repeated studies in different conditions. The most widely used blood oxygen level–dependent (BOLD) paradigm (Ogawa et al. 1990) relies on venous deoxyhemoglobin changes that accompany neuronal activity (after a 4- to 6-second delay). Other more arterially weighted perfusion techniques have also been developed (Yang et al. 1998). In particular, recently developed event-related fMRI techniques (Rosen et al. 1998), which share some of the rationale that led us originally to develop the event-related PET techniques, are relevant here. We are currently developing and applying new fMRI methods as part of our ongoing symptom capture work.

It should be noted that the fMRI techniques work more by means of direct temporal resolution, as compared with the indirect temporal discrimination provided by the PET techniques. The methodologic challenges or steps involved with fMRI are therefore a bit more straightforward, yet fMRI is also limited in terms of temporal resolution (although much less so than PET) compared with the time scale on which neuronal activity unfolds. To approach this millisecond time scale, although sacrificing direct spatial localization in the process, magnetoencephalography (MEG) (Lounasmaa et al. 1996) and new methods of electrophysiologic evoked potentials (EP) (Abdullaev and Posner 1998) can be used. Because of the relative spatial or temporal limitations of each technique, and because functional imaging techniques can provide spatial localization that can help to constrain and improve MEG and EP analyses, the combined use of PET or fMRI with MEG or EP techniques offers additional possibilities (Abdullaev and Posner 1998; Liu et al. 1998). Finally, new multivariate statistical image analysis techniques (Buchel and Friston 1997, 1998), which make it possible to study the interactions among the brain regions identified with symptom capture or other methods, will help to provide another important layer of information concerning how abnormal patterns of brain activity may lead to neuropsychiatric symptom formation.

■ References

Abdullaev YG, Posner MI: Event-related brain potential imaging of semantic encoding during processing single words. Neuroimage 7:1–13, 1998

Alexander GE, De Long MR, Strick PL: Parallel organization of functionally segregated circuits linking basal ganglia and cortex. Annu Rev Neurosci 9:357–381, 1986

Alexander GE, Crutcher MD, De Long MR: Basal ganglia-thalamocortical circuits: parallel substrates for motor, oculomotor, "prefrontal" and "limbic" functions. Prog Brain Res 85:119–146, 1990

American Psychiatric Association: Diagnostic and Statistical Manual of Mental Disorders, 4th Edition. Washington, DC, American Psychiatric Association, 1994

Arana GW, Hyman SE: Handbook of Psychiatric Drug Therapy, 2nd Edition. Boston, MA, Little, Brown, 1991

Bailey DL, Jones T, Spinks TJ, et al: Noise equivalent count measurements in a neuro-PET scanner with retractable septa. IEEE Trans Med Imaging 10:256–260, 1991

Barta PE, Pearlson GD, Powers RE, et al: Auditory hallucinations and smaller superior temporal gyral volume in schizophrenia. Am J Psychiatry 147:1457–1462, 1990

Benes FM, Vincent SL, Alsterberg G, et al: Increased GABAA receptor binding in superficial layers of cingulate cortex in schizophrenics. J Neurosci 12:924–929, 1992

Braun AR, Stoetter B, Randolph C, et al: The functional neuroanatomy of Tourette's syndrome: an FDG-PET study, I: regional changes in cerebral glucose metabolism differentiating patients and controls. Neuropsychopharmacology 9:277–291, 1993

Braun AR, Randolph C, Stoetter B, et al: The functional neuroanatomy of Tourette's syndrome: an FDG-PET study, II: relationships between regional cerebral metabolism and associated behavioral and cognitive features of the illness. Neuropsychopharmacology 13:151–168, 1995

Breiter HC, Rauch SL: Functional MRI and the study of OCD: from symptom provocation to cognitive-behavioral probes of cortico-striatal systems and the amygdala. Neuroimage 4:S127–S138, 1996

Buchel C, Friston KJ: Modulation of connectivity in visual pathways by attention: cortical interactions evaluated with structural equation modelling and fMRI. Cereb Cortex 7:768–778, 1997

Buchel C, Friston KJ: Dynamic changes in effective connectivity characterized by variable parameter regression and Kalman filtering. Hum Brain Mapp 6:403–408, 1998

Cleghorn J: Brain metabolism during auditory hallucinations. Nurs Times 87:53, 1991

Cleghorn JM, Garnett ES, Nahmias C, et al: Regional brain metabolism during auditory hallucinations in chronic schizophrenia. Br J Psychiatry 157:562–570, 1990

DeLisi LE, Buchsbaum MS, Holcomb HH, et al: Increased temporal lobe glucose use in chronic schizophrenic patients. Biol Psychiatry 25:835–851, 1989

Deiber MP, Passingham RE, Colebatch JG, et al: Cortical areas and the selection of movement: a study with positron emission tomography. Exp Brain Res 84:393–402, 1991

Devinsky O, Morrell MJ, Vogt BA: Contributions of anterior cingulate cortex to behaviour. Brain 118:279–306, 1995

Dolan RJ, Bench CJ, Liddle PF, et al: Dorsolateral prefrontal cortex dysfunction in the major psychoses: symptom or disease specificity? J Neurol Neurosurg Psychiatry 56:1290–1294, 1993

Eidelberg D, Moeller JR, Antonini A, et al: The metabolic anatomy of Tourette's syndrome. Neurology 48:927–934, 1997

Friston KJ, Frith CD: Schizophrenia: a disconnection syndrome? Clin Neurosci 3:89–97, 1995

Friston KJ, Holmes AP, Worsley KJ, et al: Statistical parametric maps in functional imaging: a general linear approach. Hum Brain Mapp 2:189–210, 1995

Goldman-Rakic PS: Working memory dysfunction in schizophrenia. J Neuropsychiatry Clin Neurosci 6:348–357, 1994

Iida H, Kanno I, Miura S: Rapid measurement of cerebral blood flow with positron emission tomography, in Exploring Brain Functional Anatomy With Positron Emission Tomography. Edited by Chadwick DJ, Whelan J. West Sussex, England, Wiley, 1991, pp 23–42

Kaplan HI, Sadock BJ: Pocket Handbook of Psychiatric Drug Treatment. Baltimore, MD, Williams & Wilkins, 1993

Liu AK, Belliveau JW, Dale AM: Spatiotemporal imaging of human brain activity using functional MRI constrained magnetoencephalography data: Monte Carlo simulations. Proc Natl Acad Sci U S A 95:8945–8950, 1998

Lounasmaa OV, Hamalainen M, Hari R, et al: Information processing in the human brain: magnetoencephalographic approach. Proc Natl Acad Sci U S A 93:8809–8815, 1996

McGuire PK, Shah GM, Murray RM: Increased blood flow in Broca's area during auditory hallucinations in schizophrenia. Lancet 342:703–706, 1993

McGuire PK, Silbersweig DA, Wright I, et al: Abnormal monitoring of inner speech: a physiological basis for auditory hallucinations. Lancet 346:596–600, 1995

McGuire PK, Silbersweig DA, Wright I, et al: The neural correlates of inner speech and auditory verbal imagery in schizophrenia: relationship to auditory verbal hallucinations. Br J Psychiatry 169:148–159, 1996

Mesulam M-M: Principles of Behavioral Neurology. Philadelphia, PA, FA Davis, 1985

Mrzljak L, Bergson C, Pappy M, et al: Localization of dopamine D4 receptors in GABAergic neurons of the primate brain. Nature 381:245–248, 1996

Ogawa S, Lee TM, Kay AR, et al: Brain magnetic resonance imaging with contrast dependent on blood oxygenation. Proc Natl Acad Sci U S A 87:9868–9872, 1990

Olney JW, Farber NB: Glutamate receptor dysfunction and schizophrenia. Arch Gen Psychiatry 52:998–1007, 1995

Pandya DN, Yeterian EH: Architecture and connections of cortical association areas, in Cerebral Cortex, Vol 4. Edited by Peters A, Jones EG. New York, Plenum, 1985

Parent A, Hazrati LN: Functional anatomy of the basal ganglia, II: the place of subthalamic nucleus and external pallidum in basal ganglia circuitry. Brain Res Brain Res Rev 20:128–154, 1995

Peterson BS, Skudlarski P, Anderson AW, et al: A functional magnetic resonance imaging study of tic suppression in Tourette syndrome. Arch Gen Psychiatry 55:326–333, 1998

Posner MI, Petersen SE, Fox PT, et al: Localization of cognitive operations in the human brain. Science 240:1627–1631, 1988

Price CJ, Friston KJ: Cognitive conjunction: a new approach to brain activation experiments. Neuroimage 5:261–270, 1997

Raichle ME: Circulatory and metabolic correlates of brain function in normal humans, in Handbook of Physiology, Vol V: The Nervous System. Edited by Mountcastle VB. Bethesda, MD, American Physiological Society, 1987, pp 643–674

Rauch SL, Savage CR, Alpert NM, et al: The functional neuroanatomy of anxiety: a study of three disorders using positron emission tomography and symptom provocation. Biol Psychiatry 42:446–452, 1997

Rauch SL, van der Kolk BA, Fisler RE, et al: A symptom provocation study of posttraumatic stress disorder using positron emission tomography and script-driven imagery. Arch Gen Psychiatry 53:380–387, 1996

Robertson MM: The Gilles de la Tourette syndrome: the current status. Br J Psychiatry 154:147–169, 1989

Rosen BR, Buckner RL, Dale AM: Event-related functional MRI: past, present, and future. Proc Natl Acad Sci U S A 95:773–780, 1998

Schneider K: Clinical Psychopathology. New York, Grune & Stratton, 1959

Silbersweig D[A], Stern E: Functional neuroimaging of hallucinations in schizophrenia: toward an integration of bottom-up and top-down approaches. Mol Psychiatry 1:367–375, 1996

Silbersweig DA, Stern E: Symptom localization in neuropsychiatry: a functional neuroimaging approach. Ann N Y Acad Sci 835:410–420, 1997

Silbersweig DA, Stern E, Frith C, et al: A functional neuroanatomy of hallucinations in schizophrenia. Nature 378:176–179, 1995

Silbersweig DA, Stern E, Frith CD, et al: Detection of thirty-second cognitive activations in single subjects with positron emission tomography: a new low-dose H2(15)O regional cerebral blood flow three-dimensional imaging technique. J Cereb Blood Flow Metab 13:617–629, 1993

Silbersweig DA, Stern E, Schnorr L, et al: Imaging transient, randomly occurring neuropsychological events in single subjects with positron emission tomography: an event-related count rate correlational analysis. J Cereb Blood Flow Metab 14:771–782, 1994

Singer HS, Walkup JT: Tourette syndrome and other tic disorders: diagnosis, pathophysiology, and treatment. Medicine (Baltimore) 70:15–32, 1991

Stern E, Silbersweig DA, Chee K-Y, et al: A functional neuroanatomy of tics in Tourette syndrome. Arch Gen Psychiatry 57:741–748, 2000

Stoetter B, Braun AR, Randolph C, et al: Functional neuroanatomy of Tourette syndrome: limbic-motor interactions studied with FDG PET, in Tourette Syndrome: Genetics, Neurobiology, and Treatment, Vol 58. Edited by Chase TN, Friedhoff HA, Cohen DJ. New York, Raven, 1992, pp 213–226

Suzuki M, Yuasa S, Minabe Y, et al: Left superior temporal blood flow increases in schizophrenic and schizophreniform patients with auditory hallucination: a longitudinal case study using 123I-IMP SPECT. Eur Arch Psychiatry Clin Neurosci 242:257–261, 1993

Volkow ND, Wolf AP, Van Gelder P, et al: Phenomenological correlates of metabolic activity in 18 patients with chronic schizophrenia. Am J Psychiatry 144:151–158, 1987

Wing JK, Cooper JE, Sartorius N: Measurement and Classification of Psychiatric Symptoms. Cambridge, England, Cambridge University Press, 1974

Wiser AK, Andreasen NC, O'Leary DS, et al: Dysfunctional cortico-cerebellar circuits cause 'cognitive dysmetria' in schizophrenia. Neuroreport 9:1895–1899, 1998

Woodruff P, Brammer M, Mellers J, et al: Auditory hallucinations and perception of external speech (letter). Lancet 346:1035, 1995

Yang YH, Frank JA, Hou L, et al: Multislice imaging of quantitative cerebral perfusion with pulsed arterial spin labeling. Magn Reson Med 39:825–832, 1998

6

NEW METHODS FOR UNDERSTANDING HOW THE BRAIN REGULATES MOOD

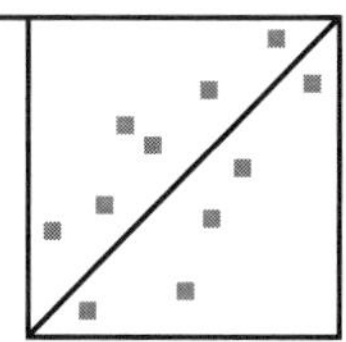

Serial Perfusion Functional Magnetic Resonance Imaging and Transcranial Magnetic Stimulation

Mark S. George, M.D.
Andrew M. Speer, M.D.
Daryl E. Bohning, Ph.D.
S. Craig Risch, M.D.
Diana J. Vincent, Ph.D.
Vidya Upadhyaya, M.D.
Laurie Stallings, Pharm.D.
Charles H. Kellner, M.D.
George W. Arana, M.D.
James C. Ballenger, M.D.

The recent revolution in functional neuroimaging has allowed profound insights into regional brain activity during normal and pathological emotions and has advanced understanding of several neuropsychiatric diseases.

The authors acknowledge Drs. Eric Wassermann, Tim Kimbrell, and Robert Post of the National Institutes of Health for help in the initial transcranial magnetic stimulation (TMS) and imaging studies. Dr. George thanks NARSAD, the Stanley Foundation, NIAAA, NIDA, DuPont Pharma, Dantec International, Picker International, Solvay, Jansenn, and Lilly for financial support of many of the imaging and repetitive TMS projects discussed in the chapter.

However, the future of the exciting field of functional neuroimaging remains unclear. Some people would suggest that, in this decade, functional neuroimaging is likely to involve continued refinement of current positron emission tomography (PET), single photon emission computed tomography (SPECT), and functional magnetic resonance imaging (fMRI) methods, as well as movement of many of these methods into more clinical settings. However, two recent developments have led others to point out that functional imaging may evolve into a different discipline, one that is even more powerful. In this chapter, two of these new developments (perfusion fMRI and transcranial magnetic stimulation [TMS]) are presented, along with a demonstration of how these new techniques are being applied to gain a better understanding of how the brain regulates mood.

Recently, several research groups developed MRI sequences that permit imaging of regional brain perfusion without the need for paramagnetic contrast agents (serial perfusion fMRI). Thus, unlike functional neuroimaging with SPECT and PET and traditional radioligands, perfusion fMRI does not involve radiation, and therefore repeated scanning is possible, as well as scanning of populations such as healthy children. With this technological advancement, functional imaging will likely change from being a pretreatment-posttreatment, snapshot mode of investigation to being a more dynamic serial tool that permits longitudinal analyses of regional brain changes. This serially scanning ability will perhaps result in a shift in the language used in imaging, from terms such as *on, off, ill,* and *well* to terms such as *half-lives, directions,* and *vectors of change.* In this chapter, we describe initial work at the Medical University of South Carolina (MUSC) in which this new tool was used to explore regional brain changes as a function of mood state in patients with rapid-cycling bipolar disorder.

The second important imaging development that will likely reshape functional neuroimaging is the new ability to stimulate brain tissue noninvasively with powerful handheld electromagnets. This technique is called *transcranial magnetic stimulation* (TMS). One of the more profound and philosophical difficulties with functional neuroimaging is determining whether a signal observed on an image is causally related to the behavior or disease in question. We discuss and describe several of the initial pilot studies in which TMS was used to induce mood changes in healthy control subjects as well as in patients with depression. We also describe exciting developments of the merging of the new technology of TMS with conventional neuroimaging. Combining TMS with neuroimaging is an important new chapter in the evolution of the understanding of brain function.

■ Serial Perfusion Functional MRI

Advances in neuroimaging with PET and SPECT have greatly increased the working knowledge of the regional brain abnormalities that accompany depression and mania (George et al. 1993, 1994a, 1996d; Ketter et al. 1996; Rubin et al. 1995; Sackeim and Prohovnik 1993). This in vivo imaging work expanded on and largely confirmed previous work in secondary depressions and manias that follow regional brain injury such as stroke (George et al. 1995c). Although there are some inconsistencies, perhaps due to differences in subject groups, varying mental activity during scanning, and use of different imaging technologies, several fairly consistent findings have emerged. During an episode of unipolar depression, the prefrontal cortex is hypometabolic (particularly on the left side), often in proportion to the degree of depression (George et al. 1994c; Ketter et al. 1994b). This finding of left prefrontal hypometabolism during depression is consistent with findings of previous studies, which showed an increased incidence of depression after left frontal strokes (Robinson and Szetela 1981).

Although fewer imaging studies of bipolar depression have been conducted, left prefrontal hypometabolism does not appear to be as consistent a finding (Baxter et al. 1989; Ketter et al. 1994a; Schwartz et al. 1987). In pilot work at the National Institute of Mental Health, depressed subjects with bipolar disorder were found to have right anterior temporal hyperactivity when depressed (Ketter et al. 1994a, 1996). Functional imaging studies conducted during acute mania are even more scarce, but several studies have shown decreased relative right anterior temporal and insular activity during acute mania (George et al. 1994a; Migliorelli et al. 1993; Starkstein et al. 1990). These same regions are often implicated in patients with secondary mania due to strokes (Robinson et al. 1988; Starkstein et al. 1987, 1988, 1989, 1991). These findings in bipolar depression and mania suggest that certain key regions—namely, the right anterior temporal cortex and insula—play an important role in mood dysregulation in bipolar disorder.

In the majority of studies of mood disorders to date, subjects have been imaged during acute episodes of depression or mania. Only a few studies have involved rescanning after treatment, with some (Baxter et al. 1985; Drevets et al. 1992; Post et al. 1987) but not all (Kimbrell et al. 1996; Nobler et al. 1994) studies showing a return toward more normal regional activity with treatment. One of the main impediments to serial functional imaging of patients with mood disorders has been the limitation, in SPECT and PET, imposed by radiation safety limits. These radiation limits have severely hampered the ability to examine the time course of regional brain activity throughout a mood cycle (Post et al. 1994).

Concepts and Methods

Several groups, including researchers at the Functional Neuroimaging Division of MUSC, have begun using the new imaging method of quantitative spin labeling and inversion recovery perfusion fMRI (Bohning et al. 1996b; Schwarzbauer et al. 1996; Ye et al. 1996). This technique has been used in preclinical models to study cerebral perfusion or regional cerebral blood flow (rCBF) (Bohning et al. 1996a) and has permitted repeated and consistent measurement of cerebral perfusion in healthy control subjects (Bohning et al. 1996b, 1997a). Perfusion fMRI offers several advantages over SPECT and PET. Perfusion fMRI involves no radiation exposure, and therefore multiple measures per subject can be done. Further, this technique can be used to measure rCBF quantitatively, which is not possible with perfusion SPECT and which requires an arterial line with PET.

Applications in Patients With Rapid-Cycling Bipolar Disorder

We have recently used perfusion fMRI to scan three patients with rapid-cycling bipolar disorder as they progress through their mood cycles. We have also scanned age- and sex-matched control subjects on the same day in the same scanner, using identical techniques. These studies will be used to test our hypothesis that bipolar subjects, when depressed, have increased activity in the right anterior temporal and insular regions and that, during mania, these same areas are relatively hypoactive. We also postulate that the same findings will be obtained when the mood disorder group is compared with healthy control subjects. Finally, we are keenly interested in determining whether there is a lag between clinical symptoms or phenomenology and changes in regional rCBF—that is, whether clinical symptoms and improvement precede rCBF changes.

The procedure we have used to date includes the following: After giving written informed consent, subjects undergo a screening interview using the Schedule for Affective Disorders and Schizophrenia—Lifetime Version modified for anxiety disorders and have their illness histories retrospectively defined and charted (Denicoff et al. 1997; George et al., in press; Squillace et al. 1984). A prospective imaging schedule based on the frequency of their cycling is composed, allowing for 14 total scans per subject (see Figure 6–1, A). (In arriving at this number, we took into account several issues, including how many scans subjects would tolerate and the economic costs of scanning, and also incorporated the requirement of a parametric comparison of the first cycle and the second cycle, as well as the desire to obtain scans during several distinct moods [e.g., depression, euthymia, and hypomania] within each set of seven scans.) Each day, regardless of cycle frequency, subjects subjectively and prospectively rate their mood using the Beck and National Institute of Mental Health life charting methods. Additionally, on each scanning day, trained clinicians administer the Hamilton Rating Scale for Depression (Hamilton 1960) and the Young Mania Scale (Young et al. 1978), as well as symptom checklists. While performing an auditory continuous performance task, subjects undergo a transverse perfusion magnetic resonance scan of the cortex in the angle of the anterior and posterior commissures (AC-PC plane plus 4 mm), a slice chosen for optimal imaging of regions previously identified in bipolar depression and mania. The entire scanning sequence initially took about 30 minutes per slice, but we recently reduced this time to 5 minutes per slice, moving closer to a scan time that would be suitable for evaluation of ischemia in an acute clinical setting (Bohning et al. 1997a).

Shown in Figure 6–1, B, are changes in mood in a 30-year-old man with rapid-cycling bipolar disorder, with a cycle frequency of 2 weeks. He entered the study unresponsive to medications (lithium and divalproex sodium) and received valproic acid for most of the study. Representative perfusion scans of this man (scans 1–3 and 5–7) are displayed in Figure 6–2. Regional data analysis is under way, and new ways of interpreting functional imaging data are being required. For example, note that scans 5 and 8 (in Figure 6–1, B, denoted by marks on the Y axis) have similar depression ratings, and the classification *depression* would have been applied in most previous functional imaging analyses. However, with serial scanning and measurement of mood, it is evident that the scans may in fact represent opposite ends of the spectrum; in scan 5, the patient is coming out of a depression (recovering), and, in scan 8, he is heading from a mania back down into a depression (relapsing).

The relationship between global gray matter perfusion and mood over time for this subject is shown in Figure 6–3. Although mood and global rCBF roughly correlated, at times changes in global perfusion preceded or lagged behind clinical ratings. These pilot studies, using a novel noninvasive technology that permits measurement of absolute brain perfusion, are perhaps yet another window into the brain of bipolar subjects, allowing serial assessment for the first time of the regional brain changes associated with mood cycling. It is to be hoped that this advance will permit better examination of regional brain changes over time and how they relate to clinical symptoms. This pilot work in carefully selected individuals will set the stage for the next generation of imaging studies in bipolar disorder, which will focus more on cyclicity and disease progression than on conventional definitions of ill and well.

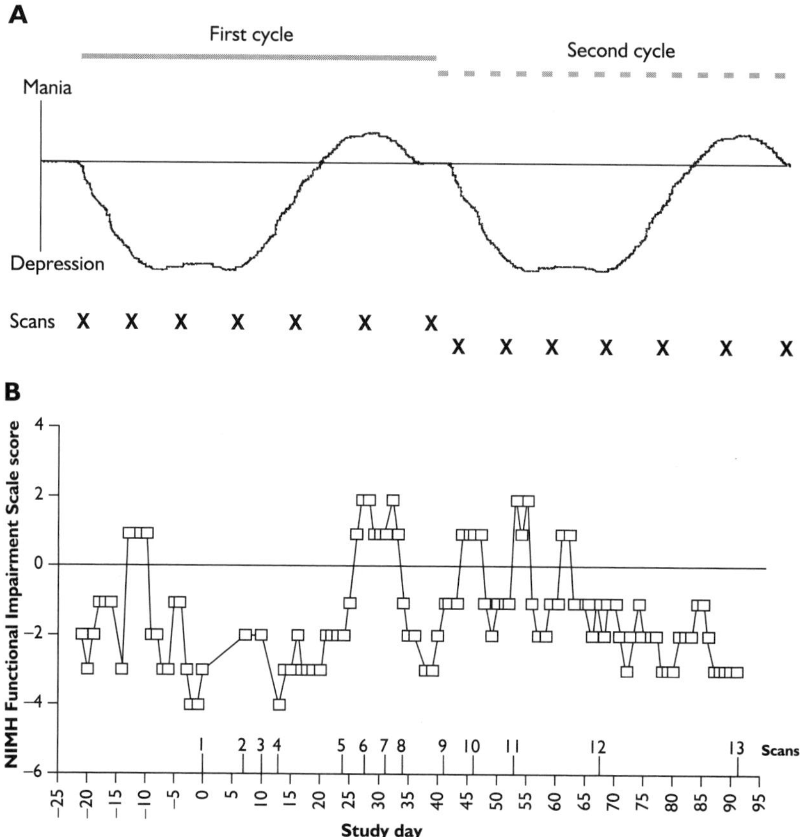

FIGURE 6–1. Serial perfusion functional magnetic resonance imaging (fMRI) in relation to mood cycling. *(A)* Theoretical and *(B)* actual life charts of a patient with rapid-cycling bipolar disorder who underwent serial perfusion fMRI over 3 months while drug therapy remained constant. Abbreviation: NIMH = National Institute of Mental Health.

■ TRANSCRANIAL MAGNETIC STIMULATION

Another recent technological development likely to have a heavy impact on the field of functional imaging is TMS (George and Belmaker 2000). The non-radiation-based perfusion scanning described in the previous section will likely allow investigators to break free of the restraints imposed by radiation, which has historically limited the number of scans per subject, particularly in special populations such as healthy children. TMS, with its ability to activate neurons noninvasively, will permit researchers to overcome the formidable

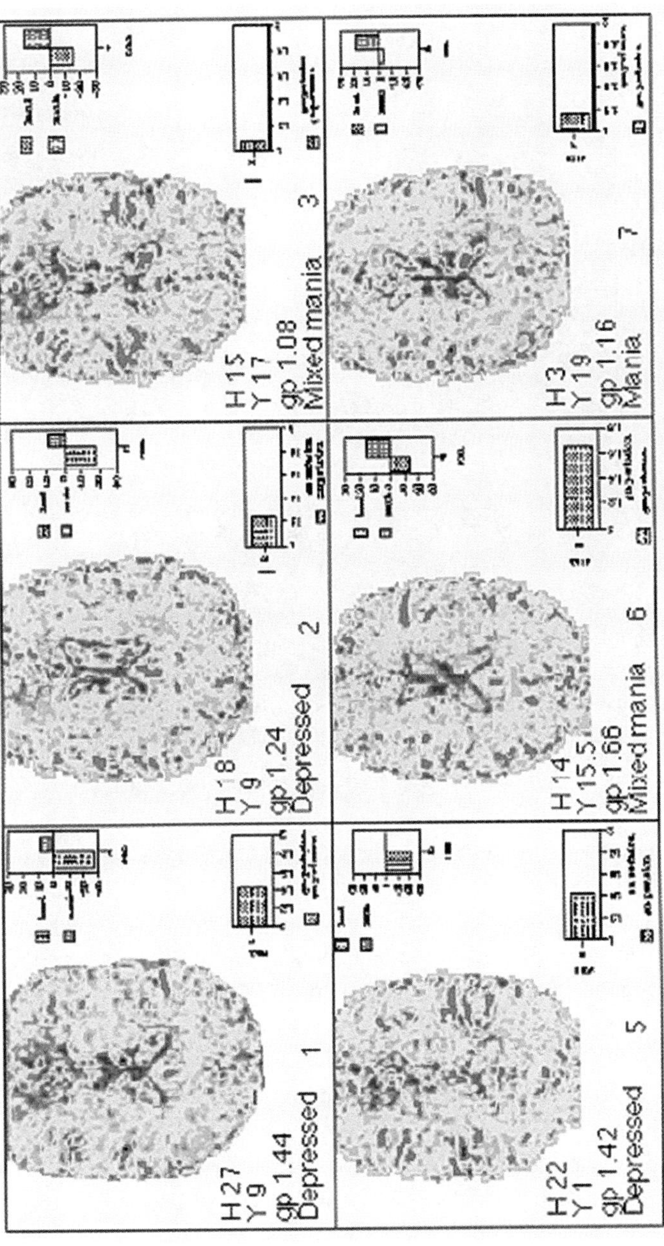

FIGURE 6–2. Serial transverse perfusion magnetic resonance scans of the patient in Figure 6–1 at the level of the anterior commissure. The Hamilton Rating Scale for Depression and Young Mania Scale ratings for the particular day are graphed in the upper right corner of each frame.

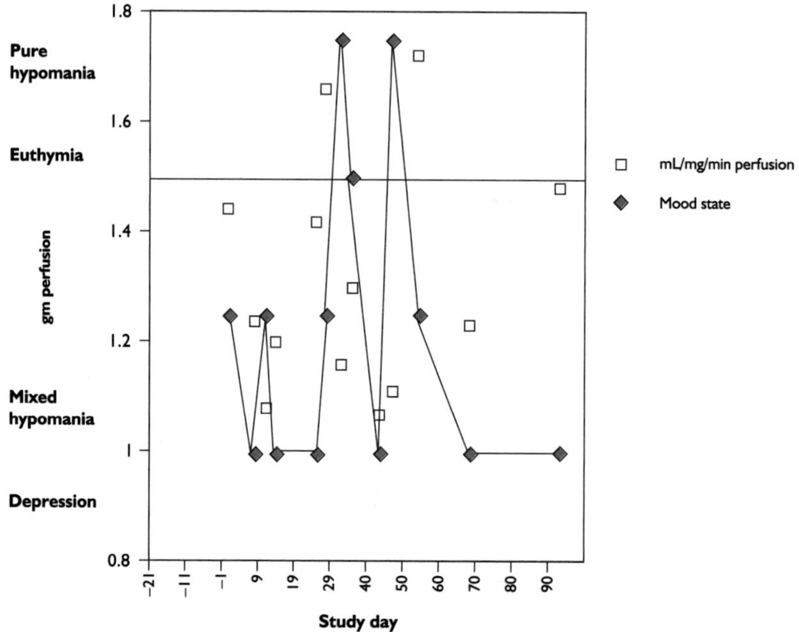

FIGURE 6–3. Graph of the relationship between global cerebral blood flow changes and mood in the patient in Figure 6–1. Mood was clinically assessed using the Young Mania Scale, Hamilton Rating Scale for Depression, and National Institute of Mental Health Self Scale.

barrier of the skull and will allow for actual probing and testing of neuronal circuits.

TMS uses the principle of inductance to convey electrical energy across the scalp and skull without the painful side effects of direct percutaneous electrical stimulation (for reviews, see George 1997; George et al. 1996b). TMS involves placing a small coil of wire on the scalp and passing a very powerful current through it (Barker et al. 1985; Roth et al. 1991b; Saypol et al. 1991). In this way, a magnetic field is produced that passes unimpeded through the tissues of the head. The magnetic field, in turn, induces a much weaker electric current in the brain. The strength of the induced current is a function of the rate of change of the magnetic field, which is in turn a function of the current in the coil. Other factors are the strength of the current and the number of windings in the coil (Cohen et al. 1990; Rothwell et al. 1991). Therefore, if enough current is to be induced to depolarize neurons in the brain, the current passed through the stimulating coil must start and stop or reverse its direction within about 300 microseconds.

The shape of the electromagnet coil is important because different coil shapes produce different magnetic fields (Cohen et al. 1990; Murro et al. 1992). The main differences are in the size and focality of the magnetic field. For instance, so-called butterfly or eight-shaped coils consist of two loops of windings that intersect in the middle. The magnetic field is strongest at the intersection and weaker elsewhere. This field allows fairly focal stimulation of the brain and has made use of the technique for cortical mapping possible (Pascual-Leone et al. 1994a, 1995; Wassermann et al. 1992; Wilson et al. 1993). The theoretical limit of spatial resolution of maps made with conventional equipment is about 5 mm (Brasil-Neto et al. 1992), although some investigators have applied deconvolutions to these maps with perhaps better spatial resolution (Bohning et al. 1997b). The stimulators and coils in production today develop about 1.5–2 tesla at the face of the coil and are capable of activating neurons 1.5–2 cm from the surface of the coil in the cortex (Bohning et al. 1997d; Epstein et al. 1990; Rudiak and Marg 1994).

The orientation of the coil with respect to the path of the axons of the target neurons appears to be important. For instance, axons appear to be particularly susceptible to TMS at points where they bend, such as the lip of a gyrus (Amassian et al. 1992). A critical fact about TMS is that, because of the orientation of the magnetic field perpendicular to the surface of the brain, under most conditions TMS has a strong tendency to activate cortical interneurons rather than cortical output cells (Gottesfeld et al. 1944; Rothwell et al. 1991). Such an activation occurs because the interneurons lie parallel to the surface of the brain, orthogonal to the magnetic field and are thus in the plane of the induced current. Activation of neurons deeper in the brain may be possible with solid core coils, formed by coiling wire around a bar of a paramagnetic material such as iron (Davey et al. 1991; Weissman et al. 1992; C.M. Epstein, personal communication, July 1997), or with other combinations of coils (D.E. Bohning, personal communication, September 1996). Even though conventional TMS can directly activate only cortical neurons, it affects cells at some distance from the stimulation site through transsynaptic connections. The fact that TMS has transsynaptic effects is obvious every time one stimulates over motor cortex and the thumb moves; obviously, TMS has acted transsynaptically in fibers exiting the central nervous system. However, preliminary evidence for transsynaptic effects within the brain comes from changes in hormones induced by stimulation (George et al. 1996a) and widespread changes in brain metabolism during TMS detected with functional imaging techniques (discussed later in this chapter) (George et al. 1995b).

Repetitive TMS

The ability to deliver multiple pulses rapidly (a technique known as *repetitive transcranial magnetic stimulation* [rTMS]) has important neurophysiological ramifications. In the first demonstration of the dramatic effects that rTMS can have on brain function, speech arrest was produced with stimulation over the motor speech (Broca's) area (Pascual-Leone et al. 1991). No such effects on neural processing had ever been produced with single TMS pulses. Some of the neurophysiology of rTMS was elucidated by Pascual-Leone and colleagues (1994a) in studies in the primary motor cortex. These researchers showed that low stimulation frequencies evoked consistent motor evoked potentials (MEPs) in the muscles targeted by the area of stimulated cortex. As the frequency of the stimulation was increased, the stimuli began to influence each other. At frequencies of about 10 Hz, the stimuli reinforced each other. At 20 Hz, every other stimulus came at a time when the corticospinal system was still inhibited by the preceding pulse. This period of inhibition after a TMS pulse usually lasts about 100 milliseconds (Valls-Sole et al. 1992). Stimulation at 20 Hz caused a high degree of synchrony of firing in the corticospinal tract; because no neurons could be recruited by every second pulse, the third pulse found many neurons free of inhibition. An alternating pattern of very small and extremely large MEPs resulted. Patterns of neuronal activity imposed by rTMS disrupt the normal function of the areas being stimulated. Sustained alterations in neural function and levels of neuronal activity are likely to underlie the ability of rTMS to produce reversible functional lesions such as those that cause speech arrest.

These diverse findings support our working theory that the frequency of stimulation may be a critical parameter in determining the effect of rTMS. For instance, trains of high-frequency stimulation produce facilitation of succeeding stimuli that last up to 4 minutes (Pascual-Leone et al. 1994a). By contrast, we have found that long trains of stimulation at 1 Hz cause suppression of the response to test stimuli. These findings bear some suggestive similarities to findings concerning the cellular neurophysiology of learning and memory in animals. High-frequency electrical stimulation of neurons can result in long-term increases in the efficiency of transmission in their synapses on other neurons (called *long-term potentiation*). This finding has been posited as a basis for certain types of learning (Gustafsson and Wigstrom 1988; Iriki et al. 1991; Sastry et al. 1986; Sil'kis et al. 1994). Electrical stimulation at frequencies in the single-hertz range produces long-term associative depression of transmission in synapses in the hippocampus (Artola et al. 1990; Stanton and Sejnowski 1989) and motor cortex (Sil'kis et al. 1994). Long-term depression may perhaps be the reciprocal of long-term potentiation and may operate naturally as a means of erasing learned associations. Weiss and co-workers (1995) showed that in rats whose seizure thresholds had been lowered (kindled) with high-frequency amygdala stimulation, daily 1-Hz stimulation for 15 minutes restored the normal seizure threshold. These investigators called this phenomenon *quenching* rather than *kindling*. These data suggest that rTMS may be capable of altering cortical function through synaptic changes that are potentially long-lasting. Not only is the rate of stimulation crucial for the ultimate effect, but different stimulus rates on the same neuron may have widely different, even antagonistic, effects.

Use of TMS to Probe Mood

An important and persistent problem with functional neuroimaging has been what some authors label the *causality problem*. Despite remarkable advances in brain imaging methods, it is still necessary, with all forms of imaging, to infer the relationship between regional brain activity and the underlying behavior. However, changes in the brain during a behavior are not necessarily causal. A brain region that is active during a behavior may be causing the behavior, may be attempting to stop the behavior, or may be incidentally activated. Short of actually stimulating the brain during surgery, it has been difficult to causally establish the link between a behavior and regional brain function or dysfunction. For example, the Wada test, in which an entire hemisphere is temporarily anesthetized by injection of amobarbital into the carotid, is a crude method of linking brain activity and a behavior (Wada and Rasmussen 1960). That is, if a patient cannot talk when his or her left hemisphere is off-line, it is reasonable to conclude that the left hemisphere is necessary for speech. However, the Wada test is invasive (requiring catheterization and radiation exposure) as well as crude (taking minutes to administer and affecting an entire hemisphere at a time). Fortunately, a new era is dawning in mapping brain-behavior relationships: TMS allows researchers temporarily to take specific brain regions off-line from a neural network and then observe whether that behavior continues to function or is modified.

TMS-Induced Changes in Normal Mood

One long-standing model of emotion regulation has been the *valence model of mood*, in which it is postulated that whereas the left hemisphere mediates positive emotions (e.g., happiness), the right mediates negative emotions (e.g., anger, fear, disgust, anxiety, and sadness) (Ross et al. 1994; Sackeim and Gur

1978; Sackeim et al. 1978, 1982). An individual's mood at any given time thus reflects the relative balance of the input of the two hemispheres. Either temporarily or permanently disabling one hemisphere would allow the other to act in an unbalanced manner. Some of the most striking evidence in support of this hypothesis comes from patients' reactions during the Wada test (Wada and Rasmussen 1960). Some observers have noted that sadness and catastrophic reactions tend to be associated with left hemisphere deactivations (Jennum et al. 1994). Conversely, when the right hemisphere is temporarily disabled with the injection, happy and euphoric responses have been observed (Christianson et al. 1993).

Generally, cortically mediated tasks such as language are associated with a high degree of hemispheric specialization. Subcortically mediated tasks such as breathing and alertness appear to be less lateralized. Despite this general rule of increasing hemispheric laterality with cortically mediated tasks, numerous studies have demonstrated the crucial role of the right brain in both understanding and expressing emotion. The left side of the face (controlled by the right hemisphere) is more expressive of emotion than the right (Sackeim and Gur 1978). Verbal and visual stimuli with an emotional content are better processed by the right hemisphere (Sackeim et al. 1978). For example, in a recent PET study, we demonstrated that the right hemisphere is activated when a subject listens to speech for the emotional tone (or prosody) rather than the content of the words (George et al. 1996c).

Other studies also support the valence theory of mood. Some PET and SPECT studies have demonstrated that clinically depressed subjects have abnormal prefrontal function, more commonly on the left than on the right (Austin et al. 1992; Baxter et al. 1989; Bench et al. 1992, 1993; Drevets et al. 1992; Mathew et al. 1980; Mayberg et al. 1994). Several studies involving poststroke subjects have found that damage to the left prefrontal cortex greatly increases the likelihood of poststroke depression (Robinson and Szetela 1981; Robinson et al. 1984, 1990). In addition, depressed patients with multiple sclerosis have more white matter lesions on the left side than do nondepressed patients with multiple sclerosis (George et al. 1994b). Also, damage to the right hemisphere, especially the right prefrontal or temporal cortex, has been linked to primary or secondary mania (Robinson et al. 1988; Starkstein et al. 1988, 1991).

Finally, in a series of studies, Davidson and colleagues (1994) found that asymmetries in prefrontal electroencephalographic activity (alpha power) correspond to selection of items (happy or sad). Healthy subjects with more left frontal activation (increased left frontal activity and relatively decreased right frontal activity) endorsed happy and euphoric items, with right frontal activation (and left frontal deactivation) corresponding to endorsement of sad items.

Compared with control subjects, depressed subjects had left frontal hypoactivation, a finding consistent with findings of other functional imaging studies and with the valence or laterality model.

The valence hypothesis, although supported by many studies, is by no means proven, and results obtained in several studies are not consistent with this theory (House et al. 1990; Sharpe et al. 1990) (for an insightful review, see Sackeim 1991). In addition, only a slim majority of functional imaging studies involving patients with mood disorders support the concept of lateralized dysfunction. In contrast, at least two PET studies involving healthy volunteers have demonstrated that there is increased left orbitofrontal and left prefrontal activity during states of transient sadness (George et al. 1995a; Pardo et al. 1993). Further work is necessary to refine this theory of differential hemispheric contribution to mood. It may prove to be the case that there is in fact a difference in hemispheric contribution or regulation of mood but that this difference also depends on differential activity within the hemispheres, the limbic system, and other subcortical structures. Conversely, it is possible that the limbic system, acting in an integrated way and spanning the two hemispheres, moderates or enhances this differential cortical regulation, producing and amplifying noise that affects findings. It may also be the case that just as the laterality of handedness does not always follow a rule, some subjects may exhibit laterality to a lesser degree, or even differently, than may the majority of individuals. Clearly, further imaging work during induced mood states in health and disease would help advance understanding in this area.

We first sought to test the valence theory of mood directly, by using rTMS to excite (and then disable) the prefrontal cortex temporarily and then observing the effects on mood (George et al. 1996a). Using rTMS over the right or left prefrontal cortex on different days in 10 adult healthy volunteers (figure-eight coil, 120% motor threshold [MT], 5 Hz for 10 seconds, 2-minute rest, on and off 10 times, a total of 20 minutes of stimulation, 500 stimuli per session), we discovered that left prefrontal stimulation caused an increase in self-rated sadness, whereas right stimulation caused increases in happiness (Figure 6–4 and Table 6–1).

In this study, the most prominent mood changes occurred in the afternoon (5 P.M.), but mood changes were also seen in the same directions at 20 minutes. This study confirmed and extended the findings of the initial study by Pascual-Leone and colleagues (1996b), who stimulated different brain regions within the same day and achieved roughly the same results, with the exception that significant mood effects were seen within 30 minutes of stimulation at a higher frequency and in shorter intertrain intervals (110% MT, 10 Hz for 5 seconds, 25 seconds apart, for 10 trains) (Table 6–1). This

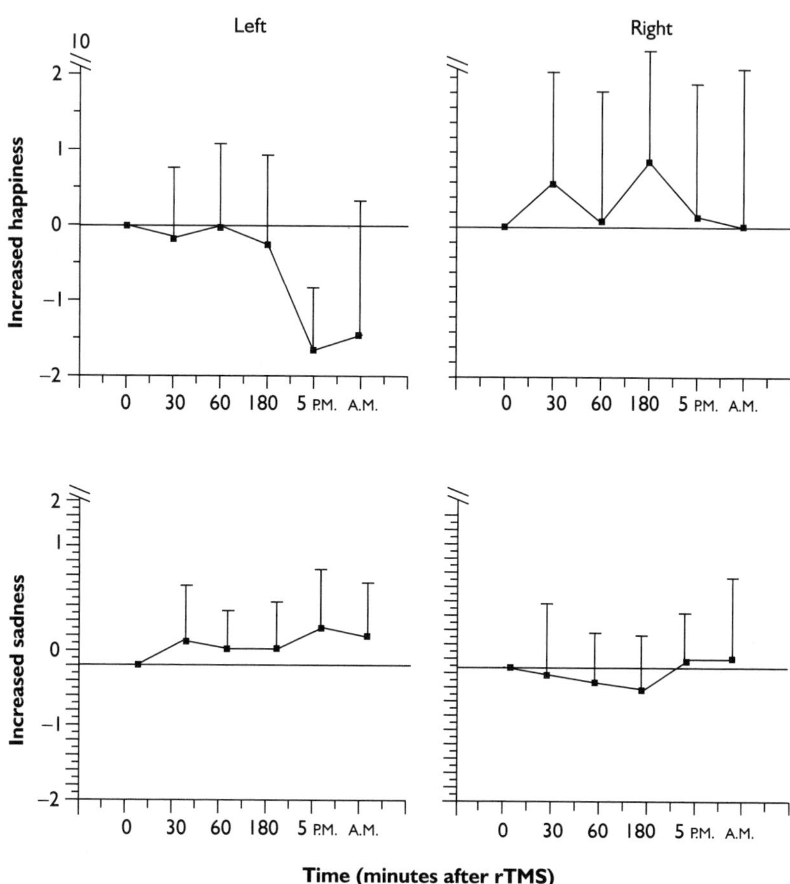

FIGURE 6–4. Graphs of changes in self-ratings of mood by 10 healthy volunteers after a morning session of repetitive transcranial magnetic stimulation (rTMS) over the left or right prefrontal cortex (120% motor threshold, 5 Hz for 10 seconds, 2-minute rest, 10 times over 20 minutes). Left prefrontal rTMS resulted in significant decreases in happiness (top) and increases in sadness (bottom) compared with right prefrontal stimulation. Visual analog scales were used. (Repeated-measures analysis of variance, $F=7.1$, $P<0.001$.)

Source. Reprinted from George MS, Wassermann EM, Williams WA, et al.: "Changes in Mood and Hormone Levels After Rapid-Rate Transcranial Magnetic Stimulation (rTMS) of the Prefrontal Cortex." *Journal of Neuropsychiatry and Clinical Neurosciences* 8:172–180, 1996a.

TABLE 6–1. Studies of laterality of repetitive transcranial magnetic stimulation and mood

Study	Frequency (Hz)	Length (seconds)	No. of trains	Intertrain interval (seconds)	Time of peak effect	No. of stimuli	Intensity (%)[a]	Mood effect: Left	Mood effect: Right
Healthy volunteers									
George et al. 1996a	5	10	10	120	8 hours	500	120	—	Increased H
Pascual-Leone et al. 1996b	10	5	10	25	20 minutes	500	110	—	Increased H
Martin et al. 1997	20	2	20	58	20 minutes	800	80	—	Increased H, increased A
Subjects with obsessive-compulsive disorder									
Greenberg et al. 1997	20	2	20	58	30 minutes	800	80	—	Increased H
Depressed subjects									
George et al. 1995b	20	2	20	58	Several days	800/day, repeated daily	80	Decreased D	NT
Pascual-Leone et al. 1996a	10	10	20	50	Several days	2,000/day, repeated daily	110	Decreased D	—
George et al. 1997	20	2	20	58	Several days	800/day, repeated daily	80	Decreased D	NT

Note. A = anxiety; D = depressive symptoms; H = happiness; NT = not tested.
[a]Percentage of motor threshold.

TMS-induced mood effect appears to be specific to prefrontal stimulation, although active nonprefrontal sites were explicitly tested in the initial study by George et al. (1996a) only.

In a recent follow-up study using a more fastidious design, we stimulated a different group of control subjects with selective prefrontal stimulation on one day and entire-hemisphere stimulation on another (Martin et al. 1997) (Table 6–1). During selective prefrontal stimulation in nine healthy control subjects over the right hemisphere (80% MT, 20 Hz for 2 seconds, 1-minute rest, 20 times over 20 minutes), self-rated happiness increased, whereas left prefrontal stimulation resulted in increased sadness (Figure 6–5). Entire-hemisphere stimulation with a larger nonfocal coil and with identical parameters and ratings caused no significant change in mood. We also found that right prefrontal stimulation caused significant increases in anxiety.

These initial findings concerning TMS-induced mood changes should be interpreted with caution because the investigations were pilot studies in a new field and involved small samples. The findings suffer from several of the current limitations in the evolving field of rTMS as a neuroinvestigative probe. First, it is unclear to what extent these findings might be specific to any of the numerous variables associated with rTMS. These variables include not only the brain region stimulated but also the type of stimulator and stimulating coil (which determine the distribution and intensity of the stimulation, both absolute and relative to each person's motor threshold), the frequency and duration of the stimuli, the duration of stimulation relative to rest time, and finally the total number of trains within a day or over a day. It is conceivable that different dosing regimens may have various effects on the underlying prefrontal cortical tissue. In motor cortex studies, different dosing regimens may be stimulative and additive, whereas others may be inhibitory with respect to motor firing (Pascual-Leone et al. 1994b). Extrapolation from findings in motor studies has led to the belief that the dosing frequency used in these studies was additive and stimulative.

Combining TMS With Functional Imaging

How does one begin to combine TMS and neuroimaging to elucidate the effects of TMS on neurons? There are many technical issues associated with performing TMS in a PET, SPECT, or magnetic resonance scanner. As a first step in this field, following on a split-dose [^{18}F]fluorodeoxyglucose (FDG)–PET scan of a depressed patient in an early TMS treatment trial (Figure 6–6 and Table 6–2) (George et al. 1995b), our group at the National Institutes of Health began to use techniques in which the tracer uptake is removed from the

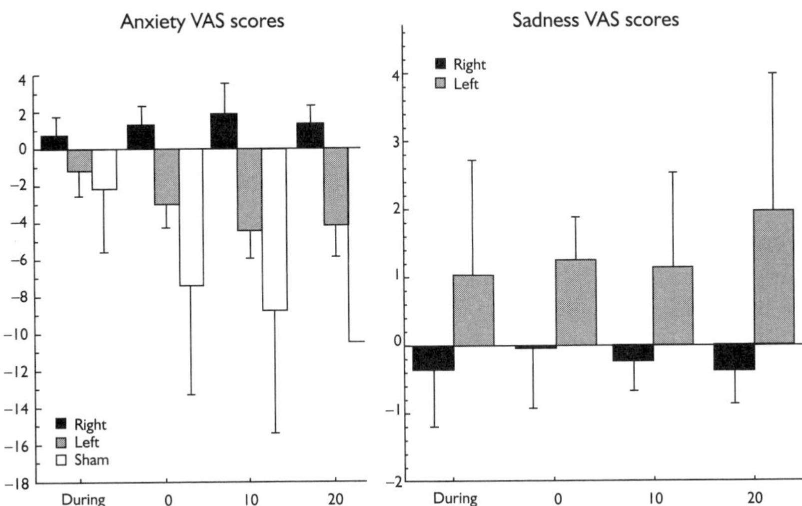

FIGURE 6–5. Graphs showing statistically significant increases, in nine healthy control subjects, in self-rated sadness 20 minutes after left prefrontal stimulation, compared with right prefrontal stimulation (paired *t* test, $t=2.38$, 8 *df*, $P<0.05$), and in self-rated anxiety 20 minutes after right prefrontal stimulation, compared with left prefrontal stimulation (paired *t* test, $t=2.5$, 8 *df*, $P<0.05$). Visual analog scales (VASs) were used.
Source. Reprinted from Martin JD, George MS, Greenberg BD, et al.: "Mood Effects of Prefrontal Repetitive High-Frequency TMS in Healthy Volunteers." *CNS Spectrums: The International Journal of Neuropsychiatric Medicine* 2:53–68, 1997.

actual scanner, with the image being "developed" later, away from the TMS coil. Our initial case study demonstrated the potential of split-dose FDG PET to elucidate the effects of TMS (George et al. 1995b).

In follow-up work at the National Institutes of Health, Wassermann and coworkers (1997) designed and carried out a split-dose FDG study looking at the effects of TMS over the motor cortex (Table 6–2). Some preliminary data from this study are shown in Figure 6–7. The time course of uptake of FDG is approximately 20–30 minutes. Thus, for an FDG scan to be obtained during rTMS, stimulation must last the entire 20–30 minutes. The risk of seizures with prolonged stimulation makes high-frequency rTMS impossible. Therefore, 1-Hz stimulation was used in the initial study with FDG (Wassermann et al. 1997). As shown in Figure 6–7, there were *decreases* at the contralateral motor site of M1 (that is, the mirror motor area) during rTMS, compared with during rest. There were also profound decreases in metabolism in prefrontal connections as well as in the ipsilateral caudate. The only increased areas of activity were in the auditory cortex, a result of the noise of the TMS machine when it fires.

TABLE 6–2. Initial studies combining functional imaging with transcranial magnetic stimulation

Time frame	Method	TMS parameters	Result	Reference
Before and after TMS (weeks)	FDG PET	Daily, left prefrontal, 80% MT, 20 Hz, 2 seconds, 20 minutes	Normalization of prefrontal deficit	George et al. 1995b
During TMS	FDG PET	100% MT over M1, 1 Hz	Decreases at mirror focus, increased auditory cortex	Wassermann et al. 1997
	Perfusion SPECT	Left prefrontal, 80% MT, 20 Hz	Left prefrontal and coil site decreases, thalamic increases	Stallings et al. 1997
	MRI	Constantly on, low voltage (low-voltage model)	Visualization of TMS magnetic field	Bohning et al. 1997d
	^{15}O PET	70% machine, 10 Hz maximum	Activation of frontal eye fields and connections	Paus et al. 1997
		120% MT over M1, 1 Hz	Significant increases in flow at coil site and at connections, "nonphysiological" response	Fox et al. 1997
Cross-modal comparison	FDG PET	Single pulse	Confirmation of MEP site	Wassermann et al. 1996
	BOLD functional MRI	Single pulse	Confirmation of MEP site	Roberts et al. 1997

Note. BOLD=blood oxygen level–dependent; FDG=[^{18}F]fluorodeoxyglucose; MEP=motor evoked potential; MRI=magnetic resonance imaging; MT=motor threshold; PET=positron emission tomography; SPECT=single photon emission computed tomography; TMS=transcranial magnetic stimulation.

In an effort to determine whether the secondary foci are, in fact, functionally real and caused by the primary stimulation, Chen and colleagues (1997) measured MEPs over the contralateral motor site before, and then after, a 20-minute train of rTMS. They found a decrease in motor activity—that is, an increase in MEPs at that site. This study demonstrates the power of coupling functional imaging with TMS. In a study that was identical except for the use of sham stimulation over M1, there were no significant changes compared with baseline (E. M. Wassermann, personal communication, July 1997). This finding demonstrates that the current "sham" method of directing the TMS coil at a 45-degree angle has no neuronal effect; the peak magnetic field is associated with superficial skin and muscle stimulation but not penetration of the brain. The FDG method has its limitations, however; stimulation for 20 minutes at high frequencies and intensities near motor threshold are likely to cause seizures.

^{15}O PET In contrast to the decreased metabolism found with FDG at 1-Hz stimulation, two recent ^{15}O-PET studies found increased rCBF immediately below a TMS coil. Paus and colleagues (1997) scanned subjects using ^{15}O PET during stimulation over the frontal eye fields (Table 6–2). Compared with rest, the subjects had increased blood flow directly under the coil as well as in the visual cortex (a projection from the frontal eye fields). It was unclear what intensity was used in this study (stimulation was performed relative to machine output and not individual motor threshold), nor is the exact frequency known (there was a complex parametric design, centered around a frequency of 10 Hz).

Fox and colleagues (1997) performed 1-Hz motor stimulation over the left M1 area for thumb and serially measured rCBF using ^{15}O PET (Table 6–2). As shown in Figure 6–8, rCBF increased locally with magnetic stimulation. Other sites with known neuroanatomical connections were also activated. Interestingly, unlike physiological changes caused by intentional thumb movement, blood flow did not immediately return to normal 10 minutes later. These preliminary data imply that TMS does not merely excite exiting cortical neurons but, rather, acts on neurons in a different manner.

Perfusion SPECT The major problem with FDG is that it takes 20 minutes or more to distribute into neurons. Thus the PET scan is a composite of activity over 20 minutes, and TMS stimulation at more than 1 Hz cannot be performed for that long because of the risk of seizures. Recently, the Functional Neuroimaging Division of MUSC combined rTMS with brain perfusion SPECT, which produces a composite picture of 1–2 minutes of activity

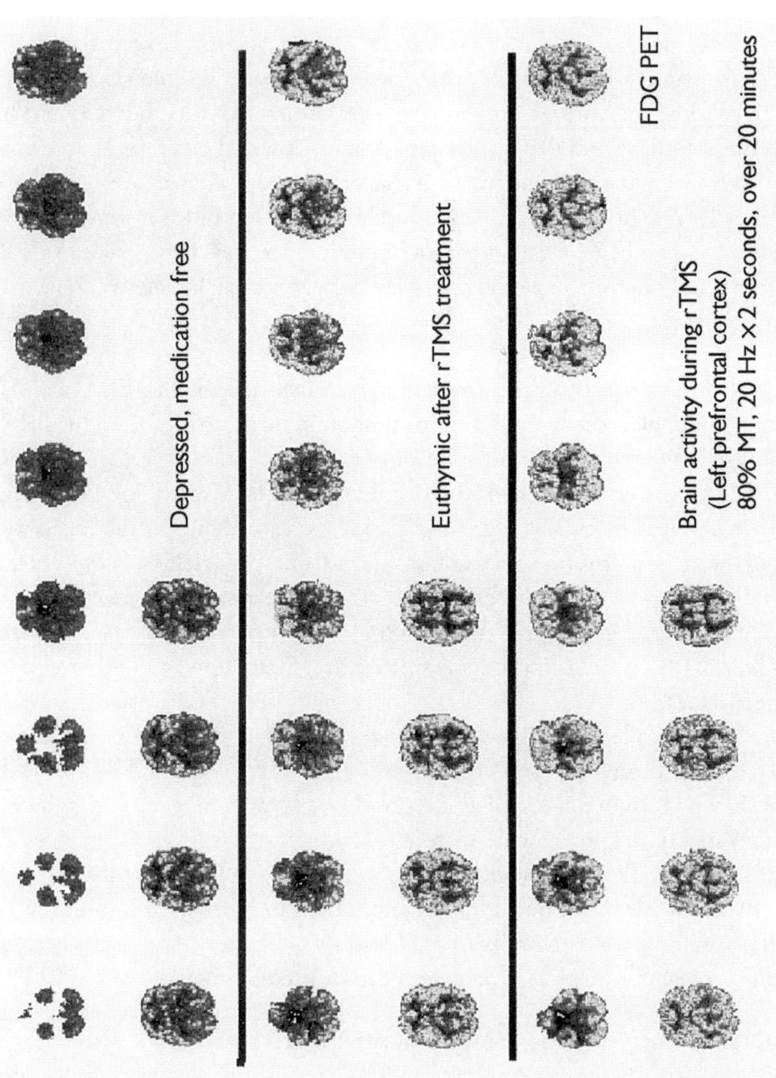
Depressed, medication free
Euthymic after rTMS treatment
Brain activity during rTMS
(Left prefrontal cortex)
80% MT, 20 Hz × 2 seconds, over 20 minutes
FDG PET

FIGURE 6–6. Progressive [^{18}F]fluorodeoxyglucose (FDG)–positron emission tomography (PET) scans, transverse plane, of a 35-year-old woman with major depression. The scans on the top represent brain activity before treatment, when the patient was actively clinically depressed and medication free. The middle scans are from 3 months later, after intermittent treatment with repetitive transcranial magnetic stimulation (rTMS) over the left prefrontal cortex. The bottom scans were performed during rTMS over the left prefrontal cortex. Note the increase in global metabolic activity, as well as increases in regional activity over the prefrontal cortex. Abbreviation: MT = motor threshold.

Source. Reprinted from George MS, Wassermann EM, Williams WA, et al.: "Daily Repetitive Transcranial Magnetic Stimulation (rTMS) Improves Mood in Depression." *NeuroReport* 6:1853–1856, 1995b.

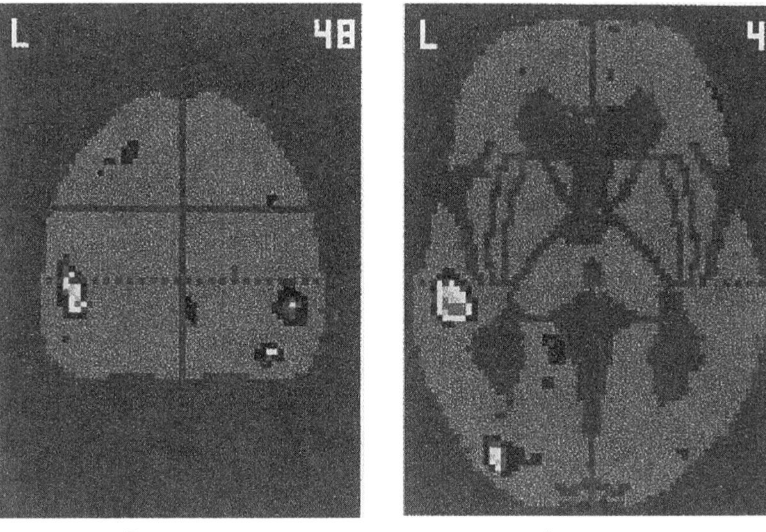

FIGURE 6–7. Statistical parametric map of the areas of brain that are decreased during 1-Hz repetitive transcranial magnetic stimulation over the right motor cortex. [^{18}F]Fluorodeoxyglucose–positron emission tomography scans were performed. Note the decreases directly beneath the coil as well as on the contralateral motor site and in diffuse prefrontal areas (left). The only increases at this frequency were in the auditory cortex, a result of the sound of the magnetic stimulation (right). The transsynaptic effects of this 1-Hz stimulation have been confirmed electrophysiologically. The remote motor regions are actually neuronally less excited by the 1-Hz stimulation to the contralateral side.

Source. Reprinted from Wassermann EM, Kimbrell TA, George MS, et al.: "Local and Distant Changes in Cerebral Glucose Metabolism During Repetitive Transcranial Magnetic Stimulation (rTMS)" (abstract). *Neurology* 48:A107–P02.049, 1997.

(Stallings et al. 1997) (Table 6–2). We administered 30 millicuries (1,110 megabecquerels) of the general perfusion tracer, NeuroliteR (DuPont Pharma, Wilmington, DE), on three occasions over a 4-week period using a triple-headed Picker camera (Cleveland, OH). Eight healthy adult subjects were scanned at baseline, during bolus tracer injection during seconds 10–20 of a train of 2 minutes of left prefrontal rTMS (60% MT; 10 Hz; 10 seconds on, 10 seconds off; a total of 600 stimuli) (referred to here as the 2-minute condition), and exactly as just described but after administration of 18 minutes of high-frequency stimulation (80% MT; 20 Hz; 2 seconds on, 28 seconds off; 1,440 and 600 stimuli, for a total of 2,040 stimuli) (20-minute condition). Scans were linearly transformed into Talairach space using

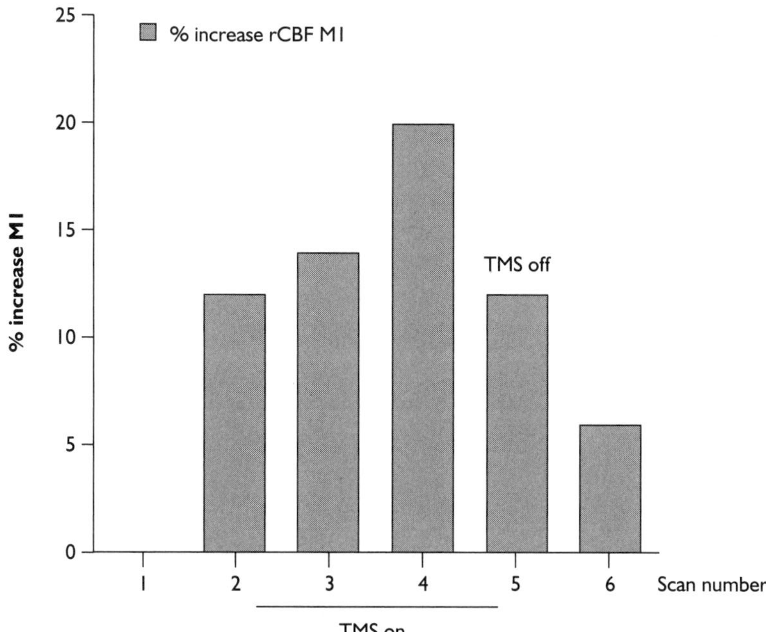

FIGURE 6–8. Graphs of the changes in relative regional cerebral blood flow (rCBF) (as measured by ^{15}O-positron emission tomography) in a region of cortex immediately below a transcranial magnetic stimulation (TMS) coil held in position to stimulate the contralateral thumb. Note the increased blood flow immediately under the TMS coil in the three healthy subjects. rCBF increased immediately after TMS (120% motor threshold, 1 Hz) was begun over the thumb area, and blood flow continued to increase over 20 minutes.
Source. Reprinted from Fox P, Ingham R, George MS, et al.: "Imaging Human Intracerebral Connectivity by PET During TMS." *NeuroReport* 8:2787–2791, 1997.

SPM96b and compared across conditions ($P<0.05$ for display).

Contrary to our prestudy hypothesis, there was no increase at the coil site during the 2-minute condition, compared with baseline, or during the 20-minute condition, compared with baseline (Figure 6–9). In fact, during the 20-minute condition, perfusion was relatively decreased at the coil site and in the surrounding left prefrontal cortex, bilateral anterior cingulate gyrus, and anterior temporal cortex. The study demonstrated an apparent TMS dose–response effect, with larger increases and decreases during the 20-minute condition (compared with baseline) than during the 2-minute condition (compared with baseline). During the 20-minute condition, compared with the 2-minute condition, there were coil site decreases and relative increases in the contralateral (right) hemisphere, because of the increase in TMS stimuli. Also, relative

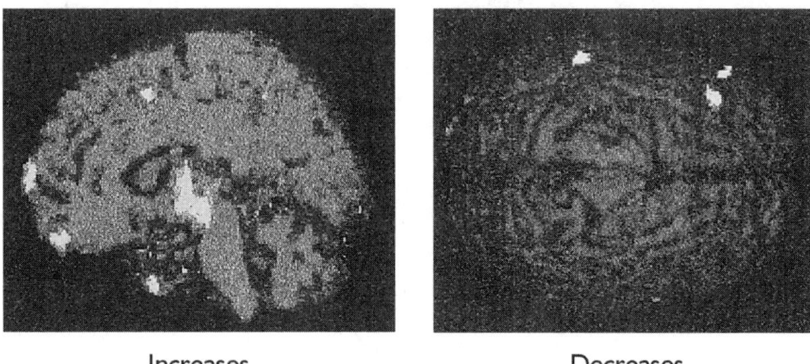

FIGURE 6–9. Images showing increases in thalamic and orbitofrontal perfusion during left prefrontal repetitive transcranial magnetic stimulation (TMS) (left) and decreases in perfusion in the left prefrontal cortex at the TMS coil site and at the anterior cingulate gyrus (right), in both cases during the 20-minute condition (see text for details), compared with baseline. This SPM output ($P<0.05$ for eight subjects) demonstrates that left prefrontal stimulation at 20 Hz likely inhibits cortical activity directly beneath the coil and that it is feasible to use split-dose single photon emission computed tomography to image the immediate and postimmediate effects of prefrontal TMS.
Source. Reprinted from Stallings LE, Speer AM, Spicer KM, et al.: "Combining SPECT and Repetitive Transcranial Magnetic Stimulation (rTMS): Left Prefrontal Stimulation Decreases Relative Perfusion Locally in a Dose Dependent Manner" (abstract). *Neuroimage* 5:S521, 1997.

perfusion was significantly increased in the orbitofrontal cortex (with the increase greater on the right than on the left) and hypothalamus during the 20-minute and 2-minute conditions, with thalamic increases occurring during the 20-minute condition (all conditions compared with baseline).

Full interpretation of these results is not possible, because of incomplete knowledge of the effect of the relative amount of stimulation compared with rest during tracer uptake, the pharmacokinetics of tracer uptake, the depth of the magnetic field, and whether different frequencies and intensities have divergent effects on neuronal tissue. Nevertheless, this pilot work demonstrates that coupling rTMS with split-dose perfusion SPECT is a promising method for elucidating the brain changes associated with rTMS. Prefrontal rTMS at high frequencies has both local and remote dose-dependent effects, and, contrary to current theories, perfusion is relatively decreased under the TMS coil, even at these high frequencies. In addition to establishing the method, these results also invite further studies in which the SPECT tracer is injected during peak TMS-induced mood changes to generate maps of regional brain activity. It is unclear what is happening 20 minutes after TMS, when mood changes begin to occur.

Functional MRI The direct magnetic path of TMS coils (and thus stimulation) is a function of coil geometry and field strength and, with the parameters used in these studies, reaches up to 4 cm below the coil or in superficial layers of cortex (Roth et al. 1991a, 1991b; Rothwell et al. 1991). Recent work at MUSC may help illuminate the issue of depth of the TMS field in vivo as well as pave the way for eventually performing TMS stimulation within a high-field magnetic resonance scanner (Bohning et al. 1997c, 1997d) (Table 6–2). An MRI-compatible model of the figure-eight rTMS coil was mounted in the head holder of a conventional magnetic resonance scanner (1.5-tesla Picker scanner) next to the temporal lobe. Two sets of phase images were acquired, the first with the coil off (as a reference) and the second with the coil energized with a 50-milliampere direct current. The two sets of phase images were then corrected for aliasing and scaled to give field intensity in gauss (Figure 6–10). These pioneering images demonstrate the potential power of blending functional imaging and TMS. Of course, although the magnetic field is not distorted by the brain tissue (see Figure 6–10), the neurobiologic effects of TMS occur only when an electric current is induced in the tissue, and probably only when the current is strong enough to depolarize a nerve (therefore just under the skull). Thus, for a full understanding of the neurobiologic effects of TMS, knowledge of the magnetic field within the brain must be integrated with functional imaging of the metabolic or blood flow effect of TMS (Roberts et al. 1997) (using SPECT, as discussed earlier; Table 6–2).

Echoplanar blood oxygen level–dependent fMRI is the functional neuroimaging tool with the best temporal resolution (except for electroencephalography [EEG] and MEG), capable as it is of sampling images on the order of milliseconds. There are, however, a host of problems involved in integrating a focal TMS coil within the constant MRI environment. Many groups are addressing these issues (Bohning et al. 1999, 1998). Another option is to integrate TMS with quantitative EEG, which has a very high temporal resolution, although spatial resolution is poor. Using MRI to determine structure and then determine the TMS field model, and then to position correctly, may be key to future integration of these two technologies, especially in clinical applications, much like gamma knife surgery has been used to focus gamma radiation on specific brain regions, with therapeutic effects.

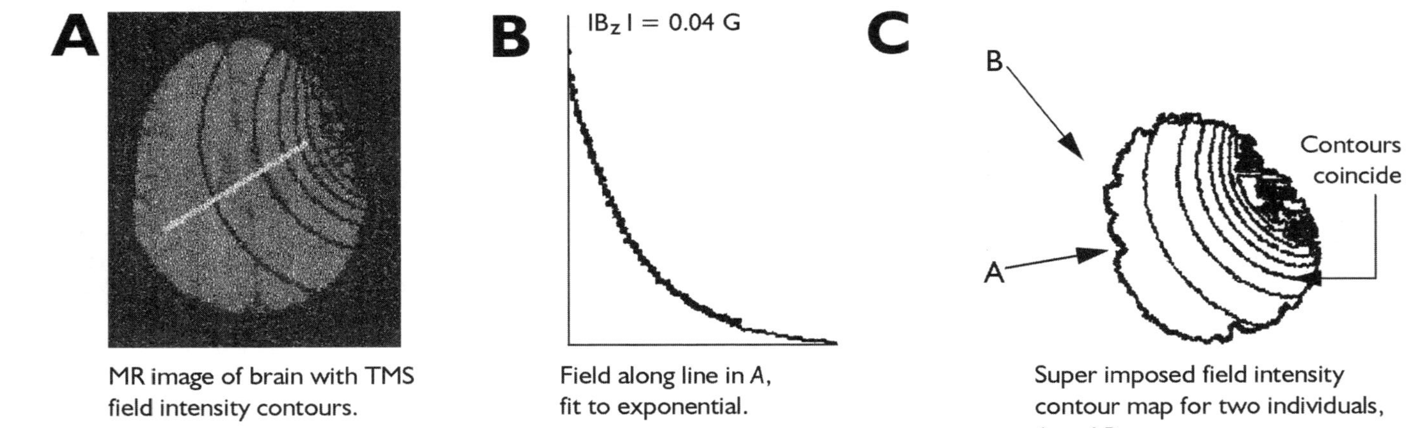

FIGURE 6–10. MRI scanners can be used to measure the magnetic fields produced by TMS. (A) Phase map of brain activity in a figure-eight butterfly coil placed over the left prefrontal cortex of a healthy volunteer. Note the waves of magnetic field produced by the coil as they intersected the cortical tissue below. (B) Field along the white line in A, fit to the exponential. The magnetic field strength of the coil along the white line in A decreased logarithmically with increased distance from the coil. (C) Superimposed field-intensity contour maps for two individuals, A and B. Because magnetic fields are not distorted by brains, the maps exactly overlap. Abbreviations: G=gauss; MR=magnetic resonance.

Source. Reprinted from Bohning DE, Pecheny AP, Epstein CM, et al.: "Mapping Transcranial Magnetic Stimulation (TMS) Fields In Vivo With MRI." *NeuroReport* 8:2535–2538, 1997.

Use of Repetitive TMS to Improve Mood in Depressed Patients

Converging evidence from SPECT, PET, and quantitative EEG studies points to hypofunction of the left prefrontal cortex in clinical depression (discussed earlier). Having considered these imaging studies, as well as studies of effects of rTMS on mood in healthy control subjects and other initial pilot treatment studies (Hoflich et al. 1993; Grisaru et al. 1994; Kolbinger et al. 1995), we wondered whether daily prefrontal rTMS could improve mood in depressed subjects (George and Wassermann 1994). We sought to determine whether stimulating subconvulsively over the prefrontal cortex would produce an antidepressant effect. We initially studied the immediate effect of right versus left prefrontal rTMS in patients with drug-resistant depression. Right prefrontal stimulation resulted in marked increases of anxiety and worsening mood. We therefore performed daily left prefrontal rTMS in six inpatients with depression that was highly drug resistant. Depression scores significantly improved for the group as a whole (Hamilton Rating Scale for Depression scores decreased from 23.8 ± 4.2 [mean ± SD]) at baseline to 17.5 ± 8.4 after treatment; $t=3.03$, 5 *df*, $P<0.02$, two-tailed paired *t* test). Two subjects showed robust mood improvement, which occurred progressively over several weeks. In one subject, depression symptoms completely remitted for the first time in 3 years. We concluded that daily left prefrontal rTMS is safe and well tolerated and might alleviate depression (George et al. 1995b).

Pascual-Leone and colleagues (1996a) next used a double-blind, placebo-controlled design and reported that left prefrontal rTMS for 5 days (90% MT, 10 Hz for 10 seconds, 1-minute rest, 20 times each morning, 2,000 stimuli per morning, 10,000 stimuli per site, a total of 40,000 per subject) significantly improved mood in 17 psychotically depressed subjects (Table 6–1). Other sites (e.g., right prefrontal and occipital sites) had no effects. rTMS even at these high doses and with these numbers of stimuli was well tolerated.

Immediately after completing our open study involving inpatients with medication-refractory depression, we undertook a double-blind, placebo-controlled crossover study of daily left prefrontal rTMS in depressed outpatients (80% MT, 20 Hz for 2 seconds, 1-minute rest, 200 times per day, 800 stimuli per morning, 8,000 stimuli per site) (George et al. 1997). There was a significant improvement in mood with TMS treatment (Figure 6–11), although the magnitude of change was not nearly as profound as in the Spanish study (Pascual-Leone et al. 1996a).

MUSC is currently engaged in a National Alliance for Research in Schizophrenia and Depression (NARSAD)-funded, parallel-design, double-blind

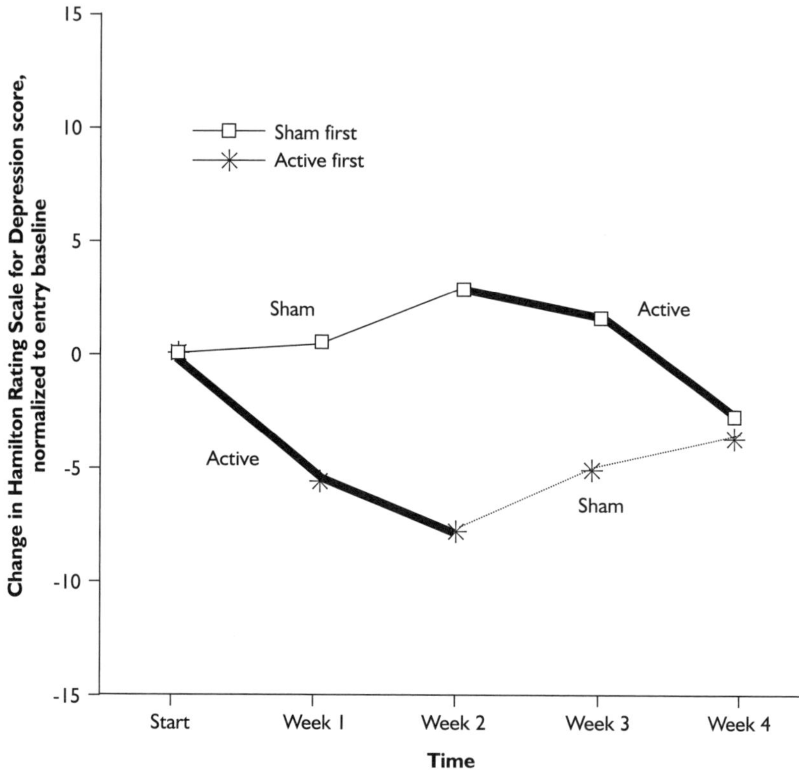

FIGURE 6–11. Changes in Hamilton Rating Scale for Depression scores with active and sham left prefrontal repetitive transcranial magnetic stimulation. Active, but not sham, stimulation significantly improved mood in 12 clinically depressed adults (two-tailed paired t test, $t=2.8$, $P<0.01$).
Source. Reprinted from George MS, Wassermann EM, Kimbrell TA, et al.: "Mood Improvement Following Daily Left Prefrontal Repetitive Transcranial Magnetic Stimulation in Patients With Depression: A Placebo-Controlled Crossover Trial." *American Journal of Psychiatry* 154:1752–1756, 1997.

study of the effects of placebo, high-frequency (20 Hz) left prefrontal stimulation, and low-frequency (5 Hz) left prefrontal stimulation on depression in outpatients (George et al., in press). Many groups in the United States and elsewhere using rTMS to understand depression formed a loose coalition at a recent rTMS safety conference in Bethesda, Maryland, maintained through an e-mail group server, and are exploring the rTMS parameters (location, intensity, frequency, dosing schedules, and diagnostic groups) in rTMS treatment trials. It is unclear what clinical role rTMS might have, if any, in the treatment of depression. Further study of normal mood regulation and how TMS affects these areas appears to be crucial for further advancement.

■ Conclusion

Advances in magnetic field technology have opened up new ways of understanding brain function. Perfusion fMRI offers the promise of using functional neuroimaging in a serial and longitudinal manner to understand the dynamic nature of neuropsychiatric diseases. Advances in the field of TMS offer the potential of going beyond functional neuroimaging to direct testing of hypotheses generated in functional neuroimaging studies. Improvements in TMS coil design, as well as active work in integrating fMRI and TMS, will likely open up new fields in biological psychiatry.

■ References

Amassian VE, Eberle L, Maccabee PJ, et al: Modelling magnetic coil excitation of human cerebral cortex with a peripheral nerve immersed in a brain-shaped volume conductor: the significance of fiber bending in excitation. Electroencephalogr Clin Neurophysiol 85:291–301, 1992

Artola A, Brocher S, Singer W: Different voltage dependent thresholds for inducing long-term depression and long-term potentiation in slices of rat visual cortex. Nature 347:69–72, 1990

Austin MP, Dougall N, Ross M, et al: Single photon emission tomography with ^{99m}Tc-exametazime in major depression and the pattern of brain activity underlying the psychotic/neurotic continuum. J Affect Disord 26:31–43, 1992

Barker AT, Jalinous R, Freeston IL: Non-invasive magnetic stimulation of the human motor cortex. Lancet 1:1106–1107, 1985

Baxter LR Jr, Phelps ME, Mazziotta JC, et al: Cerebral metabolic rates for glucose in mood disorders: studies with positron emission tomography and fluorodeoxyglucose F 18. Arch Gen Psychiatry 42:441–447, 1985

Baxter LR Jr, Schwartz JM, Phelps ME, et al: Reduction of prefrontal cortex glucose metabolism common to three types of depression. Arch Gen Psychiatry 46:243–250, 1989

Bench CJ, Friston KJ, Brown RG, et al: The anatomy of melancholia: focal abnormalities of cerebral blood flow in major depression. Psychol Med 22:607–615, 1992

Bench CJ, Friston KJ, Brown RG, et al: Regional cerebral blood flow in depression measured by positron emission tomography: the relationship with clinical dimensions. Psychol Med 23:579–590, 1993

Bohning DE, Wright AC, Pecheny AP, et al: Perfusion phantom for quantitative spin labeling and Gd tracer-based perfusion measurements (abstract). American Association of Physicists in Medicine, 1996a

Bohning DE, Wright AC, Pecheny AP, et al: Repeatability of spin label-based in vivo perfusion maps (abstract). Neuroimage 3:S128, 1996b

Bohning DE, Speer AM, Pecheny AP, et al: Acetazolamide-induced perfusion changes measured with MR spin-labeling (abstract). Neuroimage 5:S380, 1997a

Bohning DE, Epstein CM, Vincent DJ, et al: Deconvolution of transcranial magnetic stimulation (TMS) maps (abstract). Neuroimage 5:S520, 1997b

Bohning DE, Pecheny AP, Epstein CM, et al: In-vivo three dimensional transcranial magnetic stimulation (TMS) field mapping with MRI (abstract). Neuroimage 5:S522, 1997c

Bohning DE, Pecheny AP, Epstein CM, et al: Mapping transcranial magnetic stimulation (TMS) fields in vivo with MRI. Neuroreport 8:2535–2538, 1997d

Bohning DE, Shastri A, McConnell KA, et al: A combined TMS/fMRI study of intensity-dependent TMS over motor cortex. Biol Psychiatry 45:385–394, 1999

Bohning DE, Shastri A, Nahas Z, et al: Echoplanar bold fMRI of brain activation induced by concurrent transcranial magnetic stimulation. Investigative Radiology 33:336–340, 1998

Bohning DE, Shastri A, Wassermann EM, et al: fMRI response to single-pulse transcranial magnetic stimulation (TMS). J Magn Reson Imaging 11:569–574, 2000

Brasil-Neto JP, McShane LM, Fuhr P, et al: Topographic mapping of the human motor cortex with magnetic stimulation: factors affecting accuracy and reproducibility. Electroencephalogr Clin Neurophysiol 85:9–16, 1992

Chen R, Classen J, Gerloff C, et al: Depression of motor cortex excitability by low-frequency transcranial magnetic stimulation. Neurology 48:1398–1403, 1997

Christianson SA, Saisa J, Garvill J, et al: Hemispheric inactivation and mood-state changes. Brain Cogn 23:127–144, 1993

Cohen LG, Roth BJ, Nilsson J, et al: Effects of coil design on delivery of focal magnetic stimulation: technical considerations. Electroencephalogr Clin Neurophysiol 75:350–357, 1990

Davey KR, Cheng CH, Epstein CM: Prediction of magnetically induced electric fields in biologic tissue. IEEE Trans Biomed Eng 38:418–422, 1991

Davidson RJ: Asymmetric brain function, affective style, and psychopathology: the role of early experience and plasticity. Dev Psychopathol 6:741–758, 1994

Denicoff KD, Smithjackson EE, Disney ER, et al: Preliminary evidence of the reliability and validity of the prospective life-chart methodology (LCM-P). J Psychiatr Res 31:593–603, 1997

Drevets WC, Videen TO, Preskorn SH, et al: A functional anatomical study of unipolar depression. J Neurosci 12:3628–3641, 1992

Epstein CM, Schwartzenberg DG, Davey KR, et al: Localizing the site of magnetic brain stimulation in humans. Neurology 40:666–670, 1990

Fox P, Ingham R, George MS, et al: Imaging human intra-cerebral connectivity by PET during TMS. Neuroreport 8:2787–2791, 1997

George MS: Transcranial magnetic stimulation: mapping and modifying brain-behavior relationships. CNS Spectrums: The International Journal of Neuropsychiatric Medicine 2:1–68, 1997

George MS, Belmaker RH (eds): Transcranial Magnetic Stimulation in Neuropsychiatry. Washington, DC, American Psychiatric Press, 2000

George MS, Wassermann EM: Rapid-rate transcranial magnetic stimulation (rTMS) and ECT. Convulsive Therapy 10:251–253, 1994

George MS, Ketter TA, Post RM: SPECT and PET imaging in mood disorders. J Clin Psychiatry 54:6–13, 1993

George MS, Ketter TA, Kimbrell TA, et al: Brain imaging in mania, in Mania. Edited by Goodnick PJ. Washington, DC, American Psychiatric Press, 1994a

George MS, Kellner CH, Bernstein H, et al: An MRI investigation into mood disorders in multiple sclerosis: a pilot study. J Nerv Ment Dis 182:410–412, 1994b

George MS, Ketter TA, Post RM: Prefrontal cortex dysfunction in clinical depression. Depress Anxiety 2:59–72, 1994c

George MS, Ketter TA, Parekh PI, et al: Brain activity during transient sadness and happiness in healthy women. Am J Psychiatry 152:341–351, 1995a

George MS, Wassermann EM, Williams WA, et al: Daily repetitive transcranial magnetic stimulation (rTMS) improves mood in depression. Neuroreport 6:1853–1856, 1995b

George MS, Wassermann EM, Williams WA, et al: Changes in mood and hormone levels after rapid-rate transcranial magnetic stimulation (rTMS) of the prefrontal cortex. J Neuropsychiatry Clin Neurosci 8:172–180, 1996a

George MS, Wassermann EM, Post RM: Transcranial magnetic stimulation: a neuropsychiatric tool for the 21st century. J Neuropsychiatry Clin Neurosci 8:373–382, 1996b

George MS, Parekh PI, Rosinsky N, et al: Understanding emotional prosody activates right hemisphere regions. Arch Neurol 53:665–670, 1996c

George MS, Ketter TA, Post RM: What functional imaging studies have revealed about the brain basis of mood and emotion, in Advances in Biological Psychiatry. Edited by Panksepp J. Greenwich, CT, JAI Press, 1996d, pp 63–113

George MS, Wassermann EM, Kimbrell TA, et al: Mood improvement following daily left prefrontal repetitive transcranial magnetic stimulation in patients with depression: a placebo-controlled crossover trial. Am J Psychiatry 154:1752–1756, 1997

George MS, Nahas Z, Speer AM, et al: A controlled trial of daily transcranial magnetic stimulations (TMS) of the left prefrontal cortex for treating depression. Biological Psychiatry (in press)

George MS, Jones M, Post RM, et al: Chaos theory as an aid to understanding the longitudinal course of affective illness. Psychiatry Res (in press)

Gottesfeld BH, Lesse SM, Herskovitz H: Studies in electroconvulsive shock therapy of varied electrode applications. J Nerv Ment Dis 99:64, 1944

Greenberg BD, George MS, Martin JD, et al: Effect of prefrontal repetitive transcranial magnetic stimulation in obsessive-compulsive disorder: a preliminary study. Am J Psychiatry 154:867–869, 1997

Grisaru N, Yarovslavsky U, Abarbanel J, et al: Transcranial magnetic stimulation in depression and schizophrenia. Eur Neuropsychopharmacol 4:287–288, 1994

Gustafsson B, Wigstrom H: Physiological mechanisms underlying long-term potentiation. Trends in Neuroscience 11:156–162, 1988

Hamilton M: A rating scale for depression. J Neurol Neurosurg Psychiatry 23:56–62, 1960

Hoflich G, Kasper S, Hufnagel A, et al: Application of transcranial magnetic stimulation in treatment of drug-resistant major depression: a report of two cases. Human Psychopharmacology 8:361–365, 1993

House A, Dennis M, Warlow C, et al: Mood disorders after stroke and their relation to lesion location. Brain 113:1113–1129, 1990

Iriki A, Pavlides C, Keller A, et al: Long-term potentiation of thalamic input to the motor cortex induced by coactivation of thalamocortical and corticocortical afferents. J Neurophysiology 65:1435–1441, 1991

Jennum P, Friberg L, Fuglsang-Frederiksen A, et al: Speech localization using repetitive transcranial magnetic stimulation. Neurology 44:269–273, 1994

Ketter TA, George MS, Andreason PJ, et al: CMRglu in unipolar versus bipolar depression, in 1994 New Research Program and Abstracts, American Psychiatric Association 147th Annual Meeting, Philadelphia, PA, May 21–26, 1994. Washington, DC, American Psychiatric Association, 1994a

Ketter TA, George MS, Andreason PJ, et al: Depression and frontal regional cerebral metabolic rates of glucose correlate inversely (NR443), in 1994 New Research Program and Abstracts, American Psychiatric Association 147th Annual Meeting, Philadelphia, PA, May 21–26, 1994. Washington, DC, American Psychiatric Association, 1994b, p 171

Ketter TA, George MS, Kimbrell TA, et al: Functional brain imaging, limbic function, and affective disorders. The Neuroscientist 2:55–65, 1996

Kimbrell TA, Ketter TA, George MS, et al: Brain glucose metabolism in remitted mood disorder patients as measured by PET FDG, in 1994 New Research Program and Abstracts, American Psychiatric Association 149th Annual Meeting, New York, May 4–9, 1996. Washington, DC, American Psychiatric Association, 1996

Kolbinger HM, Hoflich G, Hufnagel A, et al: Transcranial magnetic stimulation (TMS) in the treatment of major depression: a pilot study. Human Psychopharmacology 10:305–310, 1995

Martin JD, George MS, Greenberg BD, et al: Mood effects of prefrontal repetitive high-frequency TMS in healthy volunteers. CNS Spectrums: The International Journal of Neuropsychiatric Medicine 2:53–68, 1997

Mathew RJ, Meyer JS, Francis DJ, et al: Cerebral blood flow in depression. Am J Psychiatry 137:1449–1450, 1980

Mayberg HS, Lewis PJ, Regenold W, et al: Paralimbic hypoperfusion in unipolar depression. J Nucl Med 35:929–934, 1994

Migliorelli R, Starkstein SE, Teson A, et al: SPECT findings in patients with primary mania. J Neuropsychiatry Clin Neurosci 5:379–383, 1993

Murro A, Smith JR, King DW, et al: A model for focal magnetic brain stimulation. Int J Biomed Comput 31:37–43, 1992

Nobler MS, Sackeim HA, Prohovnik I, et al: Regional cerebral blood flow in mood disorders, III: treatment and clinical response. Arch Gen Psychiatry 51:884–897, 1994

Pardo JV, Pardo PJ, Raichle ME: Neural correlates of self-induced dysphoria. Am J Psychiatry 150:713–719, 1993

Pascual-Leone A, Gates JR, Dhuna A: Induction of speech arrest and counting errors with rapid-rate transcranial magnetic stimulation. Neurology 41:697–702, 1991

Pascual-Leone A, Grafman J, Hallett M: Modulation of cortical motor output maps during development of implicit and explicit knowledge. Science 263:1287–1289, 1994a

Pascual-Leone A, Valls-Sole J, Wassermann EM, et al: Responses to rapid-rate transcranial magnetic stimulation of the human motor cortex. Brain 117:847–858, 1994b

Pascual-Leone A, Cammarota A, Wassermann EM, et al: Modulation of motor cortical outputs to the reading hand of braille readers. Ann Neurol 34:33–37, 1995

Pascual-Leone A, Rubio B, Pallardo F, et al: Beneficial effect of rapid-rate transcranial magnetic stimulation of the left dorsolateral prefrontal cortex in drug-resistant depression. Lancet 348:233–237, 1996a

Pascual-Leone A, Catala MD, Pascual AP: Lateralized effect of rapid-rate transcranial magnetic stimulation of the prefrontal cortex on mood. Neurology 46:499–502, 1996b

Paus T, Jech R, Thompson CJ, et al: Transcranial magnetic stimulation during positron emission tomography: a new method for studying connectivity of the human cerebral cortex. J Neurosci 17:3178–3184, 1997

Post RM, DeLisi LE, Holcomb HH, et al: Glucose utilization in the temporal cortex of affectively ill patients: positron emission tomography. Biol Psychiatry 22:545–553, 1987

Post RM, George MS, Ketter TA, et al: Mechanisms underlying recurrence and cycle acceleration in affective disorders: implications for long-term treatment, in Psychopharmacology of Depression. Edited by Montgomery S. London, Oxford University Press, 1994, pp 141–169

Roberts DR, Vincent DJ, Speer AM, et al: Multi-modality mapping of motor cortex: comparing echoplanar BOLD fMRI and transcranial magnetic stimulation. J Neural Transm 104:833–843, 1997

Robinson RG, Szetela B: Mood change following left hemisphere brain injury. Ann Neurol 9:447–453, 1981

Robinson RG, Kubos KL, Starr LB, et al: Mood disorders in stroke patients: importance of location of lesion. Brain 107 (part 1):81–93, 1984

Robinson RG, Boston JD, Starkstein SE, et al: Comparison of mania and depression after brain injury: causal factors. Am J Psychiatry 145:172–178, 1988

Robinson RG, Morris PLP, Fedoroff JP: Depression and cerebrovascular disease. J Clin Psychiatry 51:26–31, 1990

Ross ED, Homan RW, Buck R: Differential hemispheric lateralization of primary and social emotions: implications for developing a comprehensive neurology for emotions, repression and the subconscious. Neuropsychiatry Neuropsychol Behav Neurol 7:1–19, 1994

Roth BJ, Cohen LG, Hallett M: The electric field induced during magnetic stimulation, in Magnetic Motor Stimulation: Basic Principles and Clinical Experience (EEG Suppl 43). Edited by Lecy WJ, Cracco RQ, Barker AT, et al. Amsterdam, Elsevier Science, pp 268–278, 1991a

Roth BJ, Saypol JM, Hallett M, et al: A theoretical calculation of the electric field induced in the cortex during magnetic stimulation. Electroencephalogr Clin Neurophysiol 81:47–56, 1991b

Rothwell JC, Thompson PD, Day BL, et al: Stimulation of the human motor cortex through the scalp. Exp Physiol 76:159–200, 1991

Rubin E, Sackeim HA, Prohovnik I, et al: Regional cerebral blood flow in mood disorders, IV: comparison of mania and depression. Psychiatry Res 61:1–10, 1995

Rudiak D, Marg E: Finding the depth of magnetic brain stimulation: a re-evaluation. Electroencephalogr Clin Neurophysiol 93:358–371, 1994

Sackeim HA: Emotion, disorders of mood, and hemispheric functional specialization, in Psychopathology and the Brain. Edited by Carroll BJ, Barrett JE. New York, Raven, 209–242, 1991

Sackeim HA, Gur RC: Lateral asymmetry in intensity of emotional expression. Neuropsychologia 163:473–481, 1978

Sackeim HA, Prohovnik I: Brain imaging studies of depressive disorders, in The Biology of Depressive Disorders. Edited by Mann JJ, Kupfer DJ. New York, Plenum, 1993

Sackeim HA, Gur RC, Saucy MC: Emotions are expressed more intensely on the left side of the face. Science 202:434–436, 1978

Sackeim HA, Greenberg MS, Weiman AL, et al: Hemispheric asymmetry in the expression of positive and negative emotions: neurologic evidence. Arch Neurol 39:210–218, 1982

Sastry BR, Goh JW, Auyeung A: Associative induction of posttetanic and long-term potentiation in CA1 neurons of rat hippocampus. Science 232:988–990, 1986

Saypol JM, Roth BJ, Cohen LG, et al: A theoretical comparison of electric and magnetic stimulation of the brain. Ann Biomed Eng 19:317–328, 1991

Schwartz JM, Baxter LR Jr, Mazziotta JC, et al: The differential diagnosis of depression: relevance of positron emission tomography studies of cerebral glucose metabolism to the bipolar-unipolar dichotomy. JAMA 258:1368–1374, 1987

Schwarzbauer C, Morrisey SP, Haase A: Quantitative magnetic resonance imaging of perfusion using magnetic labeling of water proton spins within the detection slice. Magn Reson Med 35:540–546, 1996

Sharpe M, Hawton K, House A, et al: Mood disorders in long-term survivors of stroke: associations with brain lesion location and volume. Psychol Med 20:815–828, 1990

Sil'kis IG, Rapoport SSh, Veber NV, et al: Neurobiology of the integrative activity of the brain: some properties of long-term posttetanic heterosynaptic depression in the motor cortex of the cat. Neurosci Behav Physiol 24:500–506, 1994

Squillace K, Post RM, Savard R, et al: Life charting of the longitudinal course of recurrent affective illness, in Neurobiology of Mood Disorders. Edited by Post RM, Ballenger JC. Baltimore, MD, Williams & Wilkins, 1984, pp 38–59

Stallings LE, Speer AM, Spicer KM, et al: Combining SPECT and repetitive transcranial magnetic stimulation (rTMS): left prefrontal stimulation decreases relative perfusion locally in a dose dependent manner (abstract). Neuroimage 5:S521, 1997

Stanton PK, Sejnowski TJ: Associative long-term depression in the hippocampus induced by hebbian covariance. Nature 339:215–218, 1989

Starkstein SE, Pearlson GD, Boston J, et al: Mania after brain injury: a controlled study of causative factors. Arch Neurol 44:1069–1073, 1987

Starkstein SE, Boston JD, Robinson RG: Mechanisms of mania after brain injury: 12 case reports and review of the literature. J Nerv Ment Dis 176:87–100, 1988

Starkstein SE, Robinson RG, Honig MA, et al: Mood changes after right-hemisphere lesions. Br J Psychiatry 155:79–85, 1989

Starkstein SE, Mayberg HS, Berthier ML, et al: Mania after brain injury: neuroradiological and metabolic findings. Ann Neurol 27:652–659, 1990

Starkstein SE, Fedoroff P, Berthier ML, et al: Manic-depressive and pure manic states after brain lesions. Biol Psychiatry 29:149–158, 1991

Valls-Sole J, Pascual-Leone A, Wassermann EM, et al: Human motor evoked responses to paired transcranial magnetic stimuli. Electroencephalogr Clin Neurophysiol 85:355–364, 1992

Wada J, Rasmussen T: Intracarotid injection of sodium Amytal for the lateralization of cerebral speech dominance: experimental and clinical observations. J Neurosurg 17:266–282, 1960

Wassermann EM, McShane LM, Hallett M, et al: Noninvasive mapping of muscle representations in human motor cortex. Electroencephalogr Clin Neurophysiol 85:1–8, 1992

Wasserman E, Wang BS, Zeffiro TA, et al: Locating the motor cortex on the MRI with transcranial magnetic stimulation. Neuroimage 3:1–9, 1996

Wassermann EM, Kimbrell TA, George MS, et al: Local and distant changes in cerebral glucose metabolism during repetitive transcranial magnetic stimulation (rTMS) (abstract). Neurology 48:A107-P02.049, 1997

Weiss SRB, Li XL, Rosen JB, et al: Quenching: inhibition of development and expression of amygdala kindled seizures with low frequency stimulation. Neuroreport 6:2171–2176, 1995

Weissman JD, Epstein CM, Davey KR: Magnetic brain stimulation and brain size: relevance to animal studies. Electroencephalogr Clin Neurophysiol 85:215–219, 1992

Wilson SA, Thickbroom GW, Mastaglia FL: Transcranial magnetic stimulation mapping of the motor cortex in normal subjects: the representation of two intrinsic hand muscles. J Neurol Sci 118:134–144, 1993

Ye FQ, Pejar JJ, Jezzard P, et al: Perfusion imaging of the human brain at 1.5 T using a single-shot EPI spin tagging approach. Magn Reson Med 36:219–224, 1996

Young RC, Biggs JT, Ziegler VE, et al: A rating scale for mania: reliability, validity, and sensitivity. Br J Psychiatry 133:429–435, 1978

7

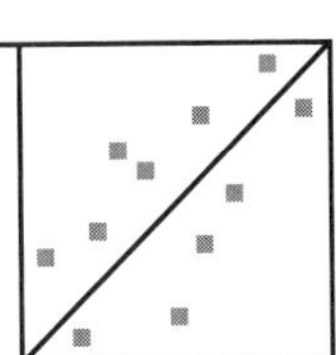

NEUROIMAGING STUDIES OF TREATMENT RESPONSE

The Example of Major Depression

Darin D. Dougherty, M.D., M.Sc.
Helen S. Mayberg, M.D., F.R.C.P.C.

The ultimate goals of all psychiatric research are better diagnosis of psychiatric illnesses and better treatment of individuals with these illnesses. Although structural and functional neuroimaging studies have contributed a great deal to our understanding of the pathophysiology of various psychiatric illnesses, few neuroimaging studies have focused on issues of treatment response. In this chapter, we review neuroimaging studies of treatment response in depression and discuss strategic issues to consider when performing these studies. Although the focus of the chapter is on neuroimaging studies of treatment response, we begin by briefly reviewing findings from a variety of neuroimaging studies involving subjects with mood disorders. Taken together, these data suggest a critical role for the anterior cingulate cortex in the pathophysiology of major depression. Moreover, neuroimaging studies of treatment response in subjects with major depression demonstrate that the baseline metabolic rate in the anterior cingulate cortex is a significant predictor of treatment response. After this review of specific findings, we conclude with a general discussion of neuroimaging studies of treatment response.

■ Neuroimaging Studies of Major Depression

Structural Neuroimaging Studies

Structural neuroimaging findings in major depression (for a review, see Soares and Mann 1997) include focal white matter hyperintensities in regions associated with the frontal cortex and basal ganglia. In addition, findings from morphometric magnetic resonance imaging studies include decreased bilateral frontal volumes in patients with unipolar depression (Coffey et al. 1993) and decreased bilateral caudate and putamen volumes in patients with depressive disorder (Husain et al. 1991; Krishnan et al. 1992). These findings are consistent with findings from lesion-induced-deficit studies of secondary depression (most notably, poststroke depression and depression associated with Parkinson's disease and Huntington's disease) showing a strong correlation between depressive symptoms and lesions of the frontal lobes and basal ganglia (Lauterbach et al. 1997; Morris et al. 1996; Robinson 1979; Robinson et al. 1984, 1988; Starkstein et al. 1987, 1988, 1990).

Functional Neuroimaging Studies

Approximately 40 neutral-state functional neuroimaging studies of affective disorder have been completed to date, and the results have been reviewed elsewhere (Dougherty and Rauch 1997). It is difficult to conclusively integrate the findings from this large number of studies because of methodological differences; techniques have included both single photon emission computed tomography and positron emission tomography (PET) using a variety of tracers and using instruments with various degrees of sensitivity and spatial resolution. Despite these methodological differences, consistent findings include decreased global metabolism with specific decreases in the frontal regions (most consistently the prefrontal cortex), basal ganglia, and cingulate cortex. Overall, neutral-state functional imaging studies have demonstrated abnormal regional cerebral blood flow (rCBF) or metabolism in components of the basal ganglia–thalamocortical circuitry postulated to mediate mood regulation and cognition (Alexander et al. 1986, 1990).

Symptom Provocation Studies to Elucidate Limbic Function in Health and Disease

Healthy Volunteers

Numerous investigations using emotion-induction paradigms in healthy control subjects have furthered our understanding of the normal functional neuroanatomy of emotions such as happiness, sadness, anger, guilt, sexual arousal, and disgust (Dougherty et al. 1999; George et al. 1995, 1996; Lane et al. 1997; Paradiso et al. 1997; Pardo et al. 1993; Phillips et al. 1997; Rauch et al. 1999;

Reimen et al. 1997; Schneider et al. 1994, 1995; Shin et al. 2000). These investigations have consistently demonstrated that activation of anterior paralimbic structures is associated with sadness in healthy control subjects. In particular, the orbitofrontal cortex, medial prefrontal cortex, anterior cingulate cortex, insular cortex, and anterior temporal poles were activated in these studies. In one study, in which healthy control subjects performed a verbal fluency task during induced elated and depressed mood states, investigators observed an attenuation of anterior cingulate cortex activation that was specific to depressed mood (Baker et al. 1997). More recent studies of normal sadness found both limbic and paralimbic activation and cortical (predominantly in prefrontal regions) deactivation that anatomically overlap changes seen in neutral-state studies involving depressed patients (Gemar et al. 1996; Mayberg et al. 1999).

Subjects With Major Depression

Symptom provocation techniques have also been used to induce emotional states in patients with anxiety disorders (see, for example, Rauch et al. 1994, 1995, 1996), and, more recently, comparable studies involving subjects with affective disorders have been performed. Three studies of sadness induction involving patients with either active or remitted major depression revealed differences between patients and healthy control subjects, as well as differences between actively depressed patients and patients with remitted depression, with disease-specific effects involving anterior paralimbic regions (Beauregard et al. 1998; Liotti et al. 1997; Mayberg et al. 1998). Although the precise localization of changes varies somewhat across studies, there is unequivocal evidence of anterior cingulate cortex and prefrontal dysfunction in different depressed states. This evidence suggests that more detailed probes of these areas could prove valuable in differentiating anterior paralimbic function in depressed patients and control subjects. To this end, one study used a Stroop interference paradigm to demonstrate that subjects with mood disorder have blunted anterior cingulate cortex activation during performance of this task, compared with control subjects (George et al. 1997). This general strategy has also been used to study prefrontal regions (i.e., tests of verbal fluency and perceptual motor performance have been administered) (Baker et al. 1997; Dolan et al. 1992; Elliott et al. 1997).

Treatment Studies in Subjects With Major Depression

Numerous functional neuroimaging studies have been conducted in depressed subjects before and after treatment. Studies of some treatments—namely, sleep deprivation (Ebert et al. 1991, 1994; Wu et al. 1992) and light therapy in subjects with seasonal affective disorder (Cohen et al. 1992)—failed to demonstrate differences in rCBF before and after treatment, despite clinical response in some subjects. However, one of these studies did find that responders to sleep deprivation showed decreased basal ganglia dopamine D_2 receptor occupancy after sleep deprivation when compared with nonresponders (Ebert et al. 1994), suggesting increased synaptic dopamine levels with treatment. Virtually all studies of the acute or subacute response to electroconvulsive therapy (ECT) have demonstrated reductions in rCBF or metabolic rate (Guze et al. 1991; Prohovnik et al. 1986; Rosenberg et al. 1988; Scott et al. 1994; Volkow et al. 1988). In addition, studies of the long-term effects of ECT have also generally demonstrated decreased rCBF or metabolic rate (Nobler et al. 1994; Silfverskiöld and Risberg 1989; Silfverskiöld et al. 1986), although one study did demonstrate increased rCBF after ECT (Bonne et al. 1996). Taken together, these data consistently demonstrate decreased rCBF or metabolic rate after both short- and long-term ECT, with some studies demonstrating global reductions and others preferential frontal lobe reductions.

Seven functional neuroimaging studies have been performed in depressed patients before and after treatment with medication. Five of these studies used measures such as global metabolism and left hemisphere to right hemisphere ratios or corticocerebellar ratios to assess differences before and after treatment: three of these studies demonstrated normalization of baseline cerebral hypometabolism after treatment (Baxter et al. 1989; Kanaya and Yonekawa 1990; Kumar et al. 1991), whereas the other two studies showed continued hypometabolism despite clinical response (Hurwitz et al. 1990; Martinot et al. 1990). Of the remaining two studies, one study used PET and [^{18}F]fluorodeoxyglucose (FDG) to study depressed patients at baseline and after 10 weeks of treatment with sertraline. Use of region-of-interest methods for statistical analyses revealed that the bilateral middle frontal gyrus, which was characterized by decreased metabolic activity at baseline, showed increased activity after treatment (Buchsbaum et al. 1997). In addition, in other areas that showed differences compared with baseline in healthy control subjects, normalization of metabolic activity occurred after treatment with sertraline; these areas included the superior medial frontal lobe, dorsal anterior cingulate gyrus, and thalamus. In particular, a correlation between change in metabolic rate and change in Hamilton Rating Scale for Depression scores indicated that the greater the normalization of the anterior cingulate cortex, the greater the improvement in the sertraline-treated group.

Lastly, one of the seven studies (and the only study to use both statistical parametric and region-of-interest-based data analyses) used PET and FDG to image depressed patients at baseline before treatment with antidepressants

(Mayberg et al. 1997). In this study, pretreatment PET data from the depressed patients were grouped according to response or nonresponse after treatment with an antidepressant. These investigators found baseline hypermetabolism in the rostral cingulate cortex in the patient group that responded to treatment with antidepressants (Figure 7–1). The authors postulated that an adaptive hypermetabolic change in the rostral cingulate cortex may be required for positive response to treatment.

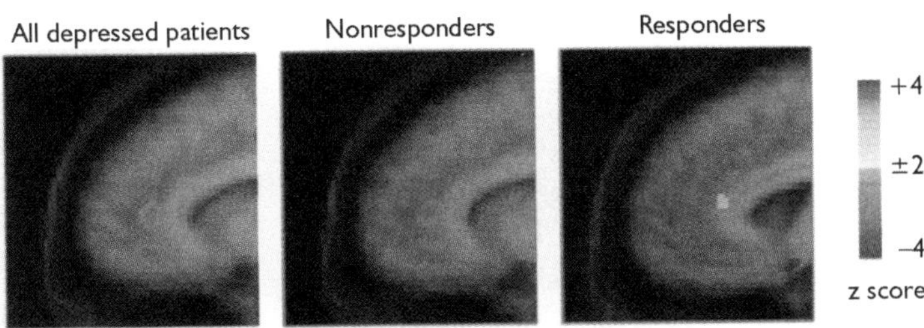

FIGURE 7–1. Superimposed sagittal positron emission tomography scans and magnetic resonance images. These z-score maps demonstrate differences in direction, magnitude, and extent of changes seen in rostral cingulate cortex glucose metabolism (BA 24a/b) in three groups of depressed patients compared with healthy control subjects. Cingulate cortex hypometabolism (negative z-scores, shown in green) characterized the nonresponder group, in contrast to hypermetabolism (positive z-scores, shown in yellow) seen in the patients who eventually responded to treatment. BA=Brodmann's area.
Source. Reprinted from Mayberg HS, Brannan SK, Mahurin RK, et al.: "Cingulate Function in Depression: A Potential Predictor of Treatment Response." *NeuroReport* 8:1057–1061, 1997. Used with permission.

Synthesis of Data From Neuroimaging Studies of Major Depression

Taken together, the existing neuroimaging data implicate components of basal ganglia–thalamocortical circuitry in the pathophysiology of major depression. Neutral-state studies consistently demonstrate abnormalities in the prefrontal cortex and basal ganglia in depressed subjects compared with healthy control subjects. Activation studies in healthy volunteers have allowed investigators to begin determining which regions of the limbic and paralimbic systems are involved in the mediating neuroanatomy of normal emotional processing. Although these paradigms have not yet been used extensively for probing limbic and paralimbic function in subjects with major depression, the studies that have sought to induce sadness in subjects with major depression have shown differences in activation of anterior paralimbic regions (i.e., the medial prefrontal cortex and anterior cingulate cortex) in depressed subjects compared with healthy control subjects (Beauregard et al. 1998; Liotti et al. 1997; Mayberg et al. 1998). These findings converge with results from neuroimaging studies of treatment response in major depression (Mayberg et al. 1999). As described in the previous section, two of the treatment studies used PET and either statistical parametric mapping or region-of-interest methods for data analyses. One study found normalization of metabolic activity in the bilateral middle frontal gyrus and medial frontal lobe after treatment (Buchsbaum et al. 1997), and findings from both studies suggest that the anterior cingulate cortex plays a role in antidepressant treatment response (Buchsbaum et al. 1997; Mayberg et al. 1997). This convergence of findings provides strong evidence of a central role for the anterior cingulate cortex in the pathophysiology of major depression (Ebert and Ebmeier 1996; Mayberg 1997).

Treatment Response Paradigms in Neuroimaging Research

The examples given earlier demonstrate how treatment response neuroimaging studies, combined with other paradigms, can contribute to an understanding of pathophysiology and perhaps provide predictors of treatment response, while offering clues to the mechanism of effective therapies. The two general types of treatment response neuroimaging studies are pretreatment studies and pretreatment-posttreatment studies. In pretreatment studies, subjects are imaged before treatment and the data obtained are analyzed in light of clinical response or nonresponse or correlated with clinical rating scale results. In pretreatment-posttreatment studies, subjects are imaged before and after treatment. Although both approaches may reveal predictors of response from pretreatment data, only pretreatment-posttreatment studies can elucidate changes in brain activity within individuals after treatment. In this section, we discuss issues specific to each of these approaches, but first we address general issues that apply to both approaches.

General Issues

As in any research study, proper phenotyping of subjects at the time of enrollment is crucial to obtaining valid results. Each psychiatric diagnosis has possible alternative diagnoses, subtypes, and specifiers that contribute to clinical heterogeneity. It is possible that these differences in clinical presentation may correspond with differences in brain function. For example, studies involving depressed patients may include subjects with unipolar depression or bipolar depression. Subjects may have characteristics of a subtype of depression, such as atypical depression or melancholic depression. In addition, specifiers such as with or without psychotic features or single episode or recurrent episodes also substantially differentiate subjects with the same core diagnosis. Thus, diligent phenotyping of subjects, subsequent selection of subjects within as narrow a diagnostic category as possible, and selection of subjects with minimal or no comorbid illness will all maximize the interpretability of the study results.

Concurrent pharmacotherapy can confound results of treatment response neuroimaging studies because such therapy likely has an additive biological effect. Ideally, subjects will all be medication free at the time of the study and all subjects will be administered the same treatment at relatively equivalent doses. These considerations will also maximize the interpretability of the study results.

Pretreatment Studies

The use of neuroimaging studies to determine predictors of response typically involves acquisition of baseline imaging data followed by a treatment intervention. At the end of the clinical trial, the baseline imaging data can be correlated with clinical response or nonresponse. An advantage of this approach is that a second scan is not required. Also, because the baseline scan is performed before the clinical trial, the therapeutic intervention will not have an effect on the imaging data. However, less information is available regarding the therapeutic intervention's mechanism of action.

The data are generally analyzed using one of two methods. One method involves a categorical approach whereby subjects are categorized as responders or nonresponders after the clinical trial. In this case, constructing group images from the imaging data and comparing the group images of the responders to those of the nonresponders may provide information regarding differences in baseline rCBF or glucose metabolism that differentiate the two groups. The other method involves covariate analyses of changes in clinical rating scale data with baseline rCBF or glucose metabolism. The use of continuous measures may elucidate more subtle predictors of response than may analyses by categorical designation (e.g., responders or nonresponders). In addition, the use of continuous measures obviates the need for an arbitrary definition of "responder." Testing for confounding mediating variables is important, however, because imaging data may appear to correlate with clinical response but actually correlate with a variable that is only partially involved or not involved in clinical response.

Pretreatment-Posttreatment Studies

Pretreatment-posttreatment neuroimaging studies typically involve baseline acquisition of imaging data followed by treatment and one or more follow-up acquisitions of imaging data. This study design is especially useful for exploring the brain changes associated with treatment response. In addition, the baseline imaging data can be correlated with clinical response to elucidate predictors of clinical response, as in pretreatment studies. A disadvantage of this study design is the necessity of repeated acquisition of imaging data. Some subjects may be lost to follow-up, or, depending on the imaging modality, greater exposure to radiation may be required.

Data may be analyzed in many ways. First, *baseline imaging data* from depressed patients and control subjects may be compared using data analytic methods such as statistical parametric mapping. In this way, baseline differences in rCBF or glucose metabolism between the two cohorts can be elucidated. Such data may inform hypotheses of the pathophysiology of major depression. It is presumed that the chosen treatment, if effective, will correct some or all of these baseline differences.

On completion of the study, summed images of depressed patients' *posttreatment scans* may be contrasted with summed pretreatment images to quantify changes in rCBF or glucose metabolism after treatment. Additionally, comparison of the depressed patients' posttreatment imaging data with the imaging data from healthy control subjects may provide information regarding the degree of "normalization" after treatment. Although the depressed patients' posttreatment data would ideally be compared with posttreatment data from a healthy control cohort, ethical concerns often preclude the collection of such data.

The *clinical data* generated from the clinical trial portion of the study can also be used in the final data analyses. Covariate analyses of the change in rating scale scores with baseline imaging data, posttreatment imaging data, and/or the differences in baseline and posttreatment imaging data can be performed. In addition to covariate analyses with continuous clinical rating scale measures, categorical division of the depressed patients' posttreatment imaging data into responders and nonresponders may help elucidate which functional changes most predict clinical response.

There are many issues to consider when designing pretreatment-posttreatment neuroimaging studies. Determining the interval between imaging data acquisition periods may be critical. Although it is possible that some functional changes may occur with only one dose of medication, clinical experience has shown that these changes are not likely to result in clinical response. Generally, the interval between pretreatment and posttreatment imaging studies should be informed by the time that the therapeutic intervention in question typically requires for clinical response. Also, patients may derive clinical benefit from different doses of the same medication or a different number of sessions of ECT, and these factors must be taken into account in the experimental design.

When designing pretreatment-posttreatment neuroimaging studies that involve medication, researchers must also decide whether subjects should be taking the medication at the time of one or both scans. The three basic choices are the following: patients are not taking medication at the time of either scan (Off-Off paradigm), patients are not taking medication at the time of the initial scan but are taking medication at the time of the follow-up scan (Off-On paradigm), and patients are taking medication during both scans (On-On paradigm). Although few pretreatment-posttreatment neuroimaging studies have been performed, those reported in the literature typically used the Off-On paradigm. A major advantage of this paradigm is that the baseline scan is not confounded by any existing treatment. However, because the patients are taking psychotropic medication at the time of the follow-up scan, it may be difficult to ascertain whether changes in rCBF or glucose metabolism are due to chronic treatment with the medication or whether these changes may be present after even one dose of the medication. Analyses targeting drug effects, response effects, and drug-response interactions can help to dissociate these issues (Mayberg et al. 2000).

In the Off-Off design, the confound of medication effect is removed. The baseline scan is not influenced by medication effects. The follow-up scan may be performed after the clinical trial and a sufficient washout period. In this manner, the follow-up scan data are not influenced by acute medication effects. However, the washout period for most antidepressant medications is 2–4 weeks. During this time, some patients may have a recurrence of symptoms. This fact raises ethical issues: placing a patient at a higher risk for relapse is contrary to the concept of treatment of the individual patient and general good clinical practice. Furthermore, if the subject has a recurrence of symptoms, the follow-up scan may not capture imaging data during true remission.

The On-On design typically includes an initial scan when the medication has just reached steady state but treatment has not yet led to a clinical response. The follow-up scan is then performed at the end of the clinical trial while the patient is still taking the medication. The interval between the patient's most recent dose of medication and the scan should be comparable for both scans. This design removes the confound of acute medication effects on brain function. Analyses of the differences between the scans should then yield information regarding the chronic beneficial effects of the medication (Mayberg et al. 2000).

■ SUMMARY

Although neutral-state functional neuroimaging studies have increased our understanding regarding the pathophysiology of major depression, studies that involve state manipulations (see Chapters 2–6 in this volume) may provide further information. Such interventions may include cognitive activation or symptom provocation paradigms or studies of the effects of acute or chronic pharmacologic treatment. In this chapter, we reviewed issues surrounding functional neuroimaging studies of treatment response. Whereas the ultimate goal of psychiatric research is improved understanding of the pathophysiology as well as treatment of psychiatric illness, the proposed contribution of these studies is the development of tests that will guide case management and thus be of clinical utility.

■ REFERENCES

Alexander GE, DeLong MR, Strick PL: Parallel organization of functionally segregated circuits linking basal ganglia and cortex. Annu Rev Neurosci 9:357–381, 1986

Alexander GE, Crutcher MD, DeLong MR: Basal ganglia-thalamocortical circuits: parallel substrates for motor, oculomotor, "prefrontal" and "limbic" functions. Prog Brain Res 85:119–146, 1990

Baker SC, Frith CD, Dolan RJ: The interaction between mood and cognitive function studied with PET. Psychol Med 27:565–578, 1997

Baxter LR Jr, Schwartz JM, Phelps ME, et al: Reduction of prefrontal cortex glucose metabolism common to three types of depression. Arch Gen Psychiatry 46:243–250, 1989

Beauregard M, Bergman S, Leroux JM, et al: The functional neuroanatomy of major depression: an fMRI study using an emotional activation paradigm. Neuroreport 9:3253–3258, 1998

Benkelfat C, Nordahl TE, Semple WE, et al: Local cerebral glucose metabolic rates in obsessive-compulsive disorder patients treated with clomipramine. Arch Gen Psychiatry 47:840–845, 1990

Bonne O, Krausz Y, Shapira B, et al: Increased cerebral blood flow in depressed patients responding to electroconvulsive therapy. J Nucl Med 37:1075–1080, 1996

Buchsbaum MS, Wu J, Siegel BV, et al: Effect of sertraline on regional metabolic rate in patients with affective disorder. Biol Psychiatry 41:15–22, 1997

Coffey CE, Wilkinson WE, Weiner RD, et al: Quantitative cerebral anatomy in depression: a controlled magnetic resonance imaging study. Arch Gen Psychiatry 50: 7–16, 1993

Cohen RM, Gross MM, Nordahl TE, et al: Preliminary data on the metabolic brain pattern of patients with winter seasonal affective disorder. Arch Gen Psychiatry 49:545–552, 1992

Dolan RJ, Bench CJ, Brown RG, et al: Regional cerebral blood flow abnormalities in depressed patients with cognitive impairment. J Neurol Neurosurg Psychiatry 55:768–773, 1992

Dougherty DD, Rauch SL: Neuroimaging and neurobiological models of depression. Harv Rev Psychiatry 5:138–159, 1997

Dougherty DD, Shin LM, Alpert NM, et al: Anger in healthy men: a PET study using script-driven imagery. Biol Psychiatry 46:466–472, 1999

Ebert D, Ebmeier KP: The role of the cingulate gyrus in depression: from functional anatomy to neurochemistry. Biol Psychiatry 39:1044–1050, 1996

Ebert D, Feistel H, Barocka A: Effects of sleep deprivation on the limbic system and the frontal lobes in affective disorders: a study with Tc-99m-HMPAO SPECT. Psychiatry Res 40:247–251, 1991

Ebert D, Feistel H, Kaschka W, et al: Single photon emission computed tomography assessment of cerebral dopamine D2 receptor blockade in depression before and after sleep deprivation: preliminary results. Biol Psychiatry 35:880–885, 1994

Elliott R, Baker SC, Rogers RD, et al: Prefrontal dysfunction in depressed patients performing a complex planning task: a study using positron emission tomography. Psychol Med 27:931–942, 1997

Gemar MC, Kapur S, Segal ZV, et al: Effects of self-generated sad mood on regional cerebral activity: a PET study in normal subjects. Depression 4:81–88, 1996

George MS, Ketter TA, Parekh PI, et al: Brain activity during transient sadness and happiness in healthy women. Am J Psychiatry 152:341–351, 1995

George MS, Ketter TA, Parekh PI, et al: Gender differences in regional cerebral blood flow during transient self-induced sadness or happiness. Biol Psychiatry 40:859–871, 1996

George MS, Ketter TA, Parekh PI, et al: Blunted left cingulate activation in mood disorder subjects during a response interference task (the Stroop). J Neuropsychiatry Clin Neurosci 9:55–63, 1997

Guze BH, Baxter LR Jr, Schwartz JM, et al: Effects of electroconvulsive therapy on brain glucose metabolism. Convulsive Therapy 7:15–19, 1991

Hurwitz TA, Clark C, Murphy E, et al: Regional cerebral glucose metabolism in major depressive disorder. Can J Psychiatry 35:684–688, 1990

Husain MM, McDonald WM, Doraiswamy PM, et al: A magnetic resonance imaging study of putamen nuclei in major depression. Psychiatry Res 40:95–99, 1991

Kanaya T, Yonekawa M: Regional cerebral blood flow in depression. Jpn J Psychiatry Neurol 44:571–576, 1990

Krishnan KRR, McDonald WM, Escalona PR, et al: Magnetic resonance imaging of the caudate nuclei in depression: preliminary observations. Arch Gen Psychiatry 49:553–557, 1992

Kumar A, Mozley D, Dunham C, et al: Semiquantitative I-123 IMP SPECT studies in late onset depression before and after treatment. Int J Geriatr Psychiatry 6:775–777, 1991

Lane RD, Reimen EM, Ahern GL, et al: Neuroanatomical correlates of happiness, sadness, and disgust. Am J Psychiatry 154:926–933, 1997

Lauterbach EC, Jackson JG, Price ST, et al: Clinical, motor, and biological correlates of depressive disorders after focal subcortical lesions. J Neuropsychiatry Clin Neurosci 9:259–266, 1997

Liotti M, Mayberg HS, Brannan SK, et al: Mood challenge in remitted depression: an ^{15}O-water PET study (abstract). Neuroimage 5:S114, 1997

Martinot JL, Hardy P, Feline A, et al: Left prefrontal glucose hypometabolism in the depressed state: a confirmation. Am J Psychiatry 147:1313–1317, 1990

Mayberg HS: Limbic-cortical dysregulation: a proposed model of depression. J Neuropsychiatry Clin Neurosci 9:471–481, 1997

Mayberg HS, Brannan SK, Mahurin RK, et al: Cingulate function in depression: a potential predictor of treatment response. Neuroreport 8:1057–1061, 1997

Mayberg HS, Liotti M, Brannan SK, et al: Disease and state-specific effects of mood challenge on rCBF (abstract). Neuroimage 7:S901, 1998

Mayberg HS, Liotti M, Brannan SK, et al: Reciprocal limbic-cortical function and negative mood: converging PET findings in depression and normal sadness. Am J Psychiatry 156:675–682, 1999

Mayberg HS, Brannan SK, Tekell JL, et al: Regional metabokic effects of fluoxetine in major depression: serial changes and relationship to clinical response. Biol Psychiatry 48:830–843, 2000

Morris PL, Robinson RG, Raphael B, et al: Lesion location and poststroke depression. J Neuropsychiatry Clin Neurosci 8:399–403, 1996

Nobler MS, Sackeim HA, Prohovnik I, et al: Regional cerebral blood flow in mood disorders, III: treatment and clinical response. Arch Gen Psychiatry 51:884–897, 1994

Paradiso S, Robinson RG, Andreasen NC, et al: Emotional activation of limbic circuitry in elderly normal subjects in a PET study. Am J Psychiatry 154:384–389, 1997

Pardo JV, Pardo PJ, Raichle ME: Neural correlates of self-induced dysphoria. Am J Psychiatry 150:713–719, 1993

Phillips ML, Young AW, Senior C, et al: A specific neural substrate for perceiving facial expressions of disgust. Nature 389:495–498, 1997

Prohovnik I, Sackeim HA, Decina P, et al: Acute reductions of regional cerebral blood flow following electroconvulsive therapy: interactions with modality and time. Ann N Y Acad Sci 462:249–262, 1986

Rauch SL, Jenike MA, Alpert NM, et al: Regional cerebral blood flow measured during symptom provocation in obsessive-compulsive disorder using oxygen 15-labeled carbon dioxide and positron emission tomography. Arch Gen Psychiatry 51:62–70, 1994

Rauch SL, Savage CR, Alpert NM: A positron emission tomographic study of simple phobic symptom provocation. Arch Gen Psychiatry 52:20–28, 1995

Rauch SL, van der Kolk BA, Fisler RE, et al: A symptom provocation study of posttraumatic stress disorder using positron emission tomography and script-driven imagery. Arch Gen Psychiatry 53:380–387, 1996

Rauch SL, Shin LM, Dougherty DD, et al: Neural activation during sexual and competitive arousal in healthy men. Psychiatry Res 91:1–10, 1999

Reimen EM, Lane RD, Ahern GL, et al: Neuroanatomical correlates of externally and internally generated human emotion. Am J Psychiatry 154:918–925, 1997

Robinson RG: Differential behavioral effects of right versus left hemispheric cerebral infarction: evidence for cerebral lateralization in the rat. Science 205:707–710, 1979

Robinson RG, Kubos KL, Starr LB, et al: Mood disorders in stroke patients: importance of location of lesion. Brain 107 (part 1):81–93, 1984

Robinson RG, Starkstein SE, Price TR: Post-stroke depression and lesion location (letter). Stroke 19:125–126, 1988

Rosenberg R, Vorstrup S, Andersen A, et al: Effect of ECT on cerebral blood flow in melancholia assessed with SPECT. Convulsive Therapy 4:62–73, 1988

Schneider F, Gur RC, Jaggi JL, et al: Differential effects of mood on cortical cerebral blood flow: a ^{133}xenon clearance study. Psychiatry Res 52:215–236, 1994

Schneider F, Gur RE, Mozley LH, et al: Mood effects on limbic blood flow correlate with emotional self-rating: a PET study with oxygen-15 labeled water. Psychiatry Res 61:265–283, 1995

Scott AI, Dougall N, Ross M, et al: Short-term effects of electroconvulsive treatment on the uptake of ^{99}Tc-exametazime into brain in major depression shown with single photon emission tomography. J Affect Disord 30:27–34, 1994

Shin LM, Dougherty DD, Orr SP, et al: Activation of anterior paralimbic structures during guilt-related script-driven imagery. Biol Psychiatry 48:43–50, 2000

Silfverskiöld P, Risberg J: Regional cerebral blood flow in depression and mania. Arch Gen Psychiatry 46:253–259, 1989

Silfverskiöld P, Gustafson L, Risberg J, et al: Acute and late effects of electroconvulsive therapy: clinical outcome, regional cerebral blood flow, and electroencephalogram. Ann N Y Acad Sci 462:236–248, 1986

Soares JC, Mann JJ: The anatomy of mood disorders: review of structural neuroimaging studies. Biol Psychiatry 41:86–106, 1997

Starkstein SE, Robinson RG, Price TR: Comparison of cortical and subcortical lesions in the production of post-stroke mood disorders. Brain 110:1045–1059, 1987

Starkstein SE, Robinson RG, Berthier ML, et al: Differential mood changes following basal ganglia vs thalamic lesions. Arch Neurol 45:725–730, 1988

Starkstein SE, Mayberg HS, Berthier ML, et al: Mania after brain injury: neuroradiological and metabolic findings. Ann Neurol 27:652–659, 1990

Volkow ND, Bellar S, Mullani N, et al: Effects of electroconvulsive therapy on brain glucose metabolism: a preliminary study. Convulsive Therapy 4:199–205, 1988

Wu JC, Gillin JC, Buchsbaum MS, et al: Effect of sleep deprivation on brain metabolism of depressed patients. Am J Psychiatry 149:538–543, 1992

8

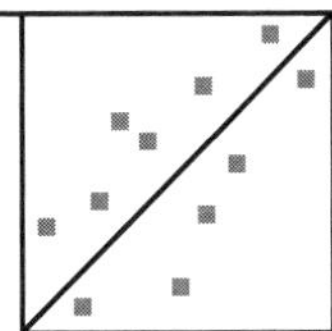

IN VIVO NEURORECEPTOR IMAGING TECHNIQUES IN PSYCHIATRIC DRUG DEVELOPMENT

Darin D. Dougherty, M.D., M.Sc.
Nathaniel M. Alpert, Ph.D.
Scott L. Rauch, M.D.
Alan J. Fischman, M.D., Ph.D.

Researchers both at academic centers and in industry are actively involved in efforts to develop new pharmacologic agents to treat psychiatric disease. Although current agents are effective for many disorders, safer and more efficacious drugs have the potential to improve treatment. However, developing a new drug can cost more than several hundred million dollars. In addition, it may take many years to develop an agent. These years of drug development delay access to a pharmaceutical agent that may help countless patients. Thus, technologies that can simplify and lower costs of drug development are being used by researchers. For example, pharmaceutical companies have developed large molecular biology branches to provide ever-increasing numbers of candidate molecules. Once a compound has been synthesized and characterized in vitro, animal and human trials are used to assess efficacy, dosing schedules, and safety. New advances in functional neuroimaging are being used to streamline this process (Farde 1996; Fowler et al. 1999).

The development of a new drug proceeds in many stages, but the process may be generalized to include the following steps: First, there is the chemical synthesis and in vitro screening of a series of compounds designed to achieve a particular biochemical objective. Second, studies are conducted in animals to determine the pharmacokinetic and pharmacodynamic profile of the drug. Then safety and efficacy are assessed in animal trials. At this point, the pharmacokinetic and pharmacodynamic profile of the drug is determined in humans. Lastly, clinical effects and side effects are characterized in well-controlled multicenter studies involving large numbers of patients.

In vivo neuroimaging is being more frequently used to assess pharmacokinetics and pharmacodynamics of candidate compounds in both animals and humans. In vivo neuroimaging can provide information regarding static and time-dependent distribution of drug in tissue, metabolites, route of excretion, and changes in cerebral blood flow and glucose metabolism as a result of drug administration (Fischman et al. 1994). In vivo neuroimaging is especially important in the development of central nervous system (CNS) drugs, because cognitive function and affective function in humans markedly differ from those in animals. In this chapter, we focus on how in vivo neuroreceptor imaging may be used in Phase I and II trials to help formulate Phase III trials. In vivo neuroreceptor imaging allows researchers to look beyond changes in regional cerebral blood flow or glucose metabolism; this type of imaging provides information regarding the site of drug action and the receptors involved.

■ DRUG-RECEPTOR INTERACTIONS

Neurotransmitter receptors, located on the surface of neurons, play an essential role in interneuronal communication (Cooper et al. 1996). Neurotransmitter systems serve different, but often overlapping, functions in neuronal communication as endogenous neurotransmitters interact with the neuroreceptors. The many types of neurotransmitter receptors include adrenergic, dopaminergic, γ-aminobutyric acid (GABA)ergic, glutamatergic, histaminergic, cholinergic, and serotonergic receptors, as well as numerous neuropeptidergic receptors. Some neurotransmitters are excitatory (e.g., glutamate), whereas others are inhibitory (e.g., GABA). Dysregulation of these neurotransmitter systems is implicated in the pathophysiology of many psychiatric illnesses (Coplan et al. 1995; Kahn and Davis 1995; Maes and Meltzer 1995; Schatzberg and Schildkraut 1995).

Most biological effects of psychotropic agents are the result of interactions with neurotransmitter receptors. Psychotropic drugs, by interacting with neuroreceptors, are hypothesized either to normalize the primary dysregulation associated with psychiatric symptoms or to mediate a compensatory mechanism to counter the dysfunction associated with the psychiatric symptoms. Psychotropic agents generally serve as agonists (potentiating the action of the neurotransmitter) or antagonists (attenuating the action of the neurotransmitter) at these receptor sites. Some psychotropic agents (e.g., benzodiazepines) exert their effects acutely, whereas others (e.g., antidepressants) exert their effects over a period of weeks, with these psychotropic agents likely modulating neuronal gene expression via intracellular second messenger systems coupled with the membrane-based neuroreceptors (Duman et al. 1997; Hyman and Nestler 1996).

The mechanism of action of psychotropic drugs arises from their effects on specific receptors. Thus, the study of receptors and their subtypes plays an increasingly important role in the development of new psychotropic drugs. The identification of receptor subtypes has led to the development of increasingly selective drugs for these receptor subtypes (Stahl 1992). Generally, receptors have been studied using autoradiographic techniques in animals or postmortem human tissue (Kuhar and Unnerstall 1990). These in vitro techniques allow characterization of the binding affinity (noted as K_d, or the dissociation constant) and receptor occupancy or density (B_{max}) of neuroreceptors. Postmortem autoradiographic techniques in animals after administration of a drug (ex vivo techniques) may also be useful. This information is useful in elucidating the pharmcodynamics and pharmacokinetics of psychotropic agents. Pharmacodynamics, at the simplest level, can be defined as the way in which an administered drug affects an organism (i.e., the effects of the drug on receptors, producing the desired therapeutic effect). Similarly, pharmacokinetics can be defined as the way in which an organism affects an administered drug (i.e., the absorption, tissue distribution, metabolism, and excretion of the drug). With the advent of neuroreceptor imaging using positron emission tomography (PET) and single photon emission computed tomography (SPECT), these properties can now be studied in vivo.

■ In Vivo Neuroreceptor Imaging

Radioligands

A detailed description of functional neuroimaging techniques such as PET and SPECT is beyond the scope of this chapter (for a review, see Malison et al. 1995). We focus here on using these functional neuroimaging modalities for neuroreceptor characterization in vivo, especially as an aid to drug development. Both PET and SPECT use radiotracer techniques to provide noninvasive, high-resolution measurements of regional cerebral blood flow and cerebral glucose metabolism. In addition, the use of specific ligands labeled with a positron-emitting radionuclide allows investigators to measure neuroreceptor binding in vivo. Ideally, the resulting radiolabeled ligand (radioligand) has high specificity for the targeted receptor (i.e., a high affinity for the targeted receptor and little or no affinity for other receptors). This property, coupled with the sensitivity of PET and SPECT, allows investigators to use doses of the radioligand in the picomolar (10^{-12} M) range; these amounts of radioligand (i.e., tracer quantities) are generally orders of magnitude lower than pharmacologic doses. For comparison, although some paramagnetic-labeled ligands have been developed for use in functional magnetic resonance imaging, the mass of tracer required is orders of magnitude higher than that needed for PET or SPECT and generally results in pharmacologic perturbation. Numerous radioligands are available for PET and SPECT imaging; the most commonly used ligands are listed in Table 8–1. Radioligands for many subtypes of neurotransmitter receptors have been developed.

Modeling

PET and SPECT data can be analyzed at three levels of sophistication. In the simplest approach, the images are inspected visually and areas of increased or decreased accumulation are qualitatively noted. At the next level of sophistication, the ratios of accumulation in receptor-rich regions to accumulation in receptor-poor regions (usually the cerebellum) are calculated. At the highest level of sophistication, dynamic data are analyzed by kinetic, or compartmental, modeling to calculate K_d and B_{max} for ligand-receptor interaction. In clinical studies, all three methods can yield useful information in conditions that produce very large changes in receptor density. However, detection of subtle changes usually requires kinetic modeling. In research studies, kinetic modeling is the rule.

TABLE 8–1. Radiolabeled ligands commonly used in positron emission tomography and single photon emission computed tomography imaging

Receptor	Ligand	Specificity	Reference
Dopamine	$[^{11}C]$SCH 23390	D_1	Halldin et al. 1986
	$[^{11}C]$Raclopride	D_2	Farde et al. 1986
	$[^{11}C]$Methylspiperone	D_2, 5-HT_2	Wagner et al. 1983
Serotonin (5-HT)	$[^{18}F]$Setoperone	5-HT_2	Blin et al. 1990
	$[^{11}C]$WAY-100635	5-HT_{1A}	Mathis et al. 1994
Benzodiazepine	$[^{11}C]$Flumazenil	BZD1, BZD2	Maziere et al. 1985
Opioid	$[^{11}C]$Carfentanil	mu	Frost et al. 1988
	$[^{11}C]$Diprenorphine	mu, kappa	Jones et al. 1988

PET and SPECT measure the concentration history of radioligand in tissue. Neither PET nor SPECT can separate the material that is bound to the receptor from that which is dissociated from the receptor or nonspecifically bound. For that reason, a less direct method is used: *kinetic modeling.* The goal of using a kinetic model of a receptor ligand study is to produce a prediction of the measured ligand concentration history as a function of a few parameters that have physiological relevance (e.g., the receptor density and equilibrium dissociation constant). The kinetic model conceptualizes the tracer as being in four states (or compartments): one state in plasma and three states in tissue (free, specific binding, and nonspecific binding). In this model, the free ligand can either bind directly to an unoccupied receptor (specific binding) or a nonspecific site (nonspecific binding) or escape from the tissue. The success of this indirect measurement procedure hinges on whether there is a unique set of model parameters that closely predict the measured data. If that set of parameters exists, it is said that the model parameters can be identified. Although many variations in modeling for the quantification of ligand-receptor interactions have been proposed, all include parameters describing the transport of free ligand from blood to tissue and receptor binding. The properties of the ligand (e.g., whether it is reversibly or irreversibly bound) must be considered in formulating the kinetic model and a measurement protocol. Additional complexity ensues when the most detailed information (B_{max} and K_d) is desired, because the biological system must be perturbed with two or more injections of ligand that significantly alter the number of free receptors.

In many cases, experiments designed to probe the pharmacodynamics of a system can feature simplified designs in which an index of receptor binding can be measured twice (with high-specific-activity injections): in a drug-naive control state and after administration of the drug of interest. In some situations, modeling can be further simplified by the use of graphical methods of analysis. Logan and colleagues (1990) described a graphical model that applies to systems in which binding of the radioligand to its receptor is reversible. Although estimates of binding potential calculated by these methods are less precise than those obtained by kinetic modeling, the techniques can be used to produce parametric images from pre- and post-drug-infusion experiments in which the voxel intensity is proportional to the binding potential. This approach can be of value for defining the regional tissue distribution; these data can also be reanalyzed using modeling techniques to calculate more precise values for binding potential.

■ NEURORECEPTOR IMAGING PARADIGMS FOR STUDYING PSYCHOTROPIC DRUGS

Because most psychotropic drugs act through interaction with neuroreceptors, PET and SPECT can be powerful tools for the development of new therapeutic agents. PET and SPECT studies of pharmacokinetics and pharmacodynamics can vary considerably in type and complexity. In general, these studies can be divided into two general categories: direct and indirect studies.

In *direct studies,* the drug of interest is radiolabeled with a radioisotope, usually ^{11}C or ^{18}F, and dynamic imaging is performed. At the most basic level, such studies can provide useful information about drug distribution. However, when it is necessary to derive specific values for the parameters of drug-receptor interaction, the imaging protocol is more complex. In the case of drugs that interact with a single class of receptors, time-activity curves from single- or multiple-injection studies can be analyzed by compartmental modeling (described earlier) to estimate B_{max}, K_d, or binding potential (B_{max}/K_d). When the drug binds to more than one type of receptor, kinetic parameters for a specific receptor can be derived from studies in which other receptors are blocked by coinjection of unlabeled ligands. Later in this chapter, we describe a use of this paradigm to assess a novel antidepressant.

In *indirect studies,* the drug under investigation is not radiolabeled. Instead, the receptor binding profile is derived from coinjection or displacement studies with radiolabeled test ligands that target specific receptors. An example of this approach is the evaluation of the dopamine D_2 and D_1 receptor–binding characteristics of conventional and atypical neuroleptics, using [^{11}C]raclopride and [^{11}C]SCH 23390 as test ligands for D_2 and D_1 receptors, respectively (Farde 1992; Farde et al. 1986, 1987, 1988, 1989, 1992). The receptor types that have been studied by this method include dopaminergic, serotonergic, cholinergic, opiate, and benzodiazepine receptors. Later in this chapter, we describe an example of this approach in assessing the pharmacokinetics of an atypical neuroleptic.

An Indirect Study: BMS-181101

BMS-181101 is a novel antidepressant that has been under clinical investigation. This agent is believed to influence CNS serotonergic neurotransmission by several mechanisms, including inhibition of 5-HT reuptake, and as a full agonist at dorsal raphe somatodendritic 5-HT_{1A} autoreceptors and presynaptic terminal 5-HT_{1D} receptors that regulate the activity of 5-HT neurons (data on file, Bristol-Myers Squibb Co., Princeton, NJ). Thus, the mechanism of action of BMS-181101 differs from that of other antidepressants currently available.

Christian and colleagues (1996) recently conducted a study designed to evaluate the pharmacokinetics and receptor binding of BMS-181101 in healthy humans. In that investigation, BMS-181101 was radioactively labeled with ^{11}C and given to six healthy subjects. First, each subject was given 10 millicuries (mCi) of high-specific-activity (approximately 1,700 mCi/μmol) [^{11}C]BMS-181101 and data were collected with a PET camera for 90 minutes. Thirty minutes after completion of this study, each subject was given 10 mCi of [^{11}C]BMS-181101 plus 3 mg of unlabeled BMS-181101 (final specific activity of approximately 1.5 mCi/μmol) and data were again collected with a PET camera for 90 minutes. Results demonstrated that the percentage of injected drug (BMS-181101) found in the brain was the same for all brain regions. In addition, there were no regional differences in volume of distribution between the high- and low-specific-activity studies (Figures 8–1 and 8–2).

These results indicate that the CNS distribution of [^{11}C]BMS-181101 is dominated by blood flow and that significant receptor-specific localization occurs in no brain region. The results also indicate that BMS-181101 does not influence CNS serotonergic neurotransmission in vivo; this finding conflicts with data from previous in vitro and animal studies of this compound. In other words, because there is no specific serotonergic binding after administration of [^{11}C]BMS-181101, it is inferred that BMS-181101 has no serotonergic receptor–mediated effects on neurotransmission. Thus, there is a marked difference between the preclinical and clinical pharmacology of the 5-HT binding profile of BMS-181101. Further development of this compound as an antidepressant by the pharmaceutical company was greatly slowed, and to our knowledge no further clinical trials have been conducted. This study greatly influenced the company's decision to stop progression into Phase III trials and most likely saved tens of millions of dollars that could be reallocated to other more promising agents.

A Direct Study: Ziprasidone

Ziprasidone is an atypical neuroleptic that is expected to become commercially available in the near future. In vitro studies have demonstrated that ziprasidone has a high affinity for both D_2 and serotonin$_2$ (5-HT$_2$) receptors, a characteristic it has in common with other currently available atypical neuroleptics (Seeger et al. 1993; Seymour et al. 1993). In one study, we assessed the

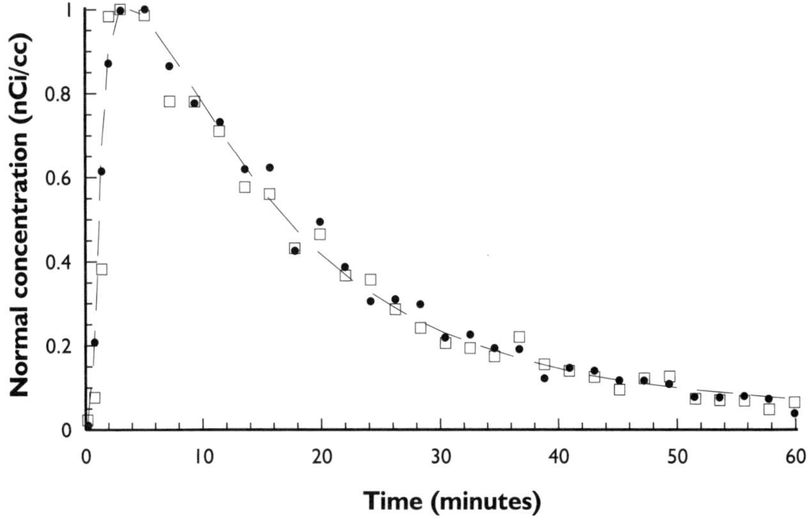

FIGURE 8–1. Tissue time-activity curve for [^{11}C]BMS-181101 in the putamen (known to have a high concentration of serotonergic receptors). The filled circles represent the first, high-specific-activity, injection (1,700 millicuries [mCi]/µmol), and the open squares represent the second, low-specific-activity, injection (1.5 mCi/µmol). The dashed line represents the curve fit to the data from the first injection. The data presented here indicate a lack of specific binding. Abbreviation: nCi=nanocuries.
Source. Reprinted with permission from Christian BT, Livni E, Babich JW, et al.: "Evaluation of Cerebral Pharmacokinetics of the Novel Antidepressant Drug, BMS-181101, by Positron Emission Tomography." *Journal of Pharmacology and Experimental Therapeutics* 279:325–331, 1996.

kinetics of 5-HT$_2$ receptor occupancy by ziprasidone in vivo (Fischman et al. 1996). Eight healthy subjects were given a single 40-mg oral dose of ziprasidone (not radioactively labeled). In addition, these subjects underwent PET with the radioligand [^{18}F]setoperone, which is specific for 5-HT$_2$ receptors, both before administration of ziprasidone and 4–18 hours after administration of the unlabeled drug. By comparing [^{18}F]setoperone receptor occupancy before and after administration of ziprasidone, we could ascertain the receptor occupancy of ziprasidone at the 5-HT$_2$ receptor.

Results indicated that ziprasidone occupancy of 5-HT$_2$ receptors was nearly (98%) complete 4 hours after ingestion of ziprasidone (Figure 8–3) and remained elevated (46%) 18 hours after administration. In addition, plasma concentrations of ziprasidone were measured concurrently and were found to decrease more rapidly and to be only weakly correlated with 5-HT$_2$ receptor occupancy. These findings are highly relevant in establishing routine clinical

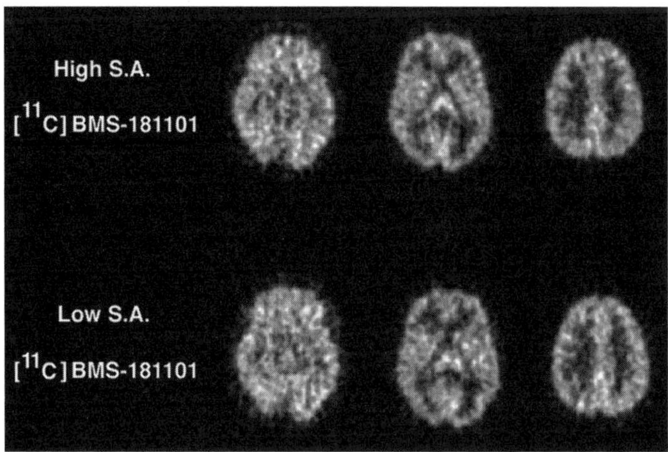

FIGURE 8–2. Distribution of [^{11}C]BMS-181101 in the brain after high- (top row) and low- (bottom row) specific-activity (S.A.) injections. These images represent the summation of the dynamic data from 10 minutes after injection to the end of acquisition (90 minutes). The three transaxial slices are at different levels in the brain, approximately 2 cm apart. These images support the finding that no significant amount of specific binding occurred.
Source. Reprinted with permission from Christian BT, Livni E, Babich JW, et al.: "Evaluation of Cerebral Pharmacokinetics of the Novel Antidepressant Drug, BMS-181101, by Positron Emission Tomography." *Journal of Pharmacology and Experimental Therapeutics* 279:325–331, 1996.

dosing schedules of ziprasidone and might suggest the need for less frequent administration to achieve therapeutic benefit than might be predicted on the basis of peripheral pharmacokinetics.

■ SUMMARY

We have provided an overview and two examples of how modern neuroimaging techniques may be used in the process of drug development. Because we use PET in such studies at our facility, we have included two examples using PET. However, SPECT is also widely used in drug development studies (Malison et al. 1995). The results of these studies clearly demonstrate the importance of PET and SPECT methods for noninvasive measurement of drug kinetics in the human CNS. Indeed, such PET and SPECT studies have become an important addition to the armamentarium of clinical pharmacologists investigating psychotropic medications. In drug development, PET and SPECT measurements generally are likely to be most useful in the following

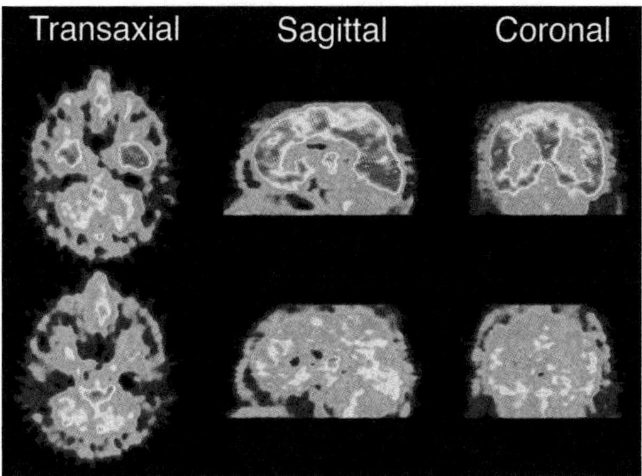

FIGURE 8–3. Transverse, sagittal, and coronal positron emission tomography images of the brain of a healthy subject before (upper row) and 4 hours after (lower row) oral administration of 40 mg of ziprasidone.
Source. Reprinted with permission from Fischman AJ, Bonab AA, Babich JW, et al.: "Positron Emission Tomographic Analysis of Central 5-Hydroxytryptamine$_2$ Receptor Occupancy in Healthy Volunteers Treated With the Novel Antipsychotic Agent, Ziprasidone." *Journal of Pharmacology and Experimental Therapeutics* 279:939–947, 1996.

situations and ways: 1) in preclinical studies, the binding profile of a new drug can be precisely compared with that of preexisting agents, or a series of analogs can be screened for further development on the basis of their in vivo binding characteristics; and 2) in Phase I and II studies, classic pharmacokinetic measurements can be coupled with imaging measurements to determine optimal dosing schedules to guide the design of Phase III studies. In general, the types of measurements that are possible can be grouped into the following categories:

- In situations in which the drug can be radiolabeled, the time course of tissue delivery can be determined noninvasively in vivo in health and disease. Such information should be useful for determining dosing schedules as well as characterizing regional distribution, which is relevant to efficacy and toxicity.
- Ligand-receptor binding can be assessed in vivo in two ways. The ability of the drug to displace standard radiolabeled ligands from their receptors can be determined; alternatively, labeled drug can be used to assess more directly the distribution and time course of binding. These measurements are particularly useful for studying drugs that are active in the CNS.

We suggest that the joining of classic clinical pharmacology with exquisite imaging measurements will help form the basis for clinical drug development in the twenty-first century.

■ References

Blin J, Sette G, Fiorelli M, et al: A method for the in vivo investigation of the serotonergic 5-HT_2 receptors in the human cerebral cortex using positron emission tomography and ^{18}F-labeled setoperone. J Neurochem 54:1744–1754, 1990

Christian BT, Livni E, Babich JW, et al: Evaluation of cerebral pharmacokinetics of the novel antidepressant drug, BMS-181101, by positron emission tomography. J Pharmacol Exp Ther 279:325–331, 1996

Cooper JR, Bloom FE, Roth RH: The Biochemical Basis of Neuropharmacology. New York, Oxford University Press, 1996, pp 82–102

Coplan JD, Wolk SI, Klein DF: Anxiety and serotonin$_{1A}$ receptor, in Psychopharmacology: The Fourth Generation of Progress. Edited by Bloom FE, Kupfer DJ. New York, Raven, 1995, pp 1301–1310

Duman RS, Heninger GR, Nestler EJ: A molecular and cellular theory of depression. Arch Gen Psychiatry 54:597–606, 1997

Farde L: Selective D1- and D2-dopamine receptor blockade both induces akathisia in humans: a PET study with [^{11}C]SCH 23390 and [^{11}C]raclopride. Psychopharmacology (Berl) 107:23–29, 1992

Farde L: The advantage of using positron emission tomography in drug research. Trends Neurosci 19:211–214, 1996

Farde L, Hall H, Ehrin E, et al: Quantitative analysis of D2 dopamine receptor binding in the living human brain by PET. Science 231:258–261, 1986

Farde L, Halldin C, Stone-Elander S, et al: PET analysis of the human dopamine receptor subtypes using ^{11}C-SCH 23390 and ^{11}C-raclopride. Psychopharmacology (Berl) 92:278–284, 1987

Farde L, Wiesel FA, Halldin C, et al: Central D2-dopamine receptor occupancy in schizophrenic patients treated with antipsychotic drugs. Arch Gen Psychiatry 45:71–76, 1988

Farde L, Wiesel FA, Nordstrom AL, et al: D1- and D2-dopamine receptor occupancy during treatment with conventional and atypical neuroleptics. Psychopharmacology (Berl) 99:S28–S31, 1989

Farde L, Nordstrom AL, Wiesel FA, et al: Positron emission tomographic analysis of central Dl and D2 dopamine receptor occupancy in patients treated with classical neuroleptics and clozapine: relation to extrapyramidal side effects. Arch Gen Psychiatry 49:538–544, 1992

Fischman AJ, Rubin RH, Strauss HW: In vivo imaging in drug discovery and design, in Handbook of Experimental Pharmacology, Vol 110: Pharmacokinetics of Drugs. Edited by Welling PG, Balant LP. New York, Springer-Verlag, 1994, pp 481–503

Fischman AJ, Bonab AA, Babich JW, et al: Positron emission tomographic analysis of central 5-hydroxytryptamine$_2$ receptor occupancy in healthy volunteers treated with the novel antipsychotic agent, ziprasidone. J Pharmacol Exp Ther 279:939–947, 1996

Fowler JS, Volkow ND, Wang G-J, et al: PET and drug research and development. J Nucl Med 40:1154–1163, 1999

Frost JJ, Mayberg HS, Fisher RS, et al: Mu-receptors measured by positron emission tomography are increased in temporal lobe epilepsy. Ann Neurol 23:231–237, 1988

Halldin C, Stone-Elander S, Farde L, et al: Preparation of ^{11}C-labelled SCH 23390 for the in vivo study of dopamine D-1 receptors using positron emission tomography. Int J Rad Appl Instrum [A] 37:1039–1043, 1986

Hyman SE, Nestler EJ: Initiation and adaptation: a paradigm for understanding psychotropic drug action. Am J Psychiatry 153:151–162, 1996

Jones AK, Luthra SK, Maziere B, et al: Regional cerebral opioid receptor studies with [^{11}C]diprenorphine in normal volunteers. J Neurosci Methods 23:121–129, 1988

Kahn RS, Davis KL: New developments in dopamine and schizophrenia, in Psychopharmacology: The Fourth Generation of Progress. Edited by Bloom FE, Kupfer DJ. New York, Raven, pp 1193–1204, 1995

Kuhar MJ, Unnerstall JR: Receptor autoradiography, in Methods in Neurotransmitter Receptor Analysis. Edited by Yamamura HI, Enna SJ, Kuhar MJ. New York, Raven, pp 177–218, 1990

Logan J, Fowler JS, Volkow ND, et al: Graphical analysis of reversible radioligand binding from time-activity measurements applied to [N-11C-methyl]-(-)-cocaine PET studies in human subjects. J Cereb Blood Flow Metab 10:740–747, 1990

Maes M, Meltzer HY: The serotonin hypothesis of major depression, in Psychopharmacology: The Fourth Generation of Progress. Edited by Bloom FE, Kupfer DJ. New York, Raven, 1995, pp 933–944

Malison RT, Laruelle M, Innis RB: Positron and single photon emission tomography: principles and applications in psychopharmacology, in Psychopharmacology: The Fourth Generation of Progress. Edited by Bloom FE, Kupfer DJ. New York, Raven, 1995, pp 865–880

Mathis CA, Simpson NR, Mahmood K, et al: [^{11}C]WAY-100635: A radioligand for imaging 5-HT$_{1A}$ receptors with positron emission tomography. Life Sci 55:403–407, 1994

Maziere B, Hantraye P, Kaijima M, et al: Visualization by positron emission tomography of the apparent regional heterogeneity of central type benzodiazepine receptors in the brain of living baboons. Life Sci 36:1609–1616, 1985

Schatzberg AF, Schildkraut JJ: Recent studies on norepinephrine systems in mood disorders, in Psychopharmacology: The Fourth Generation of Progress. Edited by Bloom FE, Kupfer DJ. New York, Raven, 1995, pp 911–920

Seeger TF, Schmidt AW, Leebel LA, et al: CP-88,059, a new antipsychotic with mixed dopamine D2 and serotonin 5-HT_2 antagonist activities, in Program and Abstracts, Society for Neuroscience 23rd Annual Meeting, New Orleans, LA, November 7–12, 1993. New Orleans, LA, Society for Neuroscience, 1993, p 1623

Seymour PA, Seeger TF, Guanowsky V, et al: Behavioral pharmacology of CP-88,059: a new antipsychotic with both 5-HT_2 and D2 antagonist activities, in Program and Abstracts, Society for Neuroscience 23rd Annual Meeting, New Orleans, LA, November 7–12, 1993. New Orleans, LA, Society for Neuroscience, 1993, p 599

Stahl SM: Serotonin neuroscience discoveries usher in a new era of novel drug therapies for psychiatry. Psychopharmacol Bull 28:3–9, 1992

Wagner HN Jr, Burns HD, Daniels RF, et al: Imaging dopamine receptors in the human brain by positron tomography. Science 221:1264–1266, 1983

9

"FUNCTIONAL" NEURORECEPTOR IMAGING

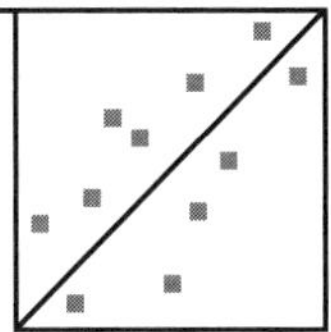

The Example of Studies of Synaptic Dopamine Activity With Single Photon Emission Computed Tomography

Ilise Lombardo, M.D.
Anissa Abi-Dargham, M.D.
Lawrence Kegeles, M.D., Ph.D.
Marc Laruelle, M.D.

Neuroreceptor imaging with positron emission tomography (PET) or single photon emission computed tomography (SPECT) is classically aimed at measuring neuroreceptor parameters in the living human brain. More recently, several groups demonstrated that, under specific conditions, in vivo neuroreceptor binding techniques can also be used to measure acute fluctuations in the concentration of the endogenous transmitters in the vicinity of radiolabeled receptors (Carson et al. 1997; Dewey et al. 1991; Innis et al. 1992; Laruelle et al. 1997b). Competition between radiotracers and transmitters for binding to neuroreceptors is the principle underlying this technique. This new application of neuroreceptor

We thank our collaborators at Yale and Columbia Universities, especially Robert Innis, M.D., Ph.D., Ronald Baldwin, Ph.D., Yolanda Zea-Ponce, Ph.D., Charles Bradberry, Ph.D., Roberto Gil, M.D., John Krystal, M.D., Dennis Charney, M.D., J. John Mann, M.D., Jack Gorman, M.D., and Ronald Van Heertum, M.D. We also acknowledge the support of the National Alliance for Research on Schizophrenia and Depression, the Stanley Foundation, the Scottish-Rite Foundation, the EJLB Foundation, and the Public Health Service (grants RO1MH54192–01, RO1DA10219–01, and K02MH01603–01).

imaging allows direct measurement of synaptic transmission in specific neurotransmitter systems in the brain, correlation of these measurements with behaviors and symptoms, and exploration of the role of neurochemical imbalances in the pathogenesis of psychiatric disorders. Applications of this new paradigm have been developed to study dopamine transmission at D_2 receptors. (In this chapter, we use the term *D_2 receptors* to denote D_2, D_3, but not D_4 receptors.)

Endogenous competition between dopamine and radiolabeled D_2 receptor ligands was initially documented in rodents. Amphetamine, which releases dopamine and thereby increases endogenous synaptic dopamine concentration (Kuczenski and Segal 1989; Sharp et al. 1987), was found to reduce in vivo binding of the D_2 receptor agonist [^{3}H]*N*-propylnorapomorphine (Köhler et al. 1981; Ross and Jackson 1989b) and the D_2 receptor antagonist [^{3}H]raclopride (Ross and Jackson 1989a; Young et al. 1991). Reduced in vivo accumulations of D_2 tracers were also reported after pretreatment with the dopamine uptake inhibitors amfonelic acid and methylphenidate and with the dopamine precursor L-dopa (De Jesus et al. 1986; Ross and Jackson 1989b). The opposite effect (i.e., increased tracer accumulation) was induced by drugs that decrease dopamine endogenous concentration, such as reserpine and γ-butyrolactone (Ross 1991; Ross and Jackson 1989b; Seeman et al. 1989; van der Werf et al. 1983; Young et al. 1991).

We developed and validated a method using SPECT and the specific D_2 receptor radiotracer [^{123}I]iodobenzamide ([^{123}I]IBZM) to measure amphetamine-induced intrasynaptic dopamine release in nonhuman primates (Innis et al. 1992; Laruelle et al. 1997b), and we adapted this method for use in humans (Laruelle et al. 1995). Using this technique, we found an increase in amphetamine-induced dopamine release in unmedicated patients with schizophrenia compared with matched control subjects, and we described a relationship between increased synaptic dopamine activity and the emergence of psychotic positive symptoms after an amphetamine challenge (Abi-Dargham et al. 1998; Laruelle et al. 1996). This finding was independently replicated, using PET and [^{11}C]raclopride (Breier et al. 1997).

More recently, we introduced a method to measure "baseline" synaptic dopamine activity (Laruelle et al. 1997a). This method allows measurement of synaptic dopamine concentration in the resting state (i.e., in the absence of pharmacologic challenge), thus enabling characterization of dopamine activity under physiological conditions.

In this chapter, we summarize the main steps in the development of these methods with SPECT, as well as initial clinical results obtained in patients with schizophrenia. Parallel developments with PET and [^{11}C]raclopride are also discussed (Breier et al. 1997; Carson et al. 1997; Dewey et al. 1993, 1995; Volkow et al. 1994).

■ The Amphetamine Challenge Test

Baboon Studies

Classically, PET and SPECT experiments are carried out after single-bolus injection of the radiotracer. With this administration protocol, the brain activity initially increases (uptake phase), reaches a peak, and then decreases (washout phase). The initial observation in this line of research was that the striatal washout rate of the SPECT D_2 receptor radiotracer [^{123}I]IBZM in baboons is significantly increased when amphetamine is injected during the washout phase (Innis et al. 1992). Given that amphetamine has negligible affinity for [^{123}I]IBZM binding (>10 μM), this effect could not be attributed to a direct displacement of [^{123}I]IBZM by amphetamine. Because amphetamine is a potent dopamine releaser, we postulated that the increased [^{123}I]IBZM washout reflected a reduction in D_2 receptor availability due to increased synaptic dopamine concentration and increased D_2 receptor occupancy by dopamine. Yet the washout rate of a tracer after single-bolus injection is also influenced by blood flow, which is affected by amphetamine. Thus, using this washout rate method, it was not possible to distinguish an effect of amphetamine on the blood flow from an effect of amphetamine on receptor availability, because both mechanisms would translate into an increased washout of the radiotracer. Because of this difficulty, we investigated the amphetamine effect under sustained equilibrium conditions like those achieved during experiments involving constant infusion of a tracer (Laruelle et al. 1997b).

In contrast to the protocol in which radiotracer is injected as a single bolus, the technique of constant infusion of a radiotracer allows establishment of a stable brain uptake, when the binding of radiotracer is in a state of sustained equilibrium. This technique, when applicable, considerably simplifies the quantitation of neuroreceptor availability and is particularly useful for measuring the effect of challenge tests on receptor availability (Abi-Dargham et al. 1994; Carson et al. 1993; Laruelle et al. 1993, 1994a, 1994b). [^{123}I]IBZM was administered as a priming bolus, and the bolus was followed by continuous infusion at a constant rate for the duration of the experiment. This method of administration induces a state of sustained binding equilibrium and a stable baseline to evaluate changes in receptor availability (Figure 9–1, A). Under these conditions, amphetamine (0.3–1 mg/kg) decreased the [^{123}I]IBZM striatal specific binding by 10%–40% (Figure 9–1, B).

Binding potential (BP) is the parameter of receptor availability (Mintun et al. 1984). BP is equal to receptor density (B_{max}) divided by affinity (K_d).

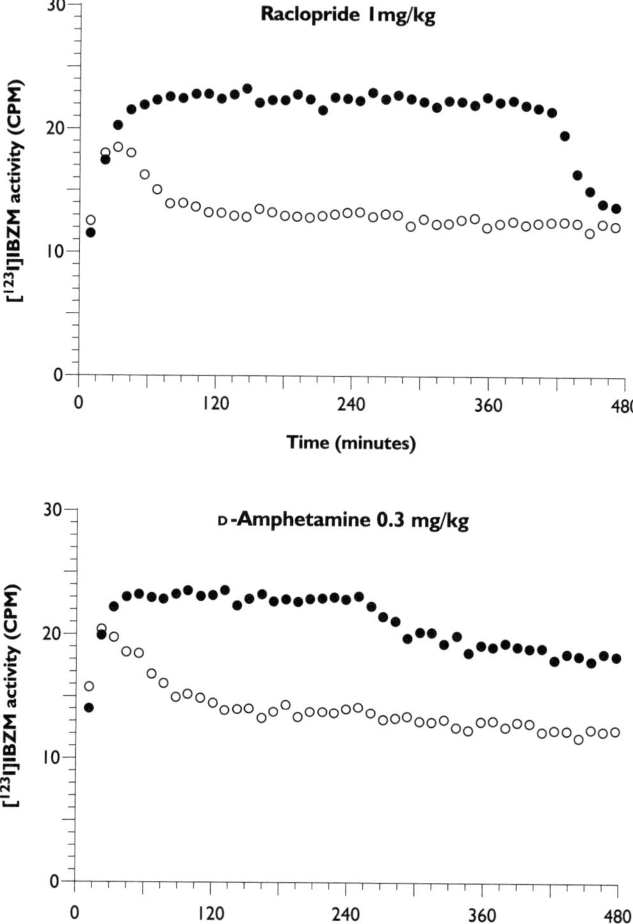

FIGURE 9–1. Striatal (closed circles) and occipital (open circles) activities during bolus plus constant infusion of [^{123}I]iodobenzamide ([^{123}I]IBZM) in a baboon. *(Top)* Constant infusion induced a state of sustained equilibrium (both striatal and occipital activities were stable over time). At the end of the experiment, the dopamine D_2 receptor antagonist raclopride was injected (arrow), resulting in a decrease in striatal activity (specific binding) to the levels observed in the occipital region (nonspecific activity). *(Bottom)* The experiment was repeated in the same baboon, under similar experimental conditions, except for the injection of D-amphetamine at 240 minutes. This injection induced a decrease in striatal activity (specific activity) but did not affect occipital activity (nonspecific activity). Abbreviation: cpm = counts per minute.
Source. Reprinted with permission from Laruelle M, Iyer RN, al-Tikriti et al.: "Microdialysis and SPECT measurements of amphetamine-induced dopamine release in nonhuman primates." *Synapse* 25:1–14, 1997.

Under sustained equilibrium conditions achieved by constant infusion of radiotracer, the decrease in the ratio of specific equilibrium to nonspecific equilibrium (in this case, the ratio of striatal activity to occipital activity) is equal to the decrease in BP (Laruelle et al. 1995). Because measurements are obtained at equilibrium, these ratios are independent of amphetamine effects on cerebral blood flow and on peripheral clearance. Thus, these experiments established that the reduction in [^{123}I]IBZM specific binding after amphetamine administration reflects a decrease in D_2 receptor BP, and not an effect of amphetamine on blood flow and peripheral clearance.

The next step was to establish that the amphetamine-induced reduction in [^{123}I]IBZM BP was mediated by dopamine release, not by some indirect effect of amphetamine unrelated to dopamine release. The mediation of the amphetamine effect by dopamine release was demonstrated by establishing that pretreatment with the dopamine depleter alpha-methyl-para-tyrosine (AMPT) blocked the effect of amphetamine on [^{123}I]IBZM BP. AMPT is a competitive inhibitor of tyrosine hydroxylase, the rate-limiting enzyme for dopamine synthesis (Spector et al. 1965; Udenfriend et al. 1965). AMPT pretreatment resulted in a significant blunting of the amphetamine effect on [^{123}I]IBZM BP, confirming that this effect was mediated by dopamine release (Laruelle et al. 1997b).

Because this method was developed to provide an indirect measure of the magnitude of dopamine release elicited by amphetamine, it was essential to study the relationship between dopamine release and the reduction of [^{123}I]IBZM BP. This comparison was accomplished in baboons by measuring amphetamine-induced dopamine release using microdialysis. We demonstrated that the reduction in [^{123}I]IBZM BP measured using SPECT after various doses of amphetamine was linearly correlated with the peak dopamine release measured using microdialysis (Figure 9–2). This observation validated the use of this noninvasive paradigm to measure changes in synaptic dopamine after amphetamine administration and provided an operational calibration of the SPECT signal. Linear correlation between microdialysis and SPECT measurements revealed that each percent decrement in [^{123}I]IBZM BP corresponded to a 40% increase in peak dopamine concentration. Similar numbers have been reported with regard to the effect of amphetamine on [^{11}C]raclopride (Breier et al. 1997). Thus, with both radiotracers, the method is relatively insensitive to changes in synaptic dopamine, to the extent that large changes in extracellular dopamine are associated with only small changes in receptor availability.

The other interesting observation was that the largest reductions in [^{123}I]IBZM or [^{11}C]raclopride BP induced by challenges aimed at increasing

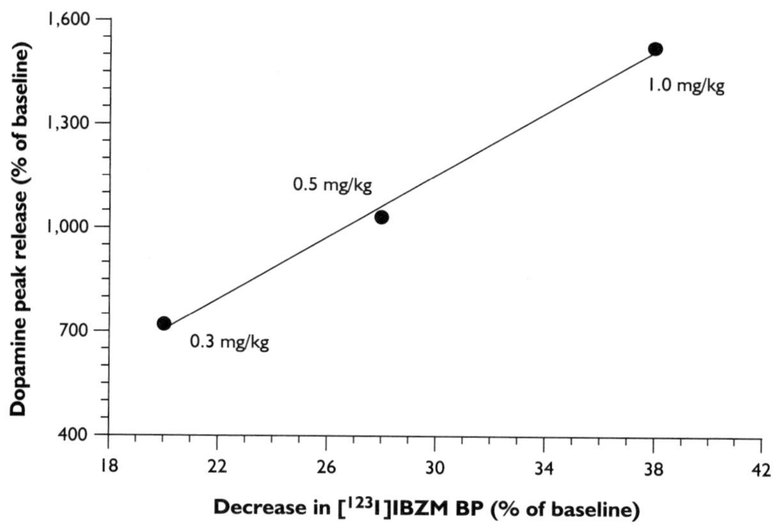

FIGURE 9–2. Correlation between amphetamine-induced peak dopamine release, measured using microdialysis (y axis), and the decrease in [^{123}I]iodobenzamide ([^{123}I]IBZM) dopamine D_2 receptor binding potential (BP), measured using single photon emission computed tomography. Each point is the mean of three experiments. This relationship was linear ($y = -190 + 44x$, $r = 0.99$). If the intercept was constrained to zero, the equation was $y = 39x$. Thus, each percent decrement in [^{123}I]IBZM BP corresponded to about a 40% increase in dopamine concentration over baseline.
Source. Reprinted with permission from Laruelle M, Iyer RN, al-Tikriti et al.: "Microdialysis and SPECT measurements of amphetamine-induced dopamine release in nonhuman primates." *Synapse* 25:1–14, 1997.

dopamine concentration were in the 30%–40% range (Breier et al. 1997; Dewey et al. 1993; Laruelle et al. 1997b). The existence of this plateau effect might be explained by several factors: 1) D_2 receptors are configured in states of high or low affinity for agonists, with approximately 50% of receptors contributing to each state (Seeman and Grigoriadis 1987; Sibley et al. 1982). The D_2 receptor antagonists [^{123}I]IBZM and [^{11}C]raclopride bind with equal affinity to both states, whereas dopamine binds mainly to receptors in the high-affinity state. Thus, dopamine does not compete efficiently with [^{123}I]IBZM or [^{11}C]raclopride binding to D_2 receptors that are in the low-affinity configuration. This factor alone would protect about 50% of the antagonist binding from competition by dopamine. 2) Endocytosis-mediated internalization of G-protein-coupled receptors in response to agonist stimulation is one of the numerous mechanisms by which cellular responses to agonists are rapidly attenuated (Grady et al. 1997; Koenig and Edwardson 1997). PET and SPECT radiotracers are lipophilic compounds capable of crossing the blood-brain barrier and cell membranes and binding to internalized as well as externalized receptors. In contrast, dopamine would not gain access to internalized receptors, and these receptors would also constitute a pool of receptors not affected by endogenous competition. 3) A substantial number of D_2 receptors are not located in the synaptic cleft, and extrasynaptic receptors might be less exposed to changes in dopamine release than might the receptors located at the synaptic level (Caille et al. 1996; Hersch et al. 1995; Levey et al. 1993; Smiley et al. 1994; Yung et al. 1995). Given all of these factors, it is not surprising that only about 40% of [^{123}I]IBZM or [^{11}C]raclopride binding is affected by changes in synaptic dopamine.

We also evaluated the reproducibility of the SPECT measurement of the amphetamine effect on D_2 receptor BP in baboons, and we found an excellent reproducibility, with an intraclass correlation coefficient of 0.97. Thus, this method was found suitable for reliably detecting differences in amphetamine-induced dopamine release between animals.

In conclusion, these experiments in primates established that measurement of reduction in [^{123}I]IBZM BP using SPECT after amphetamine challenge is a noninvasive means of measuring the magnitude of the amphetamine-induced increase in synaptic dopamine. Under sustained equilibrium conditions, the reduction in [^{123}I]IBZM specific binding induced by amphetamine is due to reduction in receptor BP and is insensitive to changes in blood flow. The reduction in [^{123}I]IBZM BP after amphetamine administration is linearly related to the magnitude of dopamine release. This effect is mediated by dopamine; the effect is blunted by inhibition of dopamine synthesis. Finally, this effect, although relatively small, can be measured with adequate reliability, at least in baboons.

Studies in Healthy Humans

After validation of the technique in baboons, we initiated feasibility studies in humans, using the constant-infusion technique and [^{123}I]IBZM (Laruelle et al. 1995). The original human studies demonstrated the feasibility of 1) obtaining a stable baseline of regional activity of [^{123}I]IBZM in the brain with a protocol of bolus plus constant infusion, 2) using this infusion schedule to measure D_2 receptor BP by equilibrium analysis, and 3) using this stable baseline to quantify the reduction in D_2 receptor availability after the D-amphetamine challenge test. Thus, this technique allows measurements, in the same experiment, of both baseline D_2 receptor BP and the amphetamine-induced dopamine release.

Eight young, healthy volunteers (mean age ± standard deviation, 26 ± 3 years) were first studied using a protocol of bolus plus constant infusion of [^{123}I]IBZM under control conditions (i.e., with no amphetamine injection). Stable levels of striatal and background (occipital) activities were maintained from 150 minutes (times are given relative to the beginning of [^{123}I]IBZM administration) to the end of the experiment (360 minutes). The experiment was repeated under similar experimental conditions, except for the injection of 0.3 mg/kg amphetamine at 240 minutes. As observed in baboons, amphetamine induced a significant decrease in [^{123}I]IBZM BP (range, 5%–20%) (Laruelle et al. 1995).

More recently, Booij et al. (1997), using a similar constant-infusion technique with [^{123}I]IBZM, found that placebo injection did not affect [^{123}I]IBZM BP but that injection of the dopamine releaser methylphenidate (0.5 mg/kg) resulted in a significant decrease in [^{123}I]IBZM BP. Similar studies have been performed in healthy volunteers with PET and [^{11}C]raclopride, using the constant-infusion technique (Breier et al. 1997) or two single-bolus injections (Volkow et al. 1994).

We also noted a significant correlation between amphetamine-induced euphoria, alertness, and restlessness and reduction in [^{123}I]IBZM BP ($r^2 = 0.84$, $P = 0.003$), confirming the role of dopamine in mediating these emotions after amphetamine administration (Laruelle et al. 1995). These experiments demonstrated that this technique can be used to study the biochemical mediation of sensation and feelings in humans.

After administration of doses of amphetamine or methylphenidate that are safe to use in humans, [^{123}I]IBZM (or [^{11}C]raclopride) BP reduction is small (in the 5%–20% range), which raises questions about the reliability of this measurement. Another important question was whether, in a given individual, the magnitude of this effect is a trait (i.e., stable over time) or a state factor (i.e., variable with time). To address these questions, Kegeles et al. (1999) studied six healthy subjects (mean age, 36 ± 10 years) twice (mean interval, 16 ± 10 days; range, 7–35 days) using the [^{123}I]IBZM SPECT and amphetamine challenge. Only male subjects were recruited, to remove the confounding effects of the menstrual cycle on results. The average amphetamine-induced [^{123}I]IBZM displacement was 8% ± 8% under test conditions and 9% ± 7% under retest conditions. No differences in [^{123}I]IBZM displacement were observed between test and retest conditions (repeated-measures analysis of variance [ANOVA], $P = 0.56$), indicating the absence of detectable tolerance or sensitization to the amphetamine effect under these conditions. The reliability of measurement of the amphetamine effect, under the null hypothesis of no difference in the amphetamine effect between test and retest conditions, was excellent, with an intraclass correlation coefficient of

0.89. In other words, the magnitude of the amphetamine effect in a given subject on the test day was a good predictor of the effect on the retest day (r^2=0.76, P=0.023). Thus, despite a small amphetamine effect, the method is dependable for measuring between-subject differences. The data also suggest that, at least in healthy subjects and over 2–3 weeks, this effect is a trait rather than a state factor.

Studies in Patients With Schizophrenia

The "classic" hypothesis concerning dopamine and schizophrenia is that hyperactivity of dopamine transmission is responsible for positive symptoms of the disorder (Carlsson and Lindqvist 1963). This hypothesis was supported by the correlation between clinical doses of antipsychotic drugs and their potency with regard to blocking D_2 receptors (Creese et al. 1976; Seeman and Lee 1975), and by the psychotogenic effects of dopamine transmission–enhancing drugs (for a review, see Angrist and van Kammen 1984; Lieberman et al. 1987b). Because positive symptoms are more sensitive than negative symptoms to direct manipulation of the dopamine system, hyperactivity of dopamine transmission is likely to be more relevant to positive than to negative symptoms (Crow 1980). These pharmacologic effects suggest, but do not establish, a dysregulation of dopamine systems in schizophrenia.

Despite decades of effort to validate this hypothesis, documentation of abnormalities of dopamine function in schizophrenia has remained elusive. Postmortem studies measuring dopamine and its metabolites in the brains of schizophrenic patients have yielded inconsistent results (for a review, see Davis et al. 1991). Increased density of striatal D_2 and D_2-like receptors, reported in most postmortem studies (Lee et al. 1978; Owen et al. 1978; for a review, see Seeman et al. 1987), has been difficult to interpret, given that neuroleptic drugs upregulate these receptors (Burt et al. 1977; Seeman 1987). PET and SPECT studies of striatal D_2 and D_2-like receptor density in neuroleptic-naive schizophrenic patients have generally yielded negative results (Breier et al. 1997; Farde et al. 1990; Hietala et al. 1994; Laruelle et al. 1996; Pilowsky et al. 1994; but also see Wong et al. 1986). The lack of clear evidence for increased dopaminergic indices in schizophrenia might indicate that dopamine transmission is enhanced only relative to other systems, such as the glutamatergic system (Carlsson 1988). On the other hand, the absence of data supporting the dopamine hypothesis of schizophrenia might be due to the difficulty in obtaining a direct measurement of dopamine transmission in the living human brain.

We used the imaging technique described to study changes in dopamine transmission after acute amphetamine challenge (0.3 mg/kg iv) in patients with schizophrenia. Patients with schizophrenia are vulnerable to psychotogenic effects of an acute challenge with amphetamine at doses that are not psychotogenic in healthy individuals (for a review, see Lieberman et al. 1987b). The aim of these studies was to explore whether this increased vulnerability to amphetamine is mediated by an increased responsiveness of striatal dopamine transmission.

Amphetamine-induced striatal synaptic dopamine activity was measured in 30 patients with schizophrenia and 30 healthy control subjects matched for age, sex, race or ethnicity, and socioeconomic background. The article describing the results of the initial 15 pairs was published in 1996 (Laruelle et al. 1996), and the report of a study involving a second cohort of 15 pairs was published in 1998 (Abi-Dargham et al. 1998). Both studies were performed using exactly the same protocol. Thus, these data can be combined, and we report here the results for the combined sample. (Subject demographics are presented in Table 9–1.)

Inclusion criteria for patients were as follows: a diagnosis of schizophrenia according to the *Diagnostic and Statistical Manual of Mental Disorders,* 4th Edition (DSM-IV; American Psychiatric Association 1994), no other DSM-IV Axis I diagnosis, no lifetime history of alcohol or substance abuse or dependence, no treatment with any psychotropic medication for at least 21 days before the study (with the exception of lorazepam, which was allowed at a maximal dose of 3 mg/day up to 24 hours before the study), no concomitant or past severe medical conditions, no pregnancy, and no current suicidal or homicidal ideation. All patients provided informed consent; assent by involved family members was also required. All patients were admitted to a research ward for the duration of the study (including the washout period).

Inclusion criteria for healthy control subjects were as follows: no past or present neurological or psychiatric illnesses, no concomitant or past severe medical conditions, and no pregnancy. All control subjects gave informed consent. Healthy control subjects were matched with patients for age, gender, race or ethnicity, and parental socioeconomic level. In the schizophrenic group, the mean duration of illness was 15 ± 7 years. All patients but three had been previously exposed to neuroleptic medication. Patients were drug free for an average of 101 ± 107 days (range, 21 to 365 days; the latter value was used for the four patients drug free for more than 1 year).

Results are presented in Table 9–2. No difference was observed in the baseline (i.e., before amphetamine administration) [^{123}I]IBZM BP between patients and control subjects, in accordance with previously published results

TABLE 9–1. Demographics of subjects in two studies of amphetamine-induced striatal dopamine activity

Parameter	Control subjects (n=30)	Schizophrenic patients (n=30)
Age (years)	41±9	42±8
Sex		
Female	4	4
Male	26	26
Race/Ethnicity		
African American	9	9
Hispanic	2	2
Caucasian	19	19
Parental SES	34±10	35±15
Subject SES	40±13	26±10*

Note. Data are presented as mean±standard deviation or n. Abbreviations: SES=socioeconomic status.
*$P<0.01$.

(Farde et al. 1990; Pilowsky et al. 1994). In contrast, the mean amphetamine-induced decrease in [^{123}I]IBZM BP was significantly greater in schizophrenic patients (–17%±13%) than in control subjects (–7%±7%; $P=0.001$) (Table 9–2 and Figure 9–3). This group difference could not be attributed to differences in amphetamine metabolism, because mean plasma amphetamine levels were similar in patients (29±10 ng/mL) and control subjects (28±11 ng/mL) and because plasma amphetamine levels were not correlated with amphetamine-induced decrease in [^{123}I]IBZM BP. In the schizophrenic group, no correlation was observed between amphetamine response and neuroleptic-free interval duration, lifetime exposure to neuroleptic medications, or use of lorazepam during the washout period.

TABLE 9–2. Results of two studies of amphetamine-induced striatal dopamine activity

Outcome measure	Control subjects (n=30)	Schizophrenic patients (n=30)	P
Baseline [^{123}I]IBZM BP (mL g^{-1})	221±63	224±92	NS
Amphetamine-induced change in [^{123}I]IBZM BP (% baseline value)	–7%±7%	–17%±13%	0.001

Note. Data are presented as mean±standard deviation. Abreviations: BP=binding potential; IBZM=iodobenzamide; NS=not significant.

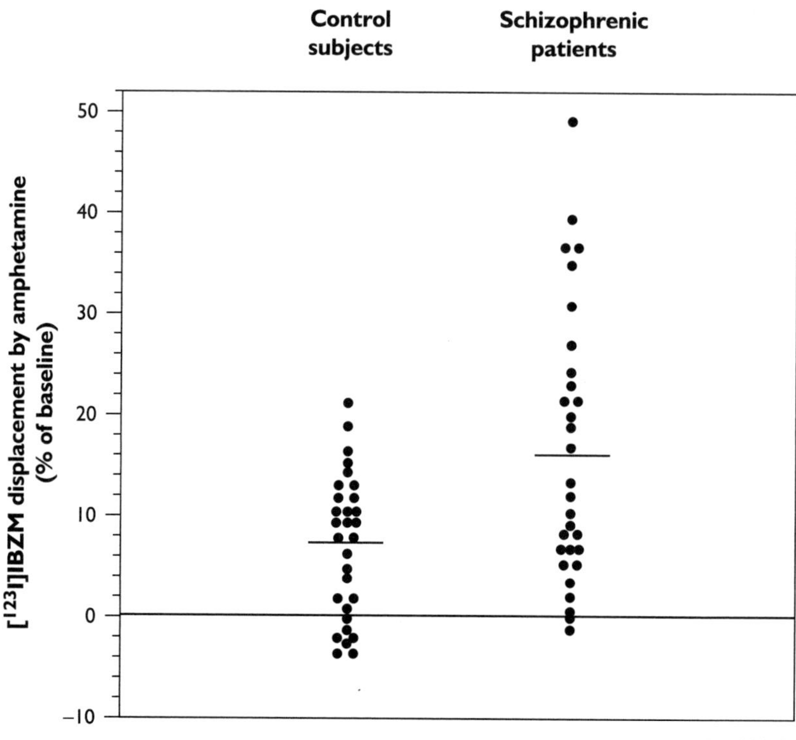

FIGURE 9–3. Amphetamine-induced relative decrease in [^{123}I]iodobenzamide ([^{123}I]IBZM) binding potential in 30 healthy control subjects and 30 patients with schizophrenia, matched for age, sex, race or ethnicity, and parental socioeconomic level.

Amphetamine-induced changes in positive psychotic symptoms were measured using the Positive and Negative Syndrome Scale (PANSS) (Kay and Opler 1986). PANSS scores were obtained just before scan session 1 and 30 minutes after amphetamine injection. A clinically significant psychotic reaction to amphetamine was defined as an increase in score of at least four points over baseline on the positive symptoms subscale of the PANSS. Amphetamine induced a transient but clinically significant worsening of positive psychotic symptoms in 12 (40%) of 30 patients. This prevalence is consistent with the previously reported prevalence of psychotic reactions to acute challenges with dopamine agonists in schizophrenia (Lieberman et al. 1987a). Psychotic reactions were characterized mostly by delusional paranoid ideation ("The CIA is watching me because I am responsible for the bombing of the U.S. Embassy in Lebanon") and hallucinations ("The angels are here; I can see them") that were not present at baseline. Amphetamine-induced psychotic reactions were transient, and all patients returned to their baseline state a few hours after the challenge. No psychotic symptoms were observed in healthy control subjects.

Schizophrenic patients who experienced worsening of positive symptoms (n=12) showed greater reductions in [^{123}I]IBZM BP (mean ± standard error of the mean, –25% ± 4%) than did schizophrenic patients whose positive symptoms did not worsen (–11% ± 3%, n = 18) and healthy control subjects (–7% ± 1%, n=30; ANOVA, P<0.001). In the schizophrenic group, the magnitude of the amphetamine effect on [^{123}I]IBZM BP was correlated with changes in positive symptoms (r=0.53, P=0.001) (Figure 9–4).

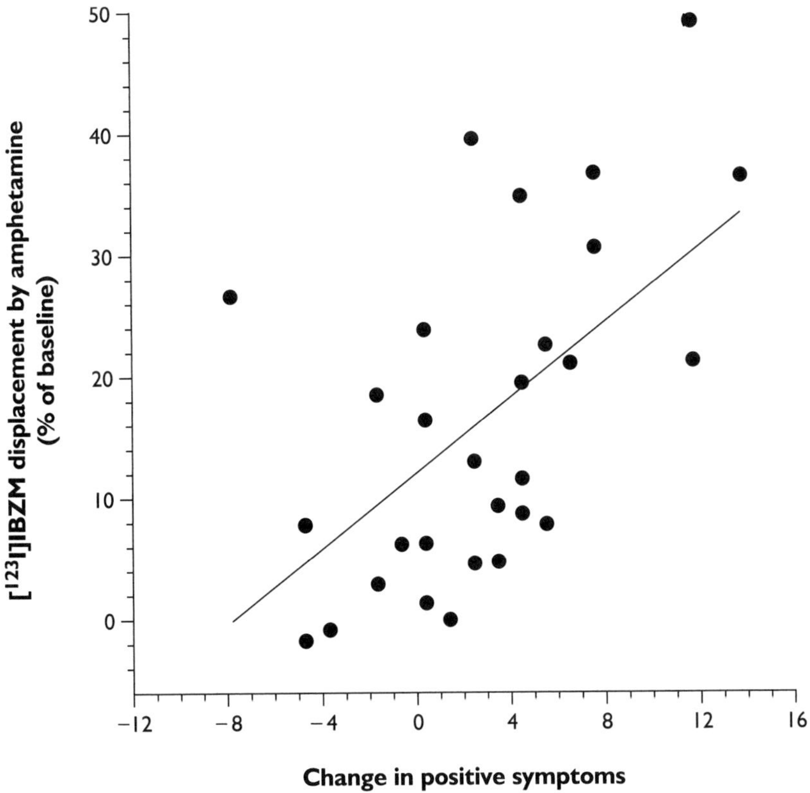

FIGURE 9–4. Relationship between amphetamine-induced changes in positive symptoms and amphetamine-induced relative decreases in [^{123}I]iodobenzamide ([^{123}I]IBZM) binding potential in 30 schizophrenic patients (r=0.53, P=0.001).

Discussion

These data suggest that schizophrenia is associated with release of excess dopamine after amphetamine challenge, and that the magnitude of this has clinical consequences for the symptomatic response to the challenge. These results were independently replicated by Breier et al. (1997), using PET, [^{11}C]raclopride, and a lower dose of amphetamine (0.2 mg/kg). Together, these results suggest the existence of increased presynaptic dopamine activity in schizophrenia, a conclusion consistent with findings of two PET studies, which showed increased accumulation of the dopamine precursor 6-[^{18}F]fluoro-L-dopa in the striatum of patients with schizophrenia (Hietala et al. 1995; Reith et al. 1994).

The increased amphetamine effect in patients with schizophrenia was not associated with previous neuroleptic exposure. However, the role of previous neuroleptic exposure cannot be excluded without the performance of studies involving neuroleptic-naive patients. So far, we have studied 7 drug-naive patients with first-episode schizophrenia (3 in the sample of 30 patients presented earlier, and 4 in an ongoing study involving drug-naive patients). The mean amphetamine-induced [^{123}I]IBZM displacement in these 7 patients was –21%±12%, a value comparable to the mean value in the schizophrenic group (–17%±13%) and higher than in the control group (–7%±7%). Likewise, in the patients studied by Breier at al. (1997), no difference was observed in amphetamine-induced [^{11}C]raclopride displacement among patients with chronic schizophrenia, drug-free schizophrenic patients, and drug-naive patients with first-break schizophrenia. These preliminary data suggest that the larger effect of amphetamine on [^{123}I]IBZM BP is present at the onset of illness and is unrelated to previous neuroleptic treatment.

This exaggerated amphetamine effect on D_2 receptor BP observed in patients with schizophrenia might reflect either an increased release of dopamine after amphetamine administration or an increased affinity of D_2 receptors for dopamine, or some combination of both factors. Available data do not support the existence of an increased affinity of D_2 receptors for agonists in schizophrenia; the sequence of the D_2 receptor gene is not altered (Gejman et al. 1994), and the binding of dopamine agonists in postmortem striata is not increased in schizophrenia (Cross et al. 1983; Lee et al. 1978). Development of D_2 receptor agonists as PET radioligands is needed to confirm these results in vivo. Thus, although a contribution by the affinity factor cannot be definitively excluded, an increased concentration of dopamine in the vicinity of the receptors is likely the predominant mechanism underlying the observed effect.

The mechanism of this putative increased dopaminergic neuronal reactivity remains to be elucidated. Corticifugal glutamatergic projections that increase the responsiveness of dopaminergic subcortical systems are inhibited by dopaminergic prefrontal projections, both directly and indirectly via GABAergic interneurons (Deutch 1993; Retaux et al. 1991). This glutamatergic cortical control occurs primarily through projections to the dopamine cell body area rather than the terminal region (Karreman and Moghaddam 1996). In nonhuman primates, selective destruction of dopamine terminals in dorsolateral, medial, and orbital regions of the prefrontal cortex does not affect striatal baseline dopamine concentration but induces a long-lasting increase in striatal potassium-induced dopamine release (Roberts et al. 1994). Given that potassium, like amphetamine, stimulates both dopamine synthesis and release (Schwarz et al. 1980), this observation is potentially relevant to the present finding. Thus, the increased responsiveness of subcortical dopamine neurons observed in this study might be secondary to prefrontal dopaminergic or GABAergic deficits; both deficits have been proposed as constituents of the "cortical pathology" in schizophrenia (Benes et al. 1991; Weinberger 1987).

The demonstration of an increased dopamine release in response to amphetamine in schizophrenia might indicate that, under these extreme and nonphysiological conditions, the modulatory feedback mechanisms regulating dopamine release are impaired. The increased striatal amphetamine-induced dopamine release observed in these studies might be a manifestation of this impaired regulation. However, a more important and fundamental question is whether the impaired regulation revealed by the amphetamine challenge is also associated with increased dopamine release in the absence of amphetamine or any pharmacologic stimulation. A pharmacologic intervention that would induce a rapid and complete depletion of synaptic dopamine could theoretically provide a measure of D_2 receptor occupancy by dopamine at baseline. To address this issue, we recently introduced the AMPT challenge test.

■ The AMPT Challenge Test

Baboon Studies

The concept of the AMPT depletion paradigm emerged from the baboon experiments in which AMPT was used primarily to document that dopamine depletion blocks the effect of amphetamine on [^{123}I]IBZM BP (Laruelle et al. 1997b). In addition to documenting the effect of AMPT on amphetamine challenge, we observed that at the end of the AMPT infusion, [^{123}I]IBZM BP was increased by 28% and 30% compared with the values measured in the same animals under control conditions. The magnitude of this effect was comparable to the increase in in vivo binding of [^{3}H]raclopride measured in rodents after acute dopamine depletion with reserpine or AMPT (Inoue et al. 1991; Ross 1991; Ross and Jackson 1989a, 1989b; Seeman et al. 1990; van der Werf et al. 1983; Young et al. 1991). Similarly, reserpine administration acutely increased [^{11}C]raclopride BP in rhesus monkeys (Ginovart et al. 1997). Together, these studies indicate that D_2 receptor occupancy by dopamine is far from negligible and that comparison of [^{123}I]IBZM BP before and after acute dopamine depletion might allow measurement of D_2 receptor occupancy by dopamine in humans.

Studies in Healthy Humans

We compared [^{123}I]IBZM BP at baseline and during dopamine depletion as achieved by oral administration of AMPT (1 g every 6 hours for 2 days) in nine healthy male subjects (mean age, 25 ± 5 years). We selected AMPT as the depleting agent because this drug is approved for human use and its effects, unlike the effects of reserpine, are rapidly reversible. This high dose and this frequency of administration were selected to rapidly induce and to maintain nearly complete inhibition of tyrosine hydroxylase activity (Engelman et al. 1968). AMPT was given for 2 days, the expectation being that this duration of treatment would be adequate to produce a nearly complete dopamine depletion (48 hours is about 10 half-lives of dopamine turnover) (Spector et al. 1965) but too short to induce significant D_2 receptor upregulation. AMPT treatment was initiated at the end of scan 1, and scan 2 was performed 2 days after scan 1 (i.e., on day 3).

Clinical examination revealed mild signs of parkinsonism in all subjects on day 3. Facial akinesia, hypokinesia or bradykinesia, and resting tremor were the extrapyramidal signs most often noted. Two subjects experienced an acute dystonic reaction (spasms of muscles of the neck and jaw) the evening of day 3. These clinical effects were consistent with profound dopamine depletion.

We observed a significant increase in [^{123}I]IBZM BP after AMPT administration (mean, 28% ± 16%; repeated-measures ANOVA, $P<0.001$) (Figure 9–5). This increase was much greater than any variability seen in our test-retest study. In a previous study (Laruelle et al. 1995), seven subjects underwent two scans, 2 weeks apart, under identical conditions ([^{123}I]IBZM constant infusion). The average difference in [^{123}I]IBZM BP between test and

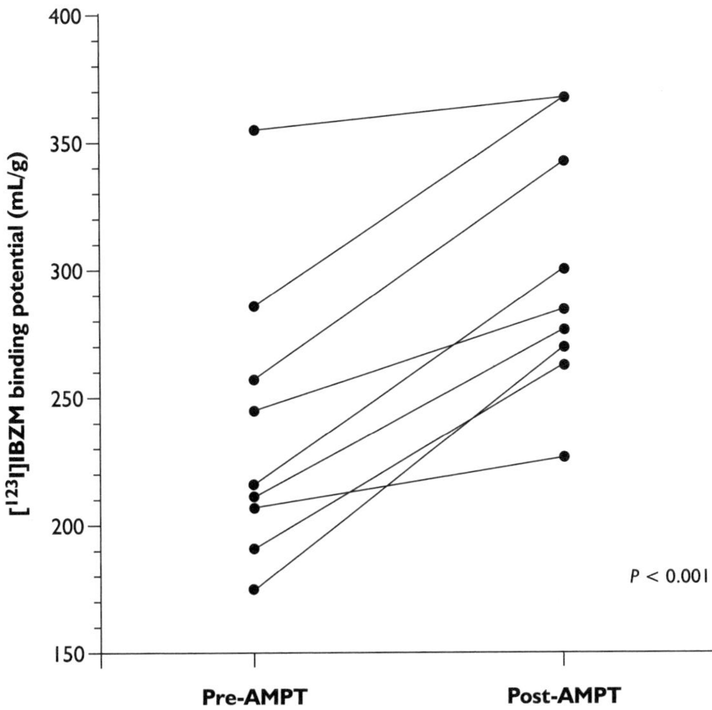

FIGURE 9–5. [^{123}I]Iodobenzamide ([^{123}I]IBZM) binding potential (BP) at baseline (before alpha-methyl-para-tyrosine [AMPT] administration) and at the end of AMPT administration (1 g four times a day for 2 days). AMPT-induced depletion of endogenous dopamine resulted in a significant increase in [^{123}I]IBZM BP (repeated-measures analysis of variance, $P<0.001$). The average increase ± standard deviation was 28% ± 16%.

Source. Reprinted with permission from Laruelle M, D'Souza CD, Baldwin RM, et al.: "Imaging D2 receptor occupancy by endogenous dopamine in humans." *Neuropsychopharmacology* 17:162–174, 1997.

retest was –0.1% ± 6.4% (range, –6.6% to +9.4%). The average absolute difference was 5.6 ± 2%. This reproducibility corresponded to an intraclass correlation coefficient of 0.96.

The between-subject variability in the AMPT effect on D_2 receptor availability could relate to differences in AMPT pharmacokinetics or differences in baseline synaptic dopamine concentration. However, plasma AMPT levels (mean, 21 ± 7 μg/mL) were not correlated with the AMPT effect on [^{123}I]IBZM BP ($r^2=0.18$, $P=0.33$). In fact, variation in plasma AMPT levels observed between subjects was not expected to have significant consequences for the pharmacodynamic effect of AMPT. Given an average plasma tyrosine level of 10 μg/mL, a tyrosine affinity constant for tyrosine hydroxylase of 62.5 μM, and an AMPT affinity constant for tyrosine hydroxylase of 17 μM (Udenfriend et al. 1965), AMPT concentrations of 13 μg/mL (the smallest value observed in this study), 21 μg/mL (mean value), and 31 μg/mL (highest value) would be expected to produce comparable degrees of enzymatic inhibition (68%, 78%, and 83%, respectively). Higher doses of AMPT would not induce significantly more blockade of the enzyme, because of the nonlinearity between inhibitor concentration and enzymatic inhibition (Engelman et al. 1968).

Rodent Studies

To verify that this AMPT regimen does not induce D_2 receptor upregulation, we treated rats with either saline or AMPT (200 mg/kg twice a day) for 2 days, and we compared in vitro D_2 receptor density between the two groups using $[^{123}I]$IBZM (Laruelle et al. 1997a). No significant increase in D_2 receptor density was observed in the AMPT group, indicating that the increase in $[^{123}I]$IBZM BP observed in vivo after 2 days' administration of AMPT was due to removal of endogenous dopamine and not to receptor upregulation. This experiment confirmed findings of an earlier study, which did not demonstrate significant D_2 receptor upregulation after 1 week of dopamine depletion induced by 6-hydroxydopamine (Narang and Wamsley 1995). Similarly, acute pretreatment of mice with reserpine (5 mg/kg) resulted in a significant increase in the in vivo specific binding of $[^3H]$raclopride, whereas no changes in D_2 receptor density were detected in vitro (Ross and Jackson 1989a). Thus, to the extent that these results can be extrapolated to humans, receptor upregulation does not contribute to the observed AMPT effect on $[^{123}I]$IBZM BP.

Discussion

These studies with AMPT demonstrate that competition by endogenous dopamine results in a 20%–30% underestimation of D_2 receptor density in vivo and suggest the possibility of taking advantage of this phenomenon to measure striatal synaptic dopamine concentration in humans. With the recently developed ability to measure extrastriatal D_2 receptors (Halldin et al. 1995), this technique might also allow measurement of dopamine activity in extrastriatal regions, such as the cerebral cortex. Such a method would be valuable for elucidating regional alterations of dopamine activity in schizophrenia and other neuropsychiatric illnesses and for relating these alterations to the clinical symptomatology. Using the AMPT paradigm, we are currently studying resting dopamine concentration in the striata of untreated schizophrenic patients.

General Discussion

The studies described here demonstrate the potential of this new application of neuroreceptor imaging to elucidate neurochemical imbalances associated with mental illness. The productivity of this line of investigation has been shown by the studies in schizophrenia described in this chapter and by the study conducted by Volkow et al. (1997), who demonstrated a decrease in methylphenidate-induced dopamine release in recently detoxified cocaine abusers. The recent demonstration that challenge by video-game playing is associated with a significant decrease in [^{11}C]raclopride BP compared with the resting state is another exciting illustration of the potential and versatility of this method (Koepp et al. 1998).

These "functional" neuroreceptor imaging studies are not limited to the study of "direct" pharmacologic challenges (i.e., challenges with drugs that directly affect synaptic dopamine concentration, such as amphetamine, methylphenidate, or AMPT). Manipulation of the GABAergic, serotonergic, and glutamatergic systems also affects [^{11}C]raclopride binding (Breier et al. 1998; Dewey et al. 1992, 1995; Smith et al. 1997, 1998). These observations open the door to the possibility of studying neurotransmitter interactions in the living human brain with these techniques.

Strong efforts are being made to extend this paradigm to, and validate it in, neuroreceptor systems other than D_2 receptors, but success has not yet been achieved. To validate the use of PET or SPECT neuroreceptor studies to assess transmitter concentration, the effect of the challenge on binding capacity must be clearly mediated by changes in transmitter concentration, and the relationship between variation in transmitter concentration and binding capacity must be documented. To our knowledge, such a validation has not yet occurred in systems other than D_2 receptors.

In addition, it is still unclear which properties of [^{11}C]raclopride or [^{123}I]IBZM are responsible for the vulnerability of their binding to competition by endogenous dopamine. Spiperone, a ligand with high affinity for D_2 receptors (K_d=0.1 nM), is known to be less vulnerable to endogenous competition than is raclopride, a ligand with relatively low affinity (K_d=1 nM) (Hartvig et al. 1997; Seeman et al. 1989; Young et al. 1991). However, the fact that several high-affinity benzamides, such as [^{123}I]iodobenzofuran (K_d=0.1 nM)

(Laruelle et al. 1997b) and [^{18}F]fallypride (K_d=0.1 nM) (Mukherjee et al. 1997; Price et al. 1997), are affected by amphetamine indicates that factors other than affinity are implicated in the well-documented differences in vulnerability to endogenous competition between spiperone and raclopride. Binding of D_1 receptor radiotracers [^{11}C]NNC 756 (K_d=0.1 nM) and [^{11}C]SCH 23390 (K_d=0.4 nM) is not affected by changes in endogenous dopamine (Abi-Dargham et al. 1999). Binding of dopamine transporter radioligands is not affected by changes in dopamine concentration (Gatley et al. 1995a, 1995b). These data indicate that factors specific to receptors (and not only to radiotracers) are implicated in this phenomenon. The elucidation of these factors will facilitate the extension of these paradigms to other neuroreceptor systems.

■ CONCLUSION

In this chapter, we showed how binding competition between the SPECT or PET radiotracers and dopamine enables measurement of synaptic dopamine activity, both at baseline and in stimulated conditions. This new application of neuroreceptor imaging goes beyond the classic measurement of receptor densities and affinities and provides a more functional and sophisticated characterization of synaptic activity. The method has been applied to the study of dopamine function in schizophrenia and cocaine addiction, providing unique insight into the pathophysiology of these illnesses. The extension of this technique to other neuroreceptor systems, and the validation of it in these systems, is a major challenge.

■ REFERENCES

Abi-Dargham A, Laruelle M, Seibyl J, et al: SPECT measurement of benzodiazepine receptors in human brain with [^{123}I]iomazenil: kinetic and equilibrium paradigms. J Nucl Med 35:228–238, 1994

Abi-Dargham A, Gil R, Krystal J, et al: Increased striatal dopamine transmission in schizophrenia: confirmation in a second cohort. Am J Psychiatry 155:761–767, 1998

Abi-Dargham A, Simpson N, Kegeles L, et al: PET studies of binding competition between endogenous dopamine and the D_1 radiotracer [^{11}C]NNC 756. Synapse 32:93–109, 1999

American Psychiatric Association: Diagnostic and Statistical Manual of Mental Disorders, 4th Edition. Washington, DC, American Psychiatric Association, 1994

Angrist B, van Kammen DP: CNS stimulants as a tool in the study of schizophrenia. Trends Neurosci 7:388–390, 1984

Benes FM, McSparren J, Bird ED, et al: Deficits in small interneurons in schizophrenic cortex. Arch Gen Psychiatry 48:996–1001, 1991

Booij J, Korn P, Linszen DH, et al: Assessment of endogenous dopamine release by methylphenidate challenge using iodine-123 iodobenzamide single-photon emission tomography. Eur J Nucl Med 24:674–677, 1997

Breier A, Su TP, Saunders R, et al: Schizophrenia is associated with elevated amphetamine-induced synaptic dopamine concentrations: evidence from a novel positron emission tomography method. Proc Natl Acad Sci U S A 94:2569–2574, 1997

Breier A, Adler CM, Weisenfeld N, et al: Effects of NMDA antagonism on striatal dopamine release in healthy subjects: application of a novel PET approach. Synapse 29:142–147, 1998

Burt DR, Creese I, Snyder SH: Antischizophrenic drugs: chronic treatment elevates dopamine receptor binding in brain. Science 196:326–328, 1977

Caille I, Dumartin B, Bloch B: Ultrastructural localization of D1 dopamine receptor immunoreactivity in rat striatonigral neurons and its relation with dopaminergic innervation. Brain Res 730:17–31, 1996

Carlsson A: The current status of the dopamine hypothesis of schizophrenia. Neuropsychopharmacology 1:179–186, 1988

Carlsson A, Lindqvist M: Effect of chlorpromazine or haloperidol on formation of 3-methoxytyramine and normetanephrine in mouse brain. Acta Pharmacol Toxicol (Copenh) 20:140–144, 1963

Carson RE, Channing MA, Blasberg RG, et al: Comparison of bolus and infusion methods for receptor quantitation: application to [^{18}F]cyclofoxy and positron emission tomography. J Cereb Blood Flow Metab 13:24–42, 1993

Carson RE, Breier A, de Bartolomeis A, et al: Quantification of amphetamine-induced changes in [^{11}C]raclopride binding with continuous infusion. J Cereb Blood Flow Metab 17:437–447, 1997

Creese I, Burt DR, Snyder SH: Dopamine receptor binding predicts clinical and pharmacological potencies of antischizophrenic drugs. Science 192:481–483, 1976

Cross AJ, Crow TJ, Ferrier IN, et al: Dopamine receptor changes in schizophrenia in relation to the disease process and movement disorder. J Neural Transm Suppl 18: 265–272, 1983

Crow TJ: Molecular pathology of schizophrenia: more than one disease process? Br Med J 280:66–68, 1980

Davis KL, Kahn RS, Ko G, et al: Dopamine in schizophrenia: a review and reconceptualization. Am J Psychiatry 148:1474–1486, 1991

De Jesus OT, Van Moffaert GJ, Dinerstein RJ, et al: Exogenous L-dopa alters spiroperidol binding, in vivo, in the mouse striatum. Life Sci 39:341–349, 1986

Deutch AY: Prefrontal cortical dopamine systems and the elaboration of functional corticostriatal circuits: implications for schizophrenia and Parkinson's disease. J Neural Transm 91:197–221, 1993

Dewey SL, Logan J, Wolf AP, et al: Amphetamine induced decreases in (^{18}F)-*N*-methylspiroperidol binding in the baboon brain using positron emission tomography (PET). Synapse 7:324–327, 1991

Dewey SL, Smith GS, Logan J, et al: GABAergic inhibition of endogenous dopamine release measured in vivo with ^{11}C-raclopride and positron emission tomography. J Neurosci 12:3773–3780, 1992

Dewey SL, Smith GS, Logan J, et al: Striatal binding of the PET ligand ^{11}C-raclopride is altered by drugs that modify synaptic dopamine levels. Synapse 13:350–356, 1993

Dewey SL, Smith GS, Logan J, et al: Serotonergic modulation of striatal dopamine measured with positron emission tomography (PET) and in vivo microdialysis. J Neurosci 15:821–829, 1995

Engelman K, Jequier E, Udenfriend S, et al: Metabolism of alpha-methyltyrosine in man: relationship to its potency as an inhibitor of catecholamine biosynthesis. J Clin Invest 47:568–576, 1968

Farde L, Wiesel F, Stone-Elander S, et al: D2 dopamine receptors in neuroleptic-naive schizophrenic patients: a positron emission tomography study with [^{11}C]raclopride. Arch Gen Psychiatry 47:213–219, 1990

Gatley SJ, Ding YS, Volkow ND, et al: Binding of D-threo-[^{11}C]methylphenidate to the dopamine transporter in vivo: insensitivity to synaptic dopamine. Eur J Pharmacol 281:141–149, 1995a

Gatley SJ, Volkow ND, Fowler JS, et al: Sensitivity of striatal [^{11}C]cocaine binding to decreases in synaptic dopamine. Synapse 20:137–144, 1995b

Gejman PV, Ram A, Gelernter J, et al: No structural mutation in the dopamine D2 receptor gene in alcoholism or schizophrenia: analysis using denaturing gradient gel electrophoresis. JAMA 271:204–208, 1994

Ginovart N, Lundin A, Farde L, et al: PET study of the pre- and post-synaptic dopaminergic markers for the neurodegenerative process in Huntington's disease. Brain 120:503–514, 1997

Grady EF, Bohm SK, Bunnett NW: Turning off the signal: mechanisms that attenuate signaling by G protein-coupled receptors. Am J Physiol 273:G586–G601, 1997

Halldin C, Farde L, Hogberg T, et al: Carbon-11-FLB 457: a radioligand for extrastriatal D2 dopamine receptors. J Nucl Med 36:1275–1281, 1995

Hartvig P, Torstenson R, Tedroff J, et al: Amphetamine effects on dopamine release and synthesis rate studied in the rhesus monkey brain by positron emission tomography. J Neural Transm 104:329–339, 1997

Hersch SM, Ciliax BJ, Gutekunst CA, et al: Electron microscopic analysis of D1 and D2 dopamine receptor proteins in the dorsal striatum and their synaptic relationships with motor corticostriatal afferents. J Neurosci 15:5222–5237, 1995

Hietala J, Syvälahti E, Vuorio K, et al: Striatal D2 receptor characteristics in neuroleptic-naive schizophrenic patients studied with positron emission tomography. Arch Gen Psychiatry 51:116–123, 1994

Hietala J, Syvälahti E, Vuorio K, et al: Presynaptic dopamine function in striatum of neuroleptic-naive schizophrenic patients. Lancet 346:1130–1131, 1995

Innis RB, Malison RT, al-Tikriti M, et al: Amphetamine-stimulated dopamine release competes in vivo for [^{123}I]IBZM binding to the D_2 receptor in non-human primates. Synapse 10:177–184, 1992

Inoue O, Kobayashi K, Tsukada H, et al: Difference in in vivo receptor binding between [^{3}H]*N*-methylspiperone and [^{3}H]raclopride in reserpine-treated mouse brain. Journal of Neural Transmission General Section 85:1–10, 1991

Karreman M, Moghaddam B: The prefrontal cortex regulates the basal release of dopamine in the limbic striatum: an effect mediated by ventral tegmental area. J Neurochem 66:589–598, 1996

Kay SR, Opler LA: Positive and Negative Syndrome Scale (PANSS) Rating Manual. New York, Department of Psychiatry, Albert Einstein College of Medicine, 1986

Kegeles LS, Zea-Ponce Y, Abi-Dargham A, et al: Stability of [^{123}I]IBZM SPECT measurement of amphetamine-induced striatal dopamine release in humans. Synapse 31:302–308, 1999

Koenig JA, Edwardson JM: Endocytosis and recycling of G protein-coupled receptors. Trends Pharmacol Sci 18:276–287, 1997

Koepp MJ, Gunn RN, Lawrence AD, et al: Evidence for striatal dopamine release during a video game. Nature 393:266–268, 1998

Köhler C, Fuxe K, Ross SB: Regional in vivo binding of [^{3}H]N-propylnorapomorphine in the mouse brain: evidence for labelling of central dopamine receptors. Eur J Pharmacol 72:397–402, 1981

Kuczenski R, Segal D: Concomitant characterization of behavioral and striatal neurotransmitter response to amphetamine using *in vivo* microdialysis. J Neurosci 9: 2051–2065, 1989

Laruelle M, Abi-Dargham A, Rattner Z, et al: Single photon emission tomography measurement of benzodiazepine receptor number and affinity in primate brain: a constant infusion paradigm with [^{123}I]iomazenil. Eur J Pharmacol 230:119–123, 1993

Laruelle M, al-Tikriti MS, Zea-Ponce Y, et al: In vivo quantification of dopamine D_2 receptor parameters in nonhuman primates with [^{123}I]iodobenzofuran and single photon emission computerized tomography. Eur J Pharmacol 263:39–51, 1994a

Laruelle M, Abi-Dargham A, al-Tikriti MS, et al: SPECT quantification of [^{123}I]iomazenil binding to benzodiazepine receptors in nonhuman primates, II: equilibrium analysis of constant infusion experiments and correlation with in vitro parameters. J Cereb Blood Flow Metab 14:453–465, 1994b

Laruelle M, Abi-Dargham A, van Dyck CH, et al: SPECT imaging of striatal dopamine release after amphetamine challenge. J Nucl Med 36:1182–1190, 1995

Laruelle M, Abi-Dargham A, van Dyck CH, et al: Single photon emission computerized tomography imaging of amphetamine-induced dopamine release in drug-free schizophrenic subjects. Proc Natl Acad Sci U S A 93:9235–9240, 1996

Laruelle M, D'Souza CD, Baldwin RM, et al: Imaging D2 receptor occupancy by endogenous dopamine in humans. Neuropsychopharmacology 17:162–174, 1997a

Laruelle M, Iyer RN, al-Tikriti MS, et al: Microdialysis and SPECT measurements of amphetamine-induced dopamine release in nonhuman primates. Synapse 25:1–14, 1997b

Lee T, Seeman P, Tourtelotte WW, et al: Binding of ^{3}H-neuroleptics and ^{3}H-apomorphine in schizophrenic brains. Nature 274:897–900, 1978

Levey AI, Hersch SM, Rye DB, et al: Localization of D1 and D2 dopamine receptors in brain with subtype-specific antibodies. Proc Natl Acad Sci U S A 90:8861–8865, 1993

Lieberman JA, Kane JM, Sarantakos S, et al: Prediction of relapse in schizophrenia. Arch Gen Psychiatry 44:597–603, 1987a

Lieberman JA, Kane JM, Alvir J: Provocative tests with psychostimulant drugs in schizophrenia. Psychopharmacology (Berl) 91:415–433, 1987b

Mintun MA, Raichle ME, Kilbourn MR, et al: A quantitative model for the in vivo assessment of drug binding sites with positron emission tomography. Ann Neurol 15:217–227, 1984

Mukherjee J, Yang ZY, Lew R, et al: Evaluation of D-amphetamine effects on the binding of dopamine D-2 receptor radioligand, ^{18}F-fallypride in nonhuman primates using positron emission tomography. Synapse 27:1–13, 1997

Narang N, Wamsley JK: Time dependent changes in DA uptake sites, D_1 and D_2 receptor binding and mRNA after 6-OHDA lesions of the medial forebrain bundle in the rat brain. J Chem Neuroanat 9:41–53, 1995

Owen F, Cross AJ, Crow TJ, et al: Increased dopamine-receptor sensitivity in schizophrenia. Lancet 2:223–226, 1978

Pilowsky LS, Costa DC, Ell PJ, et al: D2 dopamine receptor binding in the basal ganglia of antipsychotic-free schizophrenic patients: an ^{123}I-IBZM single photon emission computerised tomography study. Br J Psychiatry 164:16–26, 1994

Price JC, Mason S, Lopresti B, et al: PET measurements of endogenous neurotransmitter activity using high and low affinity radiotracers. Neuroimage 5:B77, 1997

Reith J, Benkelfat C, Sherwin A, et al: Elevated dopa decarboxylase activity in living brain of patients with psychosis. Proc Natl Acad Sci U S A 91:11651–11654, 1994

Retaux S, Besson MJ, Penit-Soria J: Synergism between D1 and D2 dopamine receptors in the inhibition of the evoked release of [^{3}H]GABA in the rat prefrontal cortex. Neuroscience 43:323–329, 1991

Roberts AC, De Salvia MA, Wilkinson LS, et al: 6-Hydroxydopamine lesions of the prefrontal cortex in monkeys enhance performance on an analog of the Wisconsin Card Sort Test: possible interactions with subcortical dopamine. J Neurosci 14: 2531–2544, 1994

Ross SB: Synaptic concentration of dopamine in the mouse striatum in relationship to the kinetic properties of the dopamine receptors and uptake mechanism. J Neurochem 56:22–29, 1991

Ross SB, Jackson DM: Kinetic properties of the accumulation of ^{3}H-raclopride in the mouse brain in vivo. Naunyn Schmiedebergs Arch Pharmacol 340:6–12, 1989a

Ross SB, Jackson DM: Kinetic properties of the in vivo accumulation of ^{3}H-(-)-*N*-n-propylnorapomorphine in mouse brain. Naunyn Schmiedebergs Arch Pharmacol 340:13–20, 1989b

Schwarz RD, Uretsky NJ, Bianchine JR: The relationship between the stimulation of dopamine synthesis and release produced by amphetamine and high potassium striatal slices. J Neurochem 35:1120–1127, 1980

Seeman P: Dopamine receptors and the dopamine hypothesis of schizophrenia. Synapse 1:133–152, 1987

Seeman P, Grigoriadis D: Dopamine receptors in brain and periphery. Neurochem Int 10:1–25, 1987

Seeman P, Lee T: Antipsychotic drugs: direct correlation between clinical potency and presynaptic action on dopamine neurons. Science 188:1217–1219, 1975

Seeman P, Bzowej NH, Guan HC, et al: Human brain D1 and D2 dopamine receptors in schizophrenia, Alzheimer's, Parkinson's, and Huntington's diseases. Neuropsychopharmacology 1:5–15, 1987

Seeman P, Guan HC, Niznik HB: Endogenous dopamine lowers the dopamine D_2 receptor density as measured by [^{3}H]raclopride: implications for positron emission tomography of the human brain. Synapse 3:96–97, 1989

Seeman P, Niznik HB, Guan HC: Elevation of dopamine D2 receptors in schizophrenia is underestimated by radioactive raclopride. Arch Gen Psychiatry 47:1170–1172, 1990

Sharp T, Zetterstrom T, Ljungberg T, et al: A direct comparison of amphetamine-induced behaviours and regional brain dopamine release in the rat using intracerebral dialysis. Brain Res 401:322–330, 1987

Sibley DR, De Lean A, Creese I: Anterior pituitary receptors: Demonstration of interconvertible high and low affinity states of the D_2 dopamine receptor. J Biol Chem 257:6351–6361, 1982

Smiley JF, Levey AI, Ciliax BJ, et al: D1 dopamine receptor immunoreactivity in human and monkey cerebral cortex: predominant and extrasynaptic localization in dendritic spines. Proc Natl Acad Sci U S A 91:5720–5724, 1994

Smith GS, Dewey SL, Brodie JD, et al: Serotonergic modulation of dopamine measured with [^{11}C]raclopride and PET in normal human subjects. Am J Psychiatry 154:490–496, 1997

Smith GS, Schloesser R, Brodie JD, et al: Glutamate modulation of dopamine measured in vivo with positron emission tomography (PET) and ^{11}C-raclopride in normal human subjects. Neuropsychopharmacology 18:18–25, 1998

Spector S, Sjoerdsma A, Udenfriend S: Blockade of endogenous norepinephrine synthesis by alpha-methyl-tyrosine, an inhibitor of tyrosine hydroxylase. J Pharmacol Exp Ther 147:86–95, 1965

Udenfriend S, Nagatsu T, Zaltzman-Nirenberg P: Inhibitors of purified beef adrenal tyrosine hydroxylase. Biochem Pharmacol 14:837–847, 1965

van der Werf JF, Sebens JB, Vaalburg W, et al: In vivo binding of *N*-n-propylnorapomorphine in the rat brain: regional localization, quantification in striatum and lack of correlation with dopamine metabolism. Eur J Pharmacol 87:259–270, 1983

Volkow ND, Wang GJ, Fowler JS, et al: Imaging endogenous dopamine competition with [^{11}C]raclopride in the human brain. Synapse 16:255–262, 1994

Volkow ND, Wang GJ, Fowler JS, et al: Decreased striatal dopaminergic responsiveness in detoxified cocaine-dependent subjects. Nature 386:830–833, 1997

Weinberger DR: Implications of normal brain development for the pathogenesis of schizophrenia. Arch Gen Psychiatry 44:660–669, 1987

Wong DF, Wagner HN, Tune LE, et al: Positron emission tomography reveals elevated D_2 dopamine receptors in drug-naive schizophrenics. Science 234:1558–1563, 1986

Young LT, Wong DF, Goldman S, et al: Effects of endogenous dopamine on kinetics of [^{3}H]methylspiperone and [^{3}H]raclopride binding in the rat brain. Synapse 9: 188–194, 1991

Yung KK, Bolam JP, Smith AD, et al: Immunocytochemical localization of D1 and D2 dopamine receptors in the basal ganglia of the rat: light and electron microscopy. Neuroscience 65:709–730, 1995

10

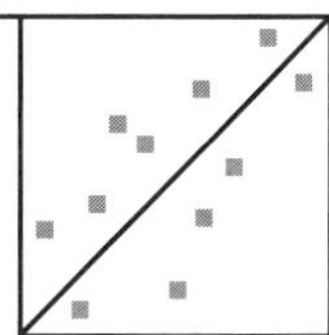

IN VIVO NEURORECEPTOR CHARACTERIZATION

The Example of [^{11}C]Flumazenil Positron Emission Tomography in the Investigation of Anxiety Disorders

Andrea L. Malizia, M.D., M.R.C.Psych., M.B.B.S., B.A.

Anxiety disorders are the commonest form of mental illness and are associated with considerable morbidity (Coryell 1988), as well as increased mortality in the most severe conditions, such as panic disorder (Katon 1996). Pharmacologic studies of these disorders have demonstrated a number of pharmacodynamic changes involving noradrenergic, serotonergic, dopaminergic, GABAergic, and cholecystokinetic systems that occur in conjunction with pathological anxiety. Among these changes, the involvement of the benzodiazepine–γ-aminobutyric acid $(GABA)_A$ receptors has been hypothesized to be central to the development of panic disorder and other, but not all, anxiety disorders, because of the specific abnormalities observed at these receptors (Malizia et al. 1995a, 1998; Nutt et al. 1990). Further, understanding the benzodiazepine site changes is likely to be helpful in designing future pharmacologic treatments, which will take advantage of selective or partial agonism.

For the experimental work described, I received a Wellcome Training Fellowship. I am grateful to John Wyeth & Brother Ltd. for financial support while this chapter was written. I am also grateful to colleagues at the Medical Research Council Cyclotron Unit, Hammersmith Hospital, London, and the Psychopharmacology Unit, University of Bristol, Bristol, United Kingdom — in particular, Sue Wilson, Ph.D., Roger Gunn, Ph.D., and David Nutt, M.D., Ph.D.

In fact, benzodiazepine ligands modulate the effects of GABA, the most abundant inhibitory transmitter in the brain, and drugs binding at this site effectively provoke or decrease anxiety in healthy volunteers and patients alike.

The benzodiazepine site is an allosteric modulatory site on the $GABA_A$ receptor (Braestrup and Squires 1977; Mohler and Okada 1997) to which benzodiazepines, cyclopyrrolones, and β-carbolines bind. These compounds modulate effects of GABA on the chloride ionophore and therefore control the influx of negative charge into neurons. The receptor-ionophore complex is made up of five components from any of the following: any of six types of α, four types of β, and three types of γ subunits and one type of δ subunit. Benzodiazepine receptor–subtype selectivity is determined by the binding to α subunits, whereas binding to γ subunits produces modulatory activity. The modulatory activity can be facilitatory (agonists) or inhibitory (inverse agonists). In addition, some compounds such as flumazenil are functionally neutral: they bind to the site but do not alter the effects of GABA. These compounds are classified as antagonists.

The evidence that modulation of the benzodiazepine-$GABA_A$ receptor affects anxiety in humans and experimental animals is overwhelming. In humans, GABA and benzodiazepine agonists are rapidly anxiolytic, whereas GABA antagonists and benzodiazepine inverse agonists produce intense and rapid anxiety (for reviews, see Kalueff and Nutt 1997; Nutt and Lawson 1992). In experimental animals such as Maudsley reactive rats, increased phylogenetic anxiety corresponds to decreased benzodiazepine binding in the brain (Robertson et al. 1978) and reduced response to agonist challenge (Commissaris et al. 1990). In mice, ontogenetic chronic stress results in global decreases in benzodiazepine binding (Mosaddeghi et al. 1993; Weizman et al. 1989), a result that seems to be dependent on the presence of intact adrenal glands (Weizman et al. 1990). Genetic manipulation in mice, which produces γ_2-subunit heterozygote knockout mice, results in rodents that are more sensitive to anxiety provocation and that have reduced flumazenil binding in most brain areas (Crestani et al. 1999). In addition, in humans, increased neuroticism as measured with the Eysenck Personality Questionnaire corresponds to decreased benzodiazepine agonist sensitivity (Glue et al. 1992). Finally, patients with panic disorder (the most severe anxiety disorder) have decreased benzodiazepine agonist sensitivity (Roy-Byrne et al. 1990) and an abnormal response to the antagonist flumazenil (Nutt et al. 1990). These observations in panic disorder can be explained either by the presence of an endogenous agonist (which would be produced only at times of intense anxiety) or by a shift in the receptor spectrum of activity. The latter may be due to alterations in the balance of subunit expression (Rudolph et al. 1999) and results in agonists behaving like partial agonists and antagonists behaving like inverse agonists (for a discussion, see Nutt et al. 1990).

Although a wealth of information exists about the interactions between benzodiazepine ligands and human anxiety, human studies were limited until quite recently because brain receptor kinetics could not be investigated in vivo. Thus it was not possible to link human pharmacodynamic studies with receptor assays, because such assays depended on the use of brains from experimental animals. However, the advent of contemporary ligand neuroimaging techniques (positron emission tomography [PET] and single photon emission computed tomography [SPECT]) has made it possible to study benzodiazepine binding in the human brain in vivo.

In this chapter, I describe the current methods for measuring benzodiazepine binding parameters in humans in vivo using [^{11}C]flumazenil and PET and discuss how these methods can be applied in various paradigms to investigate binding at the benzodiazepine site in the human brain. Although a number of methods are discussed, most of the practical information derives from the routines in place for our experiments at the Medical Research Council Cyclotron Unit in London in the mid- to late 1990s.

■ [^{11}C]FLUMAZENIL

Flumazenil (Ro 15-1788) is a benzodiazepine receptor antagonist and can be labeled with ^{11}C to produce a PET ligand for imaging the $GABA_A$ receptor. The method of production was first described by Maziere et al. (1984). Routine chemical synthesis of [^{11}C]flumazenil has been implemented in many centers; in our laboratory, high-activity flumazenil is regularly produced (up to 40,000 megabecquerels [MBq]/µmol per production), with a failure rate of less than 5%. Thus far, [^{11}C]flumazenil is one of only two PET ligands that can label this receptor, the other being Ro 15-4513 (a partial inverse agonist) (Halldin et al. 1992; Inoue et al. 1992). A number of benzodiazepine agonists, including [^{11}C]flunitrazepam (Comar et al. 1981) and [^{11}C]alprazolam (Dobbs et al. 1995), have also been synthesized, but all of these agonists are associated with poor signal-to-noise ratios (i.e., the ratio of specific binding to nonspecific binding in humans in vivo is low), and therefore they have not been used for clinical investigations.

Flumazenil binds to all types of α subunits, but there is a 100-fold difference between the affinity (K_d) for α_1, α_2, α_3, and α_5 subunits (approximately 10 nM) and the K_d for α_4 and α_6 subunits (approximately 1 µM) (Luddens et al. 1990). Therefore, the [^{11}C]flumazenil signal, when [^{11}C]flumazenil is used as a PET radioligand, does not represent binding at receptors that express α_4 and α_6 subunits.

Flumazenil is lipophilic and thus crosses the blood-brain barrier rapidly. The metabolites are hydrophilic and therefore do not cross the blood-brain barrier and do not contribute to the brain signal (Debruyne et al. 1991). Flumazenil has a brain mean residency time (half-life [$t_{1/2}$]) of 15–20 minutes (Lassen et al. 1995); therefore, there is a net efflux of flumazenil from the brain within 10–15 minutes after injection. The nonspecific binding in the brain is about 10% of the total signal. The exchange between the "free" tissue compartment and the specifically bound flumazenil is so rapid that the two compartments cannot be distinguished mathematically (Koeppe et al. 1991; Price et al. 1993) in areas of moderate to high binding.

[^{11}C]Flumazenil is widely distributed throughout the cortex, paralleling the known concentration of benzodiazepine-$GABA_A$ receptors (Pappata et al. 1988). The total signal from the basal ganglia, cerebellum, and hippocampus is about 60% of the cortical signal, whereas the total signal from the pons is 30% of the cortical signal. The pons signal is partly displaceable by "cold" intravenous flumazenil (Pappata et al. 1988) and intravenous midazolam (Malizia et al. 1996); therefore, this signal cannot be reliably used as a reference tissue (Litton et al. 1994). The PET signal from white matter (e.g., from the centrum semiovale) also represents considerable apparent specific binding, because of the partial volume effect from the cortical rim; in fact, white matter is a worse reference area than the pons (Abadie et al. 1992). Because of the absence of an adequate reference region in the brain (as obtained with the current region-of-interest [ROI] methods), [^{11}C]flumazenil studies should involve arterial sampling, so that adequate input function is obtained. Metabolite analysis must also be performed, so that metabolite concentration is subtracted from the total radioligand plasma input function.

■ METHODS

Acquisition of Dynamic PET Data

Typically, a [^{11}C]flumazenil scan consists of a number of timed frames during which the total number of counts is recorded from all the voxels in the image. The alternative is to record the events in list mode, which means that each event is tagged with the time of the event and which allows subsequent rebinning into convenient time segments. List mode has been available only recently; in most current studies, the information is acquired in predetermined frames. In our protocols, we start with a short (30-second) "background" frame just before injection of the ligand, after which we acquire a number of 10- to 60-second frames to define the delivery characteristics of the ligand. After the delivery phase, we acquire 3- to 5-minute frames for 45–60 minutes. After 1 hour, 15-minute frames are necessary to acquire enough counts, because by that time, the signal has gone through at least six half-lives from the time of the initial injection (three because of the ^{11}C $t_{1/2}$ and at least three because of the flumazenil mean residency time in tissue). Altogether, 20–25 frames are acquired. In most of our studies, conducted in three dimensions with a ECAT 953B camera (CTI, Knoxville, TN), 200–340 MBq of [^{11}C]flumazenil is injected at the beginning of the scan. Attenuation is measured with a ^{68}Ge transmission scan, and a measured scatter correction is applied after acquiring dual-energy-window counts (Grootoonk et al. 1996).

Analysis of [^{11}C]Flumazenil Scans

The sinograms acquired during the scan are reconstructed by filtered backprojection. Iterative techniques are now available, but they are still too expensive to be performed routinely; it is likely, however, that routine implementation of these techniques will considerably improve the quality of the data produced in the future. An arterial input function is obtained by calibrating the continuously recorded arterial counts (Ranicar et al. 1991) with discrete samples obtained at regular intervals during the scan and measured in a well counter. In addition, the amount of radioactively labeled metabolites at various time points is measured and is then subtracted from the total recorded counts.

A number of methods have been described for modeling [^{11}C]flumazenil data with an arterial input function. Modeling can be on a pixel-by-pixel basis or on an ROI basis. [^{11}C]flumazenil tissue signal is adequately described by a one-compartment model. Thus, both spectral analysis (Cunningham and Jones 1993) and a two-parameter kinetic model (K1 [defined in the next section] and volume of distribution [VD]) (Koeppe et al. 1991) can be used to derive binding parameters on a pixel-by-pixel basis. There is no advantage in using kinetic models with a greater number of parameters, because having more parameters does not increase the accuracy of the measurements, except perhaps in areas of low binding. Pixel-by-pixel parametric maps are preferable because they are not constrained by the bias inherent in an a priori selection of ROIs and because methods exist for the parametric comparison of these maps obtained in different populations (Frey et al. 1996; Friston et al. 1995). However, the use of statistical parametric methods may be criticized because of the necessary assumptions of normal distribution of the binding parameters. Some investigators may therefore prefer to apply nonparametric statistics, previously possible only with the use of an ROI approach. However, methods for examining pixel-based data on a nonparametric basis are emerging, and these methods should be explored and validated. Further, approaches based on the error of the parameter evaluation may herald sounder statistical analyses of these data sets (Millet et al. 1996).

By whichever method, the result of the analysis provides either a map of binding parameters or a list of ROI-based parameters. These are K1, k_2", and VD. K1 is the rate constant that describes passage of molecules from the blood into the tissue and that reflects blood flow and extraction. k_2" is the rate constant that describes efflux from the tissue and reflects blood flow, binding potential (receptor density $[B_{max}]/K_d$), and nonspecific binding (the quotation mark indicates that this constant is a composite rate constant, reflecting not only efflux from the tissue-free compartment but also binding parameters in tissue). VD is the ratio of K1 to k_2" at equilibrium and the ratio of tissue concentrations of radioligand at equilibrium to plasma concentrations of radioligand at equilibrium. Binding potential as such cannot be reliably determined for $[^{11}C]$flumazenil, because the free-tissue compartment cannot be distinguished from the specifically bound tissue. These parameters form the basis of the subsequent statistical analyses.

■ PATIENT ISSUES

One of the most important factors in successful recruitment and retention of patients for scanning is an accurate preliminary explanation of what the experiment entails. The experiment involves insertion of venous and arterial cannulas, injection of radioligand, withdrawal of blood samples, and, on the part of the subject, lying still for 2 or more hours on an uncomfortable bed with one's head in the camera. During the experiment, a number of people involved might enter the scanning or console rooms. All of these events are likely to increase the anxiety of the subject, to the extent that he or she may decide to leave. However, we have found that an explanation beforehand of all the parts of the experiment, including the most trivial details and the fact that a known experimenter will stay in the vicinity of the subject at all times, is enough to ensure full cooperation of a subject who has agreed to go ahead with the procedure.

Strict selection of patients is also important. At this point, it is not clear how present or past comorbidity affects the parameters measured. It is therefore important that a sample of patients with a "pure" form of the disease be selected. Such selection can be difficult in conditions in which comorbidity may be the norm, such as posttraumatic stress disorder or panic disorder. In addition, although it is difficult to recruit completely drug-naive patients, it is important to set firm boundaries with regard to the time since the last treatment. A period of 3 months (6 months is preferable) is selected to ensure a return to unmodified protein turnover. Further, for all studies of binding at the benzodiazepine site, it is particularly important that careful attention be paid to the clinical issue of current and previous alcohol and benzodiazepine use, and, if possible, patients and control subjects should be matched for these variables. It is advisable that subjects undergoing the scans have been benzodiazepine free for at least the previous 6 months, because prolonged downregulation of the receptor may follow prolonged or perhaps even acute use (Nutt and Costello 1988).

Finally, the characteristics of some patient populations may also affect study design. For instance, an approach that would require an equilibrium infusion of cold flumazenil is not suitable for patients with panic disorder; large doses of cold flumazenil would precipitate panic attacks in these patients (Nutt et al. 1990), who would then find it difficult to remain in the scanner. However, this paradigm can be used in studies involving patients with anxiety disorders in which flumazenil does not provoke symptoms. Flumazenil does not affect blood flow in healthy volunteers (Wolf et al. 1990).

■ PARADIGMS

Assessment of Differences in Binding Between Populations

Assessing differences in binding between populations is the simplest experimental approach. Patients and control subjects receive an injection of [^{11}C]flumazenil at the beginning of a single scan, and the data are processed to obtain maps of VD by using an arterial input function. We have used this strategy to examine differences in benzodiazepine binding between patients with panic disorder and control subjects (Malizia et al. 1998). If this type of study is being conducted in three dimensions, the scanner should be calibrated with a ^{68}Ge phantom for each scan, because small temperature variations can affect the counts, especially in the low-energy window needed for dual-energy-window scatter correction.

At least initially, data should be analyzed without covarying out the global interindividual differences in mean brain benzodiazepine binding. In fact, in our study involving panic disorder patients (Malizia et al. 1998), we found a global decrease in binding that would have been missed if in our analysis we had exclusively assessed regional relative changes in binding on a pixel-by-pixel basis. Relative analyses can, however, also yield important information. For instance, in that study (Malizia et al. 1998), relative regional analysis revealed that decreases in binding in excess of the global changes were present in the temporal pole and bilaterally in the posterior orbitofrontal cortex. These areas have been shown to be involved in the brain expression of anxiety by a number of anxiety provocation studies (see, for example, Rauch et al. 1994, 1995, 1996); therefore, this finding may be important in the appraisal of how biochemical changes can affect brain circuitry in these disorders.

Although a global binding measure can be sufficient for studying tissue receptors, there have been reports of parallel changes in number and affinity of receptors in postmortem tissue (for example, see Francis et al. 1993). In this case, separating receptor number and affinity may be important, because changes in the same direction in the numerator and denominator will minimize the apparent change in binding potential or VD. Further, separating K_d and B_{max} may be an important step in generating theories about the origin of an observed "receptor density" change. An alteration in affinity but not number could, for instance, imply a differential expression of particular receptor subunits and exclude altered levels of endogenous ligand. If this separation of K_d and B_{max} is required, an approach involving two or more scans is needed (Mintun et al. 1984). In this case, the best design is that described by Lassen (1992). In this design, one scan is performed with the radiotracer alone, and in the other scan the radiotracer is administered once an infusion of cold flumazenil has reached equilibrium. This type of study allows the estimation of K_d and B_{max} separately and has the advantage of being an equilibrium study. With this approach (taken by, for example, Lassen et al. [1995]), an a priori estimate of nonspecific binding must be used to evaluate the parameters.

A method was proposed recently for the assessment of both B_{max} and K_d using a single low-specific-activity injection of [^{11}C]flumazenil (Delforge et al. 1996, 1997a, 1997b). This method relies on kinetic modeling and the changing proportion of labeled [^{11}C]flumazenil over time, when significant amounts of cold flumazenil are coinjected. The model needs full validation before it can be used for clinical studies.

Assessment of Differences in Baseline Blood Flow

Clearly, an [^{15}O]water study can be carried out immediately before any ligand examination to record blood flow in subjects undergoing PET. An analysis of these data would show whether there are any differences in regional flow at rest between the samples studied. However, a separate scan is not necessary, because, with fully quantitative methods, K1 (delivery) can be separated from the other parameters, permitting assessment of differences in baseline flow. Delivery is the product of flow and extraction and, assuming that permeability to the molecule is not altered between conditions, changes in delivery should reflect changes in basal blood flow.

The validity of this approach was demonstrated in a test-retest study of binding parameters, in which visual activation was performed at the beginning of flumazenil scans (Holthoff et al. 1991). Using this approach in our panic disorder study, we found that patients with panic disorder had a global decrease in delivery, probably secondary to hyperventilation, but that increased state anxiety as measured with the State-Trait Anxiety Inventory (Spielberger et al. 1970) covaried with increased delivery in the dorsal anterior cingulate cortex. In conducting these analyses, it may be important to limit the comparisons to subjects who are undergoing PET for the first time, because repeated exposure may decrease anticipatory anxiety and change global metabolism (Wang et al. 1996).

Assessment of Occupancy at the Benzodiazepine Site

There are two main reasons for assessing occupancy at the benzodiazepine site. The first is to quantify the occupancy needed for clinical or specific pharmacodynamic effects and to compare this measure for different benzodiazepine ligands. For instance, measuring the regionally specific occupancy of novel benzodiazepine anxiolytics using PET is the only way of confirming selective or partial agonism in humans. The second reason is to detect production of an endogenous ligand related to brain activation in humans; assessing occupancy at the benzodiazepine site is the only method that permits such detection. Thus, this approach is likely to provide important insights into the physiological function of benzodiazepine sites.

Three methods can be used to assess endogenous or exogenous ligand occupancy at the benzodiazepine site using PET. One is equilibrium infusion of [^{11}C]flumazenil, another is a two-scan approach with administration of a pulse of radioligand for each scan, and the third involves displacement experiments in which a pulse of radioligand is followed by an endogenous or exogenous perturbation during the scan.

Equilibrium Infusion of Radioligand

Equilibrium infusion of [^{11}C]flumazenil has not been performed, but in experiments involving [^{123}I]iomazenil SPECT in humans and simians, the VD obtained by analysis of equilibrium studies correlated with the same measure obtained using bolus injections of [^{123}I]iomazenil (Laruelle et al. 1993, 1994). The technique does not seem to have been progressed further for benzodiazepine binding, but the same group (Laruelle et al. 1997) found that using [^{123}I]iodobenzamide (a SPECT dopamine D_2 receptor ligand) permits detection of endogenous release of dopamine as well as occupancy by an exogenous ligand. These experiments are laborious to set up, but this technique is probably the most robust for detection of changes in binding during a scan, because blood flow changes do not affect the signal. The main limitation of these experiments is that a large total amount of radioactive tracer is injected into subjects. Nevertheless, application of this method to [^{11}C]flumazenil experiments is likely to provide interesting data in the future.

Dual-Scan Technique

With the dual-scan technique, the VD of [^{11}C]flumazenil is assessed both during a resting state and after administration of an exogenous compound or during an "activation." In activation studies, the timing of the stimulus must be correct, to avoid artifacts due to changes in blood flow and thus delivery or washout. Using this method, Holthoff et al. (1991) demonstrated that activation of the visual cortex does not affect [^{11}C]flumazenil binding in the occipital cortex, although delivery is increased. This method has been also used to quantitate zolpidem binding in the human cortex in vivo (Abadie et al. 1996), but, probably for technical reasons, the expected differences in regional (hippocampal and temporal) binding with this selective agonist were not demonstrated. More studies with this method are needed to assess its utility, especially with reference to proof of principle with selective and partial benzodiazepine agonists. A modification of this method has been used to assess occupancy of compounds with a short plama $t_{1/2}$ (Videbaek et al. 1993).

Pulse-Chase or Displacement Technique

In pulse-chase or displacement experiments, 30 minutes after administration of [^{11}C]flumazenil a cold ligand is administered that increases the [^{11}C]flumazenil washout by occupying some of the available sites. With this method, the dose occupancy curve for cold flumazenil was determined using PET (Pappata et al. 1988) and the Multiple Organs Coincidences Counter (Malizia et al. 1995b). This method was also used in a study that demonstrated a strong correlation between PET pharmacokinetic index of human brain benzodiazepine site occupancy for midazolam (a benzodiazepine agonist) and that agent's pharmacodynamic effects as measured with electroencephalography (Malizia et al. 1996). Clearly, this method, which involves one scan only, can also be useful for investigating the endogenous release of ligands that affect [^{11}C]flumazenil binding. Ways of assessing the statistical significance of a regional increase in washout have been implemented (Friston et al. 1997; Gunn et al. 1997) and could be useful for assessing the effect of anxiety provocation on the release of putative endogenous neurotransmitters. However, a considerable drawback of this method is that local changes in blood flow midscan may affect regional washout if the change in flow results in a significant modulation of capillary surface area, in which case pharmacokinetic conclusions are limited by blood flow confounds.

■ Conclusion

The PET methodology underlying the study of benzodiazepine sites in humans is ripe for applications that should help researchers study the GABAergic correlates of human anxiety and anxiety disorders. Further methodological advances are now dependent on the synthesis of appropriate radioligands for benzodiazepine receptor subtypes.

■ References

Abadie P, Baron JC, Bisserbe JC, et al: Central benzodiazepine receptors in human brain: estimation of regional B_{max} and KD values with positron emission tomography. Eur J Pharmacol 213:107–115, 1992

Abadie P, Rioux P, Scatton B, et al: Central benzodiazepine receptor occupancy by zolpidem in the human brain as assessed by positron emission tomography. Eur J Pharmacol 295:35–44, 1996

Braestrup C, Squires RF: Specific benzodiazepine receptors in rat brain characterized by high-affinity (^{3}H)diazepam binding. Proc Natl Acad Sci U S A 74:3805–3809, 1977

Comar D, Maziere M, Cepeda C, et al: The kinetics and displacement of [^{11}C]flunitrazepam in the brain of the living baboon. Eur J Pharmacol 75:21–26, 1981

Commissaris RL, Harrington GM, Altman HJ: Benzodiazepine anti conflict effects in Maudsley reactive (MR/Har) and non reactive (MNRA/Har) rats. Psychopharmacology (Berl) 100:287–292, 1990

Coryell W: Panic disorder and mortality. Psychiatr Clin North Am 11:433–440, 1988

Crestani F, Lorez M, Baer K, et al: Decreased GABAA-receptor clustering results in enhanced anxiety and a bias for threat cues. Nat Neurosci 2:833–839, 1999

Cunningham VJ, Jones T: Spectral analysis of dynamic PET studies. J Cereb Blood Flow Metab 13:15–23, 1993

Debruyne D, Abadie P, Barre L, et al: Plasma pharmacokinetics and metabolism of the benzodiazepine antagonist [^{11}C] Ro 15-1788 (flumazenil) in baboon and human during positron emission tomography studies. Eur J Drug Metab Pharmacokinet 16:141–152, 1991

Delforge J, Spelle L, Bendriem B, et al: Quantitation of benzodiazepine receptors in human brain using the partial saturation method. J Nucl Med 37:5–11, 1996

Delforge J, Spelle L, Bendriem B, et al: Parametric images of benzodiazepine receptor concentration using a partial saturation injection. J Cereb Blood Flow Metab 17:343–355, 1997a

Delforge J, Syrota A, Bendriem B: Reaction volume concept. J Nucl Med 38:341–342, 1997b

Dobbs FR, Banks W, Fleishaker JC, et al: Studies with [^{11}C]alprazolam: an agonist for the benzodiazepine receptor. Nucl Med Biol 22:459–466, 1995

Francis PT, Pangalos MN, Stephens PH, et al: Antemortem measurement of neurotransmission: possible implications for pharmacotherapy of Alzheimer's disease and depression. J Neurol Neurosurg Psychiatry 56:80–84, 1993

Frey KA, Minoshima S, Koeppe RA, et al: Stereotaxic summation analysis of human cerebral benzodiazepine binding maps. J Cereb Blood Flow Metab 16:409–417, 1996

Friston KJ, Worsley KJ, Frackowiak RSJ, et al: Assessing the significance of focal activations using their spatial extent. Hum Brain Mapp 1:214–220, 1994

Friston KJ, Holmes AP, Worsley KJ, et al: Statistical parametric maps in functional imaging: a general linear approach. Hum Brain Mapp 2:189–210, 1995

Friston KJ, Malizia AL, Wilson S, et al: Analysis of dynamic radioligand displacement or "activation" studies. J Cereb Blood Flow Metab 17:80–93, 1997

Glue P, Wilson SJ, Ball D, et al: Benzodiazepine sensitivity in subjects with high and low trait neuroticism (abstract). Biol Psychiatry 31:149A, 1992

Grootoonk S, Spinks TJ, Sashin D, et al: Correction for scatter in 3D brain PET using a dual energy window method. Phys Med Biol 41:2757–2774, 1996

Gunn RN, Malizia AL, Rajeswaran S, et al: An application of spectral analysis to the voxel based statistical assessment of dynamic ligand displacement (abstract). Neuroimage 5:A36, 1997

Halldin C, Farde L, Litton JE, et al: [^{11}C]Ro 15-4513, a ligand for visualization of benzodiazepine receptor binding: preparation, autoradiography and positron emission tomography. Psychopharmacology (Berl) 108:16–22, 1992

Holthoff VA, Koeppe RA, Frey KA, et al: Differentiation of radioligand delivery and binding in the brain: validation of a two compartment model for [^{11}C]flumazenil. J Cereb Blood Flow Metab 11:745–752, 1991

Inoue O, Suhara T, Itoh T, et al: In vivo binding of [^{11}C]Ro15 4513 in human brain measured with PET. Neurosci Lett 145:133–136, 1992

Kalueff AV, Nutt DJ: The role of GABA in memory and anxiety. Anxiety 4:100–110, 1997

Katon W: Panic disorder: relationship to high medical utilization, unexplained physical symptoms, and medical costs. J Clin Psychiatry 57 (suppl 10):11–18, 1996

Koeppe RA, Holthoff VA, Frey KA, et al: Compartmental analysis of [^{11}C]flumazenil kinetics for the estimation of ligand transport rate and receptor distribution using positron emission tomography. J Cereb Blood Flow Metab 11:735–744, 1991

Laruelle M, Abi-Dargham A, Rattner Z, et al: Single photon emission tomography measurement of benzodiazepine receptor number and affinity in primate brain: a constant infusion paradigm with [^{123}I]iomazenil. Eur J Pharmacol 230:119–123, 1993

Laruelle M, Abi-Dargham A, al-Tikriti MS, et al: SPECT quantification of [^{123}I]iomazenil binding to benzodiazepine receptors in nonhuman primates, II: equilibrium analysis of constant infusion experiments and correlation with in vitro parameters. J Cereb Blood Flow Metab 14:453–465, 1994

Laruelle M, Iyer RN, al-Tikriti MS, et al: Microdialysis and SPECT measurements of amphetamine-induced dopamine release in nonhuman primates. Synapse 25:1–14, 1997

Lassen NA: Neuroreceptor quantitation in vivo by the steady state principle using constant infusion or bolus injection of radioactive tracers. J Cereb Blood Flow Metab 12:709–716, 1992

Lassen NA, Bartenstein PA, Lammertsma AA, et al: Benzodiazepine receptor quantification in vivo in humans using [^{11}C]flumazenil and PET: application of the steady-state principle. J Cereb Blood Flow Metab 15:152–165, 1995

Litton JE, Hall H, Pauli S: Saturation analysis in PET: analysis of errors due to imperfect reference regions. J Cereb Bllod Flow Metab 14:358–361, 1994

Luddens H, Pritchett DB, Kohler M, et al: Cerebellar GABAA receptor selective for a behavioural alcohol antagonist. Nature 346:648–651, 1990

Malizia AL, Coupland NJ, Nutt DJ: Benzodiazepine receptor function in anxiety disorders. Adv Biochem Psychopharmacol 48:115–133, 1995a

Malizia AL, Forse G, Gunn R, et al: A new human (psycho)pharmacology tool: the Multiple Organs Coincidences Counter (MOCC). J Psychopharmacol 9:294–306, 1995b

Malizia AL, Gunn RG, Wilson SJ, et al: Benzodiazepine site pharmacokinetic/pharmacodynamic quantification in man: direct measurement of drug occupancy and effects on the human brain in vivo. Neuropharmacology 35:1483–1491, 1996

Malizia AL, Cunningham VJ, Bell CJ, et al: Decreased brain GABA(A)-benzodiazepine receptor binding in panic disorder: preliminary results from a quantitative PET study. Arch Gen Psychiatry 55:715–720, 1998

Maziere M, Hantraye P, Prenant C, et al: Synthesis of ethyl 8-fluoro-5,6-dihydro-5-[^{11}C]methyl-6-oxo-4H-imidazo [1,5-a][1,4]benzodiazepine-3-carboxylate (Ro 15.1788-^{11}C): a specific radioligand for the in vivo study of central benzodiazepine receptors by positron emission tomography. Int J Appl Radiat Isot 35:973–976, 1984

Millet P, Delforge J, Pappata S, et al: Error analysis on parameter estimates in the ligand-receptor model: application to parameter imaging using PET data. Phys Med Biol 41:2739–2756, 1996

Mintun MA, Raichle ME, Kilbourn MR, et al: A quantitative model for the in vivo assessment of drug binding sites with positron emission tomography. Ann Neurol 15:217–227, 1984

Mohler H, Okada T: Benzodiazepine receptor: demonstration in the central nervous system. Science 198:849–851, 1977

Mosaddeghi M, Burke TF, Moerschbaecher JM: Chronic brief restraint decreases in vivo binding of benzodiazepine receptor ligand to mouse brain. Mol Chem Neuropathol 18:115–121, 1993

Nutt DJ, Costello MJ: Rapid induction of lorazepam dependence and reversal with flumazenil. Life Sci 43:1045–1053, 1988

Nutt D[J], Lawson C: Panic attacks: a neurochemical overview of models and mechanisms. Br J Psychiatry 160:165–178, 1992

Nutt DJ, Glue P, Lawson C, et al: Flumazenil provocation of panic attacks. Arch Gen Psychiatry 47:917–925, 1990

Pappata S, Samson Y, Chavoix C, et al: Regional specific binding of [^{11}C]RO 15 1788 to central type benzodiazepine receptors in human brain: quantitative evaluation by PET. J Cereb Blood Flow Metab 8:304–313, 1988

Price JC, Mayberg HS, Dannals RF, et al: Measurement of benzodiazepine receptor number and affinity in humans using tracer kinetic modeling, positron emission tomography, and [^{11}C]flumazenil. J Cereb Blood Flow Metab 13:656–667, 1993

Ranicar AS, Williams CW, Schnorr L, et al: The on line monitoring of continuously withdrawn arterial blood during PET studies using a single BGO/photomultiplier assembly and non stick tubing. Med Prog Technol 17:259–264, 1991

Rauch SL, Jenike MA, Alpert NM, et al: Regional cerebral blood flow measured during symptom provocation in obsessive-compulsive disorder using oxygen 15-labeled carbon dioxide and positron emission tomography Arch Gen Psychiatry 51:62–70, 1994

Rauch SL, Savage CR, Alpert NM, et al: A positron emission tomographic study of simple phobic symptom provocation. Arch Gen Psychiatry 52:20–28, 1995

Rauch SL, van der Kolk BA, Fisler RE, et al: A symptom provocation study of post-traumatic stress disorder using positron emission tomography and script-driven imagery. Arch Gen Psychiatry 53:380–387, 1996

Robertson HA, Martin IL, Candy JM: Differences in benzodiazepine receptor binding in Maudsley reactive and Maudsley non reactive rats. Eur J Pharmacol 50:455–457, 1978

Roy-Byrne PP, Cowley DS, Greenblatt DJ, et al: Reduced benzodiazepine sensitivity in panic disorder. Arch Gen Psychiatry 47:259–272, 1990

Rudolph U, Crestani F, Benke D, et al: Benzodiazepine actions mediated by specific gamma-aminobutyric acid(A) receptor subtypes. Nature 401:796–800, 1999

Spielberger CD, Gorsuch RL, Lushere R: State Trait Anxiety Inventory Manual. Palo Alto, CA, Consulting Psychologist Press, 1970

Videbaek C, Friberg L, Holm S, et al: Benzodiazepine receptor equilibrium constants for flumazenil and midazolam determined in humans with the single photon emission computer tomography tracer [^{123}I]iomazenil. Eur J Pharmacol 249:43–51, 1993

Wang GJ, Volkow ND, Overall J, et al: Reproducibility of regional brain metabolic responses to lorazepam. J Nucl Med 37:1609–1613, 1996

Weizman R, Weizman A, Kook KA, et al: Repeated swim stress alters brain benzodiazepine receptors measured in vivo. J Pharmacol Exp Ther 249:701–707, 1989

Weizman A, Weizman R, Kook KA, et al: Adrenalectomy prevents the stress-induced decrease in in vivo [^{3}H]Ro15-1788 binding to GABAA benzodiazepine receptors in the mouse. Brain Res 519:347–350, 1990

Wolf J, Friberg L, Jensen J, et al: The effect of the benzodiazepine antagonist flumazenil on regional cerebral blood flow in human volunteers. Acta Anaesthesiol Scand 34:628–631, 1990

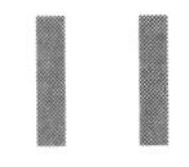

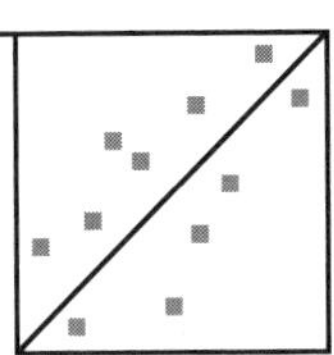

INTEGRATION OF STRUCTURAL AND FUNCTIONAL IMAGING

Examples in Depression Research

Wayne C. Drevets, M.D.

The demonstration of structural brain abnormalities in primary mood disorders is one of the greatest achievements of neuroimaging research. This evidence and converging data from postmortem neuropathological studies are effecting a paradigm shift in which mood disorders are no longer viewed simply as "functional" conditions limited to alterations of neurochemistry and neurophysiology (Drevets and Todd 1997). Instead, it appears that some subtypes of affective illness have abnormalities of both structure and function in brain systems shown by other types of evidence to be involved in emotional behavior. To elucidate more fully the neurobiologic correlates of mood disorders, researchers must therefore implement technological advances in future neuroimaging studies of depression and mania, to enable integration of anatomical and functional information.

In this chapter, I review some of the anatomical abnormalities identified by magnetic resonance imaging (MRI) and postmortem histopathological assessments of patients with mood disorders and discuss the implications of such abnormalities for the design and interpretation of physiological and receptor imaging studies. The complex interactions between neurophysiology and illness severity in prefrontal cortex areas where structural abnormalities have been identified in major depressive disorder (MDD) and bipolar disorder are addressed in light of the effects that such changes exert on physiological imaging measures. In addition, I discuss the use of neuroreceptor imaging technology to guide the development of hypotheses for postmortem histopathological studies; such an application is supported by evidence that the abnormalities of serotonin (5-HT) system morphology found in recent postmortem studies of MDD and bipolar disorder may be reflected in 5-HT receptor images acquired from clinically similar subjects. Finally, I consider the clinical correlations of the neuroimaging abnormalities evident in mood disorders, together with the results of lesion analysis, electrophysiologic studies, and other brain mapping studies and present a neural model in which dysfunction of the prefrontal cortex, basal ganglia, and brain stem monoaminergic transmitter systems that normally modulate emotional and stress responses leads to the pathological maintenance and recurrence of inappropriate cognitive-behavioral, neuroendocrine, and autonomic manifestations of emotional experience and expression (Drevets 1999).

■ Structural Imaging Abnormalities in Mood Disorders

The neuroanatomical abnormalities evident in patients with mood disorders consist of morphological lesions and morphometric reductions in gray matter volume (Drevets et al. 1999a). The former set of abnormalities are predominantly seen on magnetic resonance (MR) images acquired from patients whose mood disorders began at a late age, and these abnormalities likely reflect MRI correlates of cerebrovascular disease (Drevets et al. 1999a; Krishnan et al. 1993). Patients with late-onset depression also have morphometric changes such as reduced frontal lobe and basal ganglia volumes, enlarged cerebral ventricles, and widened cortical sulci that are thought to reflect tissue atrophy associated with ischemia (Coffey et al. 1993; Drevets et al. 1999a; Krishnan et al. 1992, 1993). In contrast, subjects with early-onset, familial mood disorders appear to have another type of neuromorphometric abnormality, evident in both in vivo MRI and postmortem neuropathological studies, involving an idiopathic reduction of gray matter volume in parts of the orbital and medial prefrontal cortex that have been shown, by other means, to play roles in modulating emotional behavior (LeDoux 1987; Neafsey et al. 1993; Price, in press).

Neuromorphological MRI Correlates of Late-Onset Depression

The most widely replicated finding of structural imaging studies of depression has been that patients whose major depression began after age 55 show more numerous and extensive MR signal hyperintensities in the deep and periventricular white matter than do both age-matched, healthy control subjects and age-matched control subjects with early-onset depression (Drevets et al. 1999a; Krishnan et al. 1993) (Figure 11–1). Tissue acquired post-mortem from elderly subjects manifesting these "patch" and "cap"-shaped areas of MR signal hyperintensity shows arteriosclerosis within the affected areas but not in the surrounding tissue where the MR signal appears normal (Awad et al. 1986b; Chimowitz et al. 1992). Larger patches of MR signal hyperintensity usually reflect myelin pallor interspersed with gliosis and dilated perivascular spaces and may also be associated with lacunar infarction, white matter necrosis, and axonal loss (Chimowitz et al. 1992). The incidence of lacunae, which reflect areas where infarcted tissue has been replaced by cerebrospinal fluid (CSF), is also increased on MR scans acquired from patients with late-onset depression (Fazekas et al. 1989; Krishnan et al. 1993). Consistent with the evidence that patches of white matter hyperintensity, large caps of white matter hyperintensity, and lacunae are associated with arteriosclerosis in elderly subjects, cerebral blood flow (CBF) has been confirmed in functional imaging studies to be decreased in the cortical and subcortical areas where patches or large caps of white matter hyperintensity are evident on MR images (Chimowitz et al. 1992; Fazekas et al. 1989; Lesser et al. 1994).

The risk factors for developing patches of white matter hyperintensity are also risk factors for cerebrovascular disease, such as advancing age, hypertension, diabetes, and ischemic stroke (Awad et al. 1986a, 1986b; Chimowitz et al. 1992; Fazekas et al. 1989). Moreover, elderly depressed patients with white matter hyperintensity are more likely than control subjects to have family histories of hypertension and less likely than patients with early-onset depression to have family histories of depression (the major risk factor for early-onset mood disorders) (Fujikawa et al. 1994). Such MRI findings are associated with an increased risk of psychotic features, cognitive impairment, and treatment-related adverse reactions (e.g., delirium), which are also more prevalent in subjects with known cerebrovascular disease (Drevets 1994; Fujikawa et al. 1996; Lesser et al. 1996). Finally, the areas where cerebral infarction has been associated with an increased incidence of major depression—namely, the left frontal lobe and the striatum—are the areas most commonly affected by white matter hyperintensity in late-onset MDD (Greenwald et al. 1996, 1998; Starkstein and Robinson 1989). Thus, in patients with late-onset depression who have MRI evidence of white matter hyperintensity and lacunae, cerebrovascular disease may play a role in the pathogenesis of MDD (Drevets 1994, 1999; Krishnan et al. 1993).

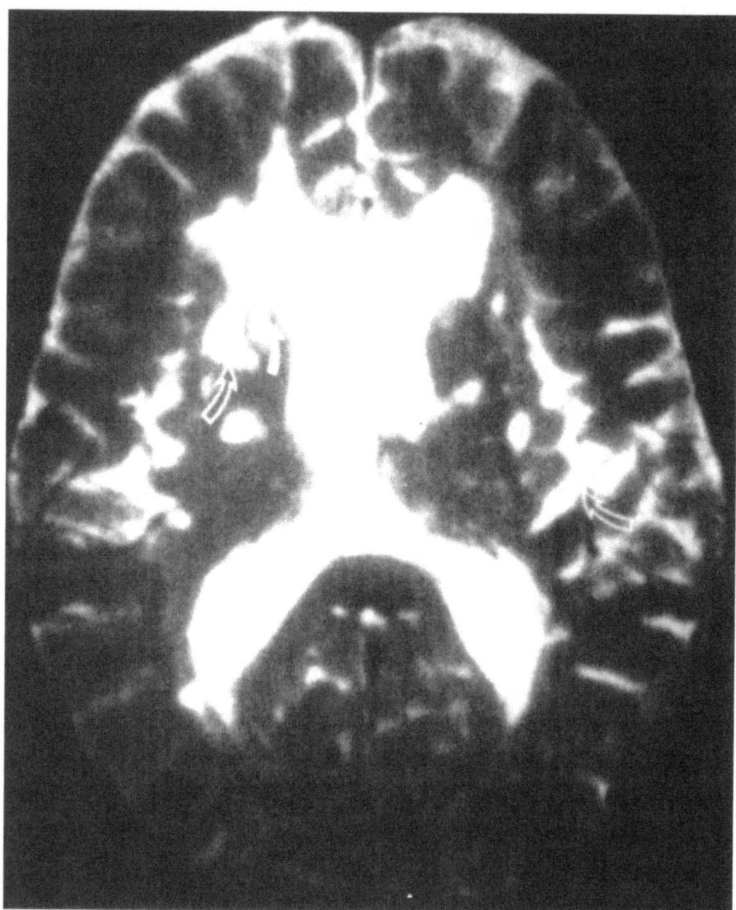

FIGURE 11–1. Brain magnetic resonance image (axial view through the base of lateral ventricles) showing large, confluent, deep white matter hyperintensities (open arrows) and hyperintensity in the right caudate head (arrow) in an elderly depressed patient.
Source. Courtesy of G.S. Figiel; reproduced with permission from Drevets WC: "Brain Imaging in Psychiatry," in *Behavioral Science for Medical Students.* Edited by Sierles FS. Baltimore, MD, Williams & Wilkins, 1993, pp. 212–235. Used with permission.

Implications for Functional Imaging Studies of Late-Life Mood Disorders

Atherosclerotic changes in the cerebral vasculature reduce radiotracer delivery to affected tissues (e.g., as evidenced by the reductions in resting CBF in affected regions [Chimowitz et al. 1992; Fazekas et al. 1989; Lesser et al.

1994]) and alter relationships between neuronal activity, hemodynamic regulation, and oxygen extraction. For example, in early cerebrovascular disease the diminished capacity to increase CBF is compensated by a reciprocal increase in the oxygen extraction fraction to permit continued neuronal activity (Derdeyn et al. 1998). During this phase, neural activity can still increase to subserve sensory, behavioral, or cognitive processing, but the corresponding changes in the regional positron emission tomography (PET)–CBF or functional MRI–blood oxygen level–dependent signal will be attenuated or absent. As cerebrovascular disease progresses, ischemia becomes associated with a reduction in oxygen and glucose utilization, and local neuronal function becomes impaired.

Advanced cerebrovascular disease is ultimately associated with atrophy of the affected tissue, which can further reduce the apparent magnitude of PET and single photon emission computed tomography (SPECT) measures of CBF and metabolism via "partial volume averaging" effects (Mazziotta et al. 1981). These effects result from the low spatial resolution of PET and SPECT images, in which measurements reflect an averaging of the radioactive emissions originating from the gray matter, white matter, and CSF contained within a volume of interest (VOI). Partial volume averaging also results in some activity from tissue adjacent to but outside a VOI being included in the averaged value measured for the VOI. As the proportion of gray matter decreases within or around a VOI, the partial volume averaging effect of emphasizing CSF (which is metabolically inactive) and white matter (which is one-fourth as metabolically active as gray matter) reduces the apparent CBF and metabolism from that area in the PET or SPECT image (Links et al. 1996; Mazziotta et al. 1981). The apparent binding potential (BP) of neuroreceptor radioligands is also reduced in atrophic or hypoplastic tissue if the neural processes expressing the target receptors decrease in concert with the gray matter volume.

In summary, because the white matter hyperintensity and lacunae evident in 70%–90% of patients with late-onset depression appear to reflect cerebrovascular disease, physiological or receptor pharmacologic images from such subjects cannot be interpreted in the same way as image data from patients with early-onset depression or healthy control subjects. Elucidating the pathophysiology of depression associated with such neuromorphological lesions may instead require application of magnetic resonance spectroscopy or PET approaches that permit specific characterization of the metabolic status of ischemic tissue. In addition, it may be feasible to study late-onset depression using longitudinal studies in which subjects are imaged before and after treatment. In previous studies of depression in elderly patients, differences between the pretreatment-depressed and posttreatment-remitted conditions were similar to those found in younger subjects (Nobler et al. 1994; Rubin et al. 1994) (Table 11–1).

Neuromorphometric Abnormalities in Early-Onset Mood Disorders

Early-onset, familial mood disorders appear to be associated with a distinct type of neuromorphometric abnormality involving a reduction in gray matter volume in limbic or paralimbic areas of the orbital and medial prefrontal cortex and the ventral temporal lobe (Bowen et al. 1989; Öngür et al. 1998; Rajkowska et al. 1997, 1999). Researchers using neuroimaging results to guide microscopic assessments in histopathological studies have obtained evidence that these reductions in cortical volume are associated with decreased glial cell counts and increased neuronal density in MDD and bipolar disorder (Drevets et al. 1998; Öngür et al. 1998; Rajkowska et al. 1997, 1999). Although the etiology and biological significance of these abnormalities remain unclear, their apparent specificity for areas implicated in emotional behavior suggests they are relevant to the pathogenesis of mood disorders (Drevets et al. 1998; Price, in press).

These abnormalities may affect functional imaging results by a variety of mechanisms and must be considered in the design and interpretation of PET, SPECT, functional MRI, and magnetic resonance spectroscopy studies of MDD and bipolar disorder. Although it is conceivable that reductions in cortical volume may be state dependent in some subjects (e.g., effects of severe hypercortisolemia), in the prefrontal cortex these abnormalities instead appear traitlike, insofar as they exist independent of mood state (Drevets et al. 1997b). It remains unclear whether these neuromorphometric abnormalities may normalize to some extent in response to the increased expression of neurotrophic factors (e.g., brain-derived neurotrophic factor) and neuroprotective factors (e.g., bcl-2) induced by chronic treatment with antidepressant and mood-stabilizing drugs, respectively (Chen et al. 1999; Nibuya et al. 1995). It also appears that such abnormalities will prove specific to mood disorder subtypes, possibly accounting for discrepant findings across studies within the neuroimaging and postmortem study literature.

■ Delineating the Anatomical Correlates of Depression Using PET

Longitudinal PET studies of major depression have found some CBF and metabolic abnormalities that appear traitlike, insofar as they persist in spite of

TABLE 11–1. Antidepressant treatment effects on ventral prefrontal cortical cerebral blood flow and metabolism in depression

Reference	Treatment(s)	Change in CBF or glucose metabolism[a]
Bonne et al. 1996	ECT	Increase in anterior cingulate cortex in responders, no significant changes in ventral anterolateral PFC
Buchsbaum et al. 1997	Sertraline therapy	Decrease in dorsal anterior cingulate cortex and subgenual PFC
Cohen et al. 1992	Phototherapy	Decrease in medial orbital cortex[a]
Drevets and Raichle 1992	Desipramine therapy	Decrease in left lateral orbital PFC
Drevets et al. 1996	Sertraline therapy	Decrease in subgenual PFC and posterior orbital or anterior insular cortex
Ebert et al. 1991	Sleep deprivation	Decrease in orbital cortex in responders[a]
Goodwin et al. 1993	Various antidepressant drug treatments	Increase in anterior cingulate cortex, no significant changes in ventral anterolateral cortex
Mayberg et al. 1999	Fluoxetine therapy	Decrease in subgenual PFC and posterior orbital or anterior insular cortex
Nobler et al. 1994	ECT	Decrease in left ventrolateral PFC in responders[c]
Rubin et al. 1994	Nortriptyline or sertraline therapy	Decrease in left ventrolateral PFC in responders[c]
Wu et al. 1992	Sleep deprivation	Decrease in anterior cingulate cortex in responders

Note. Not all studies examined the same regions, and the absence of a listed result for a specific region indicates that no image data were provided for that region. Abbreviations: CBF = cerebral blood flow; ECT = electroconvulsive therapy; PFC = prefrontal cortex.
[a]Posttreatment scan vs. pretreatment scan.
[b]Treatment-associated change not shown by paired statistical tests.
[c]Studies performed using ^{133}Xe, which provides CBF measures only near the scalp.

symptom remission, and other abnormalities that are instead mood state dependent. The former abnormalities have proven to be of greatest importance for guiding structural neuroimaging and postmortem histopathological studies (Drevets et al. 1997b, 1998; Öngür et al. 1998). In contrast, abnormalities that are mood state dependent likely reflect areas where physiological activity increases or decreases to mediate or respond to the emotional and cognitive manifestations of the depressive syndrome (Drevets and Raichle 1998). The return of activity to normal levels after symptom remission likely indicates that the brain regions supporting such physiological responses are morphologically normal in mood disorders.

One obstacle to using functional imaging data to guide the more time-consuming neuromorphometric MRI and histopathological measurements has been that the abnormality findings in rigorously designed imaging experiments appear in some cases to disagree with published results of other studies. If taken at face value, the extensive functional imaging literature concerning MDD would appear to implicate most areas of the brain in the pathophysiology of depression, to disagree across studies regarding the specific location and the direction relative to normal of such abnormalities, and thus to offer little clear localizing information for postmortem studies. Therefore, the selection of neuroimaging data likely to guide histopathological assessments fruitfully requires critical assessment of the psychiatric imaging literature. Recognition of when apparent discrepancies across studies reflect technical issues related to scanner technology, image analysis strategy, sample size, or confounding drug effects thus becomes essential to employing physiological imaging results for effective hypothesis generation. In contrast, knowledge of the extent to which differences in results across studies instead reflect dissimilarities in the depressive subtype studied may prove invaluable in determining the specific clinical conditions under which abnormalities can be detected and characterized by further studies (Drevets et al. 1999a).

Image Acquisition and Analysis Issues Influencing Type I and II Error

The technical issues that affect sensitivity for identifying abnormalities in a clinical sample using neuroimaging techniques are reviewed elsewhere (Drevets et al. 1999a; Frackowiak et al. 1997; Links et al. 1996; Mazziotta et al. 1981; Poline et al. 1997; Raichle 1987), but some principles relevant to interpreting apparent discrepancies across mood disorder studies are introduced here. Many imaging studies of MDD do not reproduce other studies' results, simply because of differences in the imaging technology or analysis strategy used. For example, CBF images acquired using ^{133}Xe inhalation and SPECT or nontomographic multidetector systems provide measures limited to the cortical gray matter lying near the scalp, and the medial and orbital prefrontal cortex, mesiotemporal cortex, and basal ganglia are not sampled (Drevets et al. 1999a; Raichle 1987). In addition, most published PET studies used tomographs that had an axial field of view that did not result in sampling of the entire brain, and when such images were converted to statistical parametric maps (e.g., SPM [Frackowiak et al. 1997]), comparisons across groups were further restricted (to 6 or 7 cm) because such techniques exclude voxels not sampled by all subjects from analysis. Thus, in our initial study of familial pure depressive disease, areas excluded from analysis included the posterior orbital surface (where we subsequently found the largest percent difference in CBF between depressed patients and control subjects [Drevets and Raichle 1998; Price et al. 1996]) and the dorsomedial or dorsal anterolateral prefrontal cortex (where we and others found decreased CBF and metabolism in MDD in other studies [Baxter et al. 1989; Bell et al. 1999; Ring et al. 1994]). More recent studies have used state-of-the-art PET cameras with an axial field of view of 15 cm and that sample the entire brain, reducing the likelihood of sampling differences across studies.

Even when newer tomographs are used, image analysis approaches require trade-offs between the sensitivity for detecting abnormalities and the likelihood of reporting statistical artifact (type I error). For example, the capabilities of anatomical localization in PET images have been enhanced by improvements in sensitivity and spatial resolution [now 4–5 mm for state-of-the-art PET cameras] and the development of techniques for coregistering PET and MR images. Yet researchers availing themselves of these advantages when conducting region-of-interest (ROI) analyses may define an ROI that leads to either inadequate sampling (e.g., by mispositioning the ROI) or excessive dilution (e.g., by choosing an ROI that is too large) of an area of abnormal radiotracer uptake in a clinical sample. To address the likelihood of type II error, investigators employ omnibus image analysis strategies that permit surveying of large areas of brain via voxel-by-voxel statistical comparisons that reveal inherent differences between samples (Drevets et al. 1992; Frackowiak et al. 1997). Such omnibus approaches typically involve blurring of images before analysis, to minimize the effects of interindividual anatomical variability and decrease the number of computations performed (Frackowiak et al. 1997; Poline et al. 1997), negating the higher spatial resolution otherwise afforded by state-of-the art tomographs.

In most of the recent studies of depression, researchers relied exclusively on statistical parametric mapping methods (e.g., SPM) and blurred their primary tomograms to resolutions of 20–30 mm before analysis. Although this practice may lead to identification of abnormalities in relatively large cortical areas, the sensitivity for detecting abnormalities in small structures is decreased. For example, Abercrombie et al. (1996) showed that the abnormal increase in amygdala metabolism in MDD previously found by Drevets et al. (1992) using ROI analysis was replicable by MRI-based ROI analysis but not

SPM. Similarly, the abnormal reduction of metabolism in the subgenual prefrontal cortex proved highly reproducible with the use of targeted ROI analysis (Drevets et al. 1997b) but was identified in some (e.g., Drevets et al. 1997b; Kegeles et al. 1999) and not other (e.g., Drevets et al. 1992) studies in which SPM or other omnibus approaches were applied. Finally, brain surfaces characterized by a high degree of anatomical variability (e.g., the orbital frontal cortex) are difficult to evaluate in intergroup comparisons with SPM because this variability increases the standard deviation of corresponding PET measures, reducing the magnitude of statistical parametric values in SPM images.

The application of SPM and other image analysis strategies that involve large numbers of intergroup statistical comparisons has also increased type I error in psychiatric imaging research, because the resulting significance values have rarely been appropriately corrected. Thus, in most studies of depression, intergroup differences were identified through comparison of image data between depressed patients and control subjects either in dozens of ROIs or in several thousand resolution elements (the independent sampling unit of a statistical parametric image). Yet in most of these studies, researchers neither corrected reported *P* values for the number of comparisons (Poline et al. 1997) nor replicated findings in independent subject samples. The literature has consequently been diluted by results that cannot be distinguished from multiple-comparison artifact. This practice is at times defended by the argument that a difference that otherwise would not reach an appropriately corrected significance threshold is reportable because it replicates an earlier finding. Whereas true replications merit such consideration, in most of these cases the differences alleged to constitute replication occurred too distantly from a previously reported abnormality to reasonably implicate the same area. For example, areas of apparently reduced flow or metabolism located anywhere in the prefrontal cortex have been alleged to constitute replications of the earlier finding by Baxter et al. (1989) in the dorsal anterolateral prefrontal cortex, even when such areas lie several centimeters away in functionally distinct portions of the prefrontal cortex (which constitutes one-half of the human brain). This problem has created substantial confusion regarding the specific location of metabolic abnormalities in the prefrontal cortex in depression.

When constrained by appropriate statistical considerations and followed by rigorous replication using targeted ROI analyses in independent subject samples, omnibus image analysis approaches involving statistical parametric mapping have proven invaluable for delineating areas where differences exist between depressed patients and control subjects (Drevets et al. 1992, 1997b;

Poline et al. 1997). For all of the regions where both abnormal metabolism and reduced gray matter volume were identified in mood disorders, omnibus approaches were used repeatedly to detect and localize abnormalities, and higher-resolution ROI analyses followed to confirm the significance of such abnormalities in independent samples (Bell et al. 1999; Drevets et al. 1992, 1995a, 1997b).

Sample Selection Issues Critical to Identifying Neuroimaging Abnormalities in Depression

The ability to consistently identify abnormalities of structure and function in depression has also depended on sample selection issues. Sample size is the most straightforward of these issues: the magnitude of difference in mean neuroimaging measures between depressed patients and control subjects is typically small relative to these measures' variability (effect sizes of reported abnormalities typically range from 1 to 2). The sample sizes in most neuroimaging studies have been too small to provide adequate statistical sensitivity (power) to detect previously reported abnormalities in MDD, so many nonreplications of findings across studies likely reflect type II error.

Another obvious, but commonly overlooked, issue in the design of functional imaging studies is the likelihood that image data are confounded by medication effects. Antidepressant, antipsychotic, and benzodiazepine anxiolytic drugs have been shown to decrease regional CBF and glucose metabolism in many areas of the frontal, parietal, and temporal cortices (see, for example, Drevets et al. 1999a; Maes et al. 1993; Silfverskiöld and Risberg 1989). Researchers conducting studies involving depressed patients taking psychotropic drugs at the time of scanning have usually failed to detect the areas of hypermetabolism identified in samples of unmedicated patients with depression and have frequently reported areas of reduced flow or metabolism not evident in unmedicated samples (Drevets et al. 1999a). Findings of the majority of published functional neuroimaging studies of depression have been confounded by medication effects and must be excluded when a functional anatomy of mood disorders is being developed.

A more challenging issue to address in depression imaging studies is the possibility that abnormalities of brain structure and function are specific to mood disorder subtypes. Reviewed earlier was MRI evidence that patients with late-onset depression have neuromorphological correlates of cerebrovascular disease (Krishnan et al. 1993). In imaging studies of mood disorders, therefore, late-onset cases or cases with MRI evidence of lacunae and white matter hyperintensity must be considered separately from early-onset cases, given the effects of cerebrovascular disease on radiotracer delivery, hemodynamic responses, and metabolic activity described earlier (Drevets et al. 1999a).

Early-onset MDD is also likely to encompass a group of disorders that are heterogeneous with respect to etiology and pathophysiology and that may thus be characterized by an assortment of distinct functional brain imaging abnormalities (Drevets and Todd 1997). The only laboratories that have reported clear replications of their own previous functional imaging results in independent subject samples used some means of "enriching" samples of MDD patients (i.e., using entrance criteria that enhanced the likelihood of identifying psychobiological markers of depression). In the studies by Drevets and colleagues described here, the variability of image data in samples of MDD patients was reduced by selecting subjects who were unmedicated; had primary (i.e., arising before other psychiatric or medical conditions), recurrent MDD that began before age 45; and met criteria for familial pure depressive disease (Winokur 1982). Familial pure depressive disease is primary MDD in a subject who has a first-degree relative with MDD and no first-degree relatives with mania, alcoholism, or antisocial personality disorder. Depressed subjects with familial pure depressive disease or bipolar disorder were previously shown to be more likely than subjects with depression spectrum disease (subjects with primary MDD who have first-degree relatives with alcoholism or sociopathy) or sporadic depressive disease (subjects with primary MDD who have no first-degree relatives with MDD, alcoholism, or sociopathy) to have abnormal suppression by dexamethasone of cortisol secretion (Arana et al. 1985; Winokur 1982), blunted hypoglycemic response to insulin (Lewis et al. 1983), reduced platelet [^{3}H]imipramine binding sites (Lewis and McChesney 1985), decreased latency to rapid eye movement sleep (Kupfer et al. 1992), and a response to electroconvulsive therapy (Coryell and Zimmerman 1984). The familial pure depressive disease and bipolar disorder–depression subtypes may thus be more likely to have biological abnormalities than some other depressive subtypes. In PET studies, depressed patients with familial pure depressive disease or bipolar disorder have been more likely than depression spectrum disease subjects matched for sex, age, and Hamilton Rating Scale for Depression scores to have increased CBF or metabolism in the orbital cortex, amygdala, and medial thalamus; decreased metabolism in the subgenual prefrontal cortex; and decreased 5-HT$_{1A}$ receptor BP in the mesiotemporal cortex and raphe (Drevets et al. 1995a, 1997a, 1999b) (Figures 11–2, 11–3, and 11–4). Studies involving alternative means for selecting MDD patient samples enriched for the likelihood of having biological markers for depression, such as responsiveness to sleep deprivation (Ebert et al. 1991; Wu et al. 1992) or phototherapy (Cohen et al. 1992) or criteria for the melancholic subtype (Abercrombie et al. 1996), have also found increased metabolism in the amygdala and orbital cortex and reduced metabolism in the subgenual prefrontal cortex.

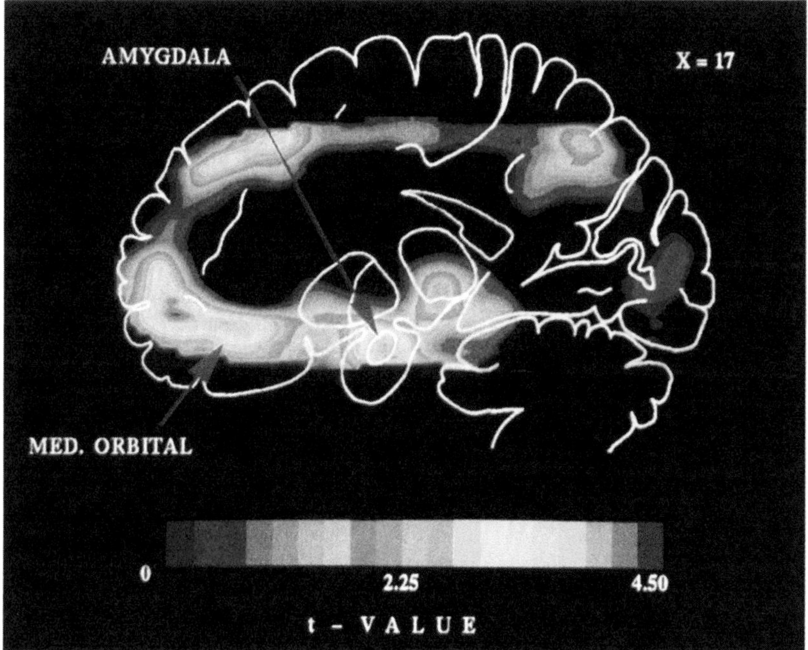

FIGURE 11–2. Areas of abnormally increased blood flow in familial major depressive disorder (MDD). The image section shown is from an image of *t* values, produced by a voxel-by-voxel computation of the unpaired *t* statistic to compare cerebral blood flow (CBF) between depressed patients and control subjects (Drevets et al. 1992). The positive *t* values in this sagittal section at 17 mm to the left of midline show areas of increased CBF in the depressed patients, relative to the control subjects, in the amygdala and the medial posterior orbital cortex (MED. ORBITAL). Abnormal activity in these regions in MDD has been confirmed in other studies, using higher-resolution, glucose metabolism measurements (Drevets 1999). Anterior is to the left.
Source. Reprinted from Price JL, Carmichael ST, Drevets WC: "Networks Related to the Orbital and Medial Prefrontal Cortex: A Substrate for Emotional Behavior?" *Progress in Brain Research* 107:523–536, 1996. Used with permission.

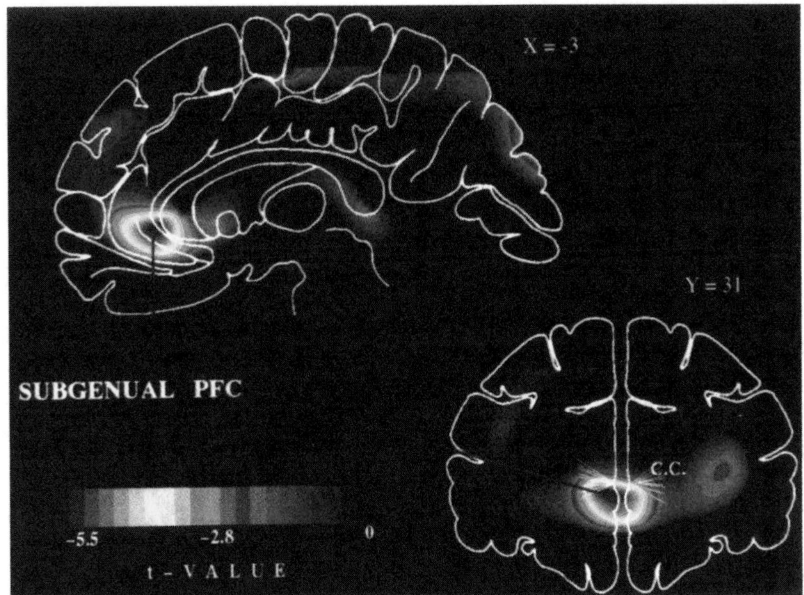

FIGURE 11–3. Coronal (y=31 mm anterior to the anterior commissure) and sagittal (x=–3 mm left of midline) sections showing negative voxel t values where glucose metabolism is decreased in depressed patients relative to control subjects. Abbreviations: CC=corpus callosum.

Source. Reprinted from Drevets WC, Price JL, Simpson JR, et al.: "Subgenual Prefrontal Cortex Abnormalities in Mood Disorders." *Nature* 386:824–827, 1997b. Used with permission.

■ RELATIONSHIPS BETWEEN FUNCTIONAL AND STRUCTURAL ABNORMALITIES IN DEPRESSION

Subgenual Prefrontal Cortex

The prototypical example of an area where the integration of functional and structural imaging technology informed science about the pathophysiology of mood disorders is the prefrontal cortex ventral to the genu of the corpus callosum (subgenual prefrontal cortex; Figure 11–3). This region was initially shown to have reduced CBF in a statistical parametric image in which PET images from depressed patients with bipolar disorder were compared with PET images from healthy control subjects (Drevets et al. 1995a, 1997b). The statistical significance of this difference was subsequently established using a targeted ROI approach to compare image data from independent samples of

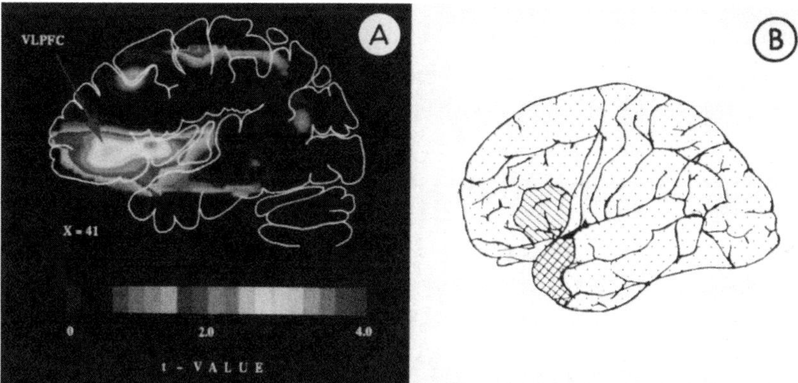

FIGURE 11–4. Site of gray matter loss in a group of elderly subjects with major depression is similar to the site of abnormally increased cerebral blood flow (CBF), correlating inversely with illness severity, in a group of young patients with unipolar major depression. *(A)* Sagittal section from an image composed of voxel *t* values at 41 mm left of midline showing abnormally increased CBF in the left ventrolateral prefrontal cortex (VLPFC), lateral posterior orbital cortex, and anterior insula in young depressed patients, relative to healthy control subjects (Drevets et al. 1992). *(B)* Map of gray matter wet weight loss from regions of the cerebral cortex in elderly depressed subjects compared with control subjects (Bowen et al. 1989). Shaded areas indicate significant reductions.

Source. Reprinted from Drevets WC: "Geriatric Depression: Brain Imaging Correlates and Pharmacologic Considerations." *Journal of Clinical Psychiatry* 55:71–81, 1994. Used with permission.

depressed patients with bipolar disorder and control subjects. The finding was then extended: PET measures of glucose metabolism were shown to be decreased, relative to control subjects, in both a third, independent set of depressed patients with bipolar disorder and a set of patients with unipolar depression and familial pure depressive disease (Drevets et al. 1997b). The abnormal reduction in subgenual prefrontal cortex metabolism was later replicated by Buchsbaum et al. (1997) (who referred to the same region as the "rectal gyrus") in patients with MDD and by Kegeles et al. (1999) in a mixed sample of familial MDD patients and bipolar disorder patients.

When metabolism failed to normalize in this area after otherwise effective treatment (Drevets 1997), a neuromorphometric MRI study was conducted to assess the possibility that partial volume averaging effects associated with a corresponding reduction in cortical volume contribute to the reduction of CBF and metabolism in familial pure depressive disease and bipolar disorder. These MRI-based neuromorphometric measures showed a left-lateralized, mean gray matter volume reduction of 39% and 48% in the patients with familial bipolar disorder and the patients with MDD, respectively (Drevets et al. 1997b). This volumetric difference persisted during treatment and was present in various mood states. These MRI-based findings were replicated and extended by Hirayasu et al. (1999), who confirmed the left-lateralized abnormality in patients with familial bipolar disorder but not in patients with nonfamilial bipolar disorder; and by Botteron et al. (1999), who showed this abnormality was present in both affected and unaffected co-twins from monozygotic twin pairs (ages 18–24 years) discordant for MDD.

Postmortem assessments of subgenual prefrontal cortex tissue from patients with bipolar disorder or MDD confirmed the abnormal reduction in cortical volume (Drevets et al. 1998; Öngür et al. 1998). In these studies, the reduction in gray matter was associated with a reduction in glia (without an equivalent loss of neurons) in familial MDD and bipolar disorder patients, relative to psychiatrically healthy and schizophrenic control subjects. Although it is not expected that the reduction in glial cells alone accounts for the reduction in cortical volume, it is conceivable that a reduction in the number of astrocytes may lead to underdevelopment of the neuropil (Araque 1999; Magistretti et al. 1995), which potentially explains both the decreased cortical volume and the increased neuronal density found in these samples of mood disorder patients. Within the group of patients with bipolar disorder, both the neuromorphometric MRI and postmortem histopathological abnormalities were most prominent in subjects who had first-degree relatives with MDD or bipolar disorder. In addition, within the samples of patients with bipolar disorder, subjects who had first-degree relatives with bipolar disorder but tended to remain psychotic between mood episodes (i.e., patients with schizoaffective disorder) appeared to have the most prominent reduction in cortex and glia.

The reduction in glia appeared to extend ventrally down the ventromedial prefrontal cortex wall and laterally into the posterior orbital cortex. In a complementary study, Rajkowska et al. (1997, 1999) demonstrated a reduction in cortical volume in the posterior and rostral orbital cortex lateral to the area we examined. In addition, the posterior orbital cortex and the dorsal anterolateral prefrontal cortex (where we also found abnormally reduced metabolism in patients with MDD [Bell et al. 1999]) had an abnormal reduction of glia in MDD and bipolar disorder patients. These findings may be regionally specific to limbic and paralimbic cortical areas, however, because glial counts were not abnormally reduced in the rostral orbital cortex, somatosensory cortex, or dorsolateral prefrontal cortex (Brodmann's area 46) (Öngür et al. 1998; Rajkowska et al. 1997, 1999).

Implications for Functional Imaging Studies

In the case of the subgenual prefrontal cortex, the identification of apparent reductions in local glucose metabolism, with the metabolism failing to normalize during otherwise effective treatment, and the recognition that such differences may be accounted for by corresponding reductions in cortical volume guided investigators conducting subsequent neuromorphometric MRI and postmortem studies to the discovery of neuropathological abnormalities in MDD and bipolar disorder (Drevets et al. 1997b; Mazziotta et al. 1981). Questions raised by these results were whether partial volume averaging effects entirely accounted for the apparent reduction in CBF and metabolism in depression and whether physiological activity was abnormal per unit of tissue volume. Addressing these issues was of particular interest in interpreting the additional observation that effective antidepressant treatment resulted in a further decrease in glucose metabolism in the subgenual prefrontal cortex (Buchsbaum et al. 1997; Drevets et al. 1997b; Mayberg et al. 1999), and in determining whether the reduction in glia may be associated with altered metabolic activity in major depression (Drevets et al. 1998).

Techniques for correcting PET data for partial volume effects have been developed that involve the use of MRI data to scale PET values by the amount of brain tissue contributing radioactive counts to a VOI (Meltzer et al. 1999). Such methods require acquisition of MR images with high spatial and tissue contrast resolution and homogeneous MR signal intensity to permit segmentation of the anatomical image into brain tissue and CSF voxels (Meltzer et al. 1999). When registered with the PET image, this binary image provides a tissue scaling factor for each VOI, one that represents the fraction of the three-dimensional volume that is composed of neural tissue rather than CSF. Dividing the PET VOI value by this corrected tissue volume scales the PET activity to PET counts per volume of tissue rather than PET counts per volume of space (as in the original PET image). The major source of error involved in this correction is the automated separation of brain and CSF signals based on threshold MR signal intensities. Although this error source can be effectively addressed when "two-compartment" corrections that stratify neural tissue versus CSF are performed, it remains an obstacle with "three-compartment" techniques that correct PET values for the relative proportions of gray matter, white matter, and CSF (Meltzer et al. 1999).

Computer simulations performed to correct the PET measures for the effects of a reduction in cortical volume led to the conclusion that glucose metabolism in the remaining subgenual prefrontal cortex tissue is actually abnormally increased in depressed patients relative to control subjects (W.C.

Drevets, J.R. Simpson, M.E. Raichle, unpublished data, July 1999). This finding is compatible with observations that effective antidepressant treatment results in a further decrease in glucose metabolism in the subgenual prefrontal cortex (Buchsbaum et al. 1997; Drevets et al. 1997b; Mayberg et al. 1999) and that, in healthy subjects, CBF increases in the subgenual prefrontal cortex during sadness induced by contemplation of sad autobiographical material (Damasio et al. 1998; George et al. 1995; Mayberg et al. 1999). The finding is also compatible with the finding of Mayberg et al. (1999) that effective fluoxetine treatment decreases subgenual prefrontal cortex glucose metabolism to a level below normal in MDD. This result would be expected if metabolism in this region reflected both mood-independent partial volume effects of reduced tissue (which decrease apparent metabolism to below normal) and mood-dependent hypermetabolism in the remaining cortex in the unmedicated-depressed phase of MDD.

Mayberg et al. (1997) also reported that CBF in the subgenual prefrontal cortex does not increase in subjects with remitted MDD when they perform a sadness-induction task (using contemplation of sad autobiographical material) that activates this region in healthy control subjects (Damasio et al. 1998; George et al. 1995; Mayberg et al. 1999). Because this region has decreased cortical volume in both the depressed and remitted phases of MDD (Drevets et al. 1997b) and decreased glucose metabolism in the medicated-remitted phase of MDD, compared with the unmedicated-depressed phase of MDD, the lack of significant CBF response during sadness induction may reflect attenuation of the CBF response by partial volume effects of reduced cortical volume (assuming that this lack of response does not instead reflect pharmacologic effects of antidepressant drugs or a behavioral performance difference between groups).

Alternatively, the reason that regional CBF does not increase in the left subgenual prefrontal cortex might be that the relationship between neuronal activity, energy utilization, and CBF is pathologically altered by abnormal glial function in MDD (Drevets et al. 1998; Öngür et al. 1998; Rajkowska et al. 1999). Preliminary postmortem assessments of the type of glia that is reduced in this region in MDD and bipolar disorder suggest that this abnormality includes astroglia (a conclusion based on preliminary glial fibrillary acidic protein–staining results [Makkos et al. 2000]), which play a role in establishing the relationship between neuronal activity, glucose metabolism, and oxygen utilization (Araque 1999; Magistretti et al. 1995). Reduced astroglial function could thus alter the relationship between neuronal activity and the physiological parameters measured in PET and functional MRI brain mapping studies. Characterizing such a phenomenon may require iterative experimental approaches involving PET and magnetic resonance spectroscopy during performance of well-characterized neurobehavioral tasks that probe the function of the subgenual prefrontal cortex, together with parallel postmortem histochemical studies that more specifically illuminate the nature of the reduction in cortex and glia in mood disorders.

Clinical Implications of Subgenual Prefrontal Cortex Dysfunction

The functions of glia (i.e., astroglia) in providing trophic factors and energy substrates to neurons, maintaining potassium homeostasis, and transporting glutamate and γ-aminobutyric acid (GABA) from the extracellular fluid suggest mechanisms by which glial hypofunction may disturb synaptic activity within the subgenual prefrontal cortex (Araque 1999; Magistretti et al. 1995). Although it remains unclear whether the reduction in glial number in the subgenual prefrontal cortex is associated with glial hypofunction in MDD and bipolar disorder, the finding that the proportion of high-affinity, glycine-displaceable [^{3}H]CGP 39653 binding to *N*-methyl-D-aspartate (NMDA) glutamatergic receptors is reduced in the prefrontal cortex in individuals who commit suicide is potentially consistent with this hypothesis (Nowak et al. 1995). This finding conceivably could reflect a compensatory shift away from the high-affinity state of these receptors associated with an impairment of glia-mediated glutamate transport. Notably, repeated electroconvulsive therapy and chronic antidepressant drug administration desensitize glutamatergic-NMDA receptors in the frontal cortex of rats, and anticonvulsant agents that putatively inhibit glutamate release appear effective in treating and preventing abnormal mood episodes in bipolar disorder (see, for example, Post et al. 1992; Sporn and Sachs 1997). Antidepressant and mood-stabilizing treatments may thus compensate for a reduction in astroglial function in MDD and bipolar disorder (Nowak et al. 1993; Paul et al. 1994).

In humans, the subgenual prefrontal cortex comprises Brodmann's area 24b and, to a lesser extent, 24a on the prelimbic portion of the anterior cingulate gyrus (the reduction in cortex may also extend caudally into infralimbic cortex ([area 25] and rostrally into the pregenual portions of the anterior cingulate cortex and medial prefrontal cortex; Öngür et al. 1998]. This region is known to play important roles in modulating autonomic, neuroendocrine, and monoamine neurotransmitter responses to stressful and emotionally provocative stimuli (reviewed by Drevets et al. [1998]). The findings of abnormal cortical volume, glucose metabolism, and glial cell counts within the subgenual prefrontal cortex in MDD and bipolar disorder thus suggest intriguing hypotheses regarding the mechanisms by which such responses become abnormal in mood disorders.

The synaptic interactions that may be affected by glial hypofunction in the subgenual prefrontal cortex involve the extensive reciprocal projections between this region and the amygdala, lateral hypothalamus, nucleus accumbens, ventral tegmental area (VTA), substantia nigra, dorsal raphe nucleus (DRN), locus coeruleus, periaqueductal gray (PAG), and nucleus solitarius of the vagus nerve (Carmichael and Price 1995; Frysztak and Neafsey 1994; Neafsey et al. 1993; Sesack and Pickel 1992; Sesack et al. 1989). Humans with lesions that include the subgenual prefrontal cortex demonstrate abnormal autonomic responses to emotional experiences, an inability to experience emotion related to concepts that ordinarily evoke emotion, and an inability to use information regarding the likelihood of punishment and reward in guiding social behavior (Damasio et al. 1990). Rats with experimental lesions of the prelimbic cortex (the apparent homologue of the primate subgenual prefrontal cortex) demonstrate altered autonomic, neuroendocrine, and behavioral responses to stress that in some cases resemble changes in these systems in humans with mood disorders.

Bilateral lesions of the dorsal prelimbic and anterior cingulate cortices increase freezing behavior and heart rate elevations during exposure to fear-conditioned stimuli, whereas bilateral lesions of the infralimbic and ventral prelimbic cortices reduce heart rate responses to fear-conditioned stimuli, suggesting that the latter regions play a role in increasing heart rate during stress (Frysztak and Neafsey 1994; Morgan and LeDoux 1995). The drive on sympathetic autonomic arousal and corticosterone release during stress was more specifically linked to the right ventromedial prefrontal cortex, because of evidence that, during restraint stress, rats with lesions of the left infralimbic, prelimbic, and anterior cingulate cortices show heightened sympathetic arousal and corticosterone secretion, whereas animals with lesions on the right show reduced corticosterone secretion and gastric stress pathology (Sullivan and Gratton 1999). These data were interpreted as indicating that left ventromedial prefrontal cortex lesions disinhibit a drive on sympathetic and hypothalamic-pituitary-adrenal–axis arousal that is stimulated by the right ventromedial prefrontal cortex (Sullivan and Gratton 1999). Given the left lateralization of the neuroimaging abnormalities in the subgenual prefrontal cortex (Drevets et al. 1997b; Hirayasu et al. 1999), it might be hypothesized that left subgenual prefrontal cortex dysfunction contributes to the heightened sympathetic autonomic arousal and cortisol release seen in MDD (Carroll 1994; Diorio et al. 1993; Veith et al. 1994).

The subgenual prefrontal cortex may influence neuroendocrine and sympathetic autonomic responses through its connections to the hypothalamus, amygdala, PAG, and locus coeruleus. Diorio et al. (1993) demonstrated that lesions of the prelimbic and infralimbic cortices increase plasma adrenocorticotropic hormone and corticosterone responses to restraint stress and hypothesized that this finding reflected disconnection of projections between glucocorticoid receptor–expressing cells in the prelimbic or infralimbic cortex and the hypothalamus. Diorio et al. (1993) proposed that the glucocorticoid receptors located in the prelimbic and infralimbic cortices are involved in the negative feedback of adrenal steroids on stress-related limbic-hypothalamic-pituitary-adrenal–axis activity. It is thus conceivable that subgenual prefrontal cortex dysfunction contributes to the abnormal feedback inhibition of cortisol secretion in MDD and bipolar disorder (Barden et al. 1995; Carroll 1994).

The subgenual prefrontal cortex may also play a role in modulating the parasympathetic tone on the heart rate. Frysztak and Neafsey (1994) showed that lesions of the prelimbic and infralimbic cortices reduce heart rate variability at rest and during exposure to fear-conditioned stimuli. This result was hypothesized to reflect disruption of the connections between the nucleus solitarius and cells in the ventral prelimbic and infralimbic cortices (Frysztak and Neafsey 1994; Neafsey et al. 1986), because heart rate variability is thought to reflect parasympathetic control of the sinus node via vagal nerve transmission (Pagani et al. 1986). Dysfunction of the left subgenual prefrontal cortex may thus relate to both the increased resting heart rate and the reduced heart rate variability reported in depressed subjects relative to nondepressed subjects (Carney et al. 1988; Veith et al. 1994). The increased sympathetic-to-parasympathetic tone or balance suggested by these electrocardiographic findings is hypothesized to contribute to the increased risk of ventricular tachycardia, myocardial infarction, and sudden death in depressed relative to nondepressed subjects with cardiovascular disease (Carney et al. 1988, 1993; Frasure-Smith et al. 1995).

Finally, the subgenual prefrontal cortex may play a role in evaluating the behavioral significance of stimuli through its projections to neurons in the VTA (Crino et al. 1993; Leichnetz and Astruc 1976; Sesack and Pickel 1992; Sesack et al. 1989). In rats, electrical or glutamatergic stimulation of medial prefrontal cortex areas that include the subgenual prefrontal cortex elicits burst firing patterns from dopamine cells in the VTA and increases dopamine release in the nucleus accumbens (Chergui et al. 1993; Murase et al. 1993; Roth and Elsworth 1995; Taber and Fibiger 1993). The increase in dopamine release mediated by this phasic burst-firing of dopamine neurons appears to modulate the encoding of information regarding stimuli that predict reward and deviations between such predictions and the actual occurrence of reward (Schultz 1997). In mood disorders, subgenual prefrontal cortex dysfunction may thus interfere with hedonic perception and motivated behavior by altering the electrophysiologic responses of VTA neurons.

Posterior Orbital Cortex

The posterior orbital cortex is another prefrontal cortex area where gray matter volume and glial counts are abnormally reduced in MDD, yet physiological activity is increased in the unmedicated-depressed state relative to the medicated-remitted state (Drevets et al. 1999a; Rajkowska et al. 1999) (Figures 11–2 and 11–4). Cross-sectional studies involving unmedicated patients with MDD found increased CBF and metabolism, relative to healthy control subjects, in these regions (Baxter et al. 1987; Biver et al. 1994; Cohen et al. 1992; Drevets et al. 1992, 1995a; Ebert et al. 1991). Longitudinal studies in which depressed patients were imaged before and during treatment showed that orbital cortex CBF and metabolism decrease after effective antidepressant therapy, electroconvulsive therapy, phototherapy, repetitive transcranial magnetic stimulation, and sleep deprivation (Table 11–1). The increased physiological activity in these regions in the unmedicated-depressed phase of MDD relative to the remitted phase of MDD is compatible with evidence that the posterior orbital CBF increases during a variety of emotion-related conditions in humans (reviewed by Drevets and Raichle [1998]). For example, flow increases in the lateral and medial posterior orbital cortex and the anterior insular cortex during experimentally induced sadness or anxiety in healthy subjects (Drevets and Raichle 1998; George et al. 1995, Pardo et al. 1993; Schneider et al. 1995) and during induced anxiety and/or obsessional states in subjects with obsessive-compulsive disorder (Rauch et al. 1994), posttraumatic stress disorder (Rauch et al. 1996), or simple animal phobia (Drevets et al. 1995b; Rauch et al. 1995).

Nevertheless, the posterior and lateral orbital areas where we and others found abnormally increased CBF or metabolism in unmedicated subjects with primary MDD implicated areas where Bowen et al. (1989) and Rajkowska et al. (1999) found abnormally reduced gray matter wet weight and cortical thickness, respectively, in postmortem studies of MDD and bipolar disorder (Figure 11–4). As in the case of the subgenual prefrontal cortex, this reduction in volume was associated with a reduction in glia but no equivalent reduction of neurons (Drevets et al. 1998; Rajkowska et al. 1997, 1999).

Implications for Functional Imaging Studies of Depression

Because the orbital areas where gray matter volume is reduced in MDD are sites where CBF increases in response to sad and anxious mood in healthy, anxiety disorder subjects and in depressed subjects, the partial volume averaging effects resulting from reduced cortical volume may produce complex interactions between illness severity and PET measures of neurophysiological activity (Drevets et al. 1992, 1994, 1995a; Mazziotta et al. 1981). In these regions, the PET measure comprises a summation of increased CBF or metabolism in response to the emotive state and concomitantly reduced CBF or metabolism caused by partial volume effects (Links et al. 1996). The complexity of detecting physiological activation in brain regions functionally related to emotional processing in regions where cortical volume is abnormally decreased may partly account for the paradoxical relationship between Hamilton Rating Scale for Depression scores and orbital cortex CBF or metabolism in MDD (Drevets et al. 1992, 1994, 1995a, 1999a). That is, if the gray matter volume reduction in this area correlates with illness severity, then net CBF or metabolic values may be lower in the most severe cases than in milder cases. Such a complex relationship between illness severity and physiological activity may also give rise to discrepant results across subject samples with distinct illness severity. Estimating the relative contributions of the competing effects of abnormal cortical volume and increased physiological activity to the relationship between depression severity and CBF or metabolism may thus depend on correction of PET measures for partial volume effects (Meltzer et al. 1999).

Clinical Correlates of Posterior Orbital Cortex Dysfunction

The negative correlations between posterior orbital physiological activity and ratings of depression severity and depressive ideation in MDD may additionally reflect this region's functional role in emotional behavior (Drevets et al. 1992, 1995a). The inverse relationship between posterior orbital activity and emotion ratings is evident not only in MDD during depression but also in obsessive-compulsive disorder and simple phobia in response to phobic stimuli and in healthy subjects during induced sadness. Posterior orbital CBF increases in each case, yet the magnitude of the CBF change correlates inversely with concomitant changes in obsessive thinking, anxiety, and sadness, respectively (Drevets et al. 1995b; Rauch et al. 1994; Schneider et al. 1995). These observations are consistent with evidence from electrophysiologic and lesion analysis studies that the posterior orbital cortex plays roles in modulating defensive, autonomic, and behavioral responses and in redirecting psychological and behavioral response patterns as reward contingencies change (Iversen and Mishkin 1970; Rolls 1995; Rosenkilde et al. 1981; Thorpe et al. 1983; Timms 1977). For example, humans with lesions of the orbital cortex exhibit difficulty in shifting intellectual strategies in response to changing demands (i.e., they perseverate in strategies that become inappropriate [Fuster 1989]), and monkeys with surgical lesions of the lateral orbital or ventrolateral prefrontal cortex demonstrate "perseverative interference," characterized by difficulty in learning to withhold responses to nonrewarding stimuli (Iversen and Mishkin 1970).

During depressive episodes, activation of the posterior orbital cortex may reflect endogenous attempts to break perseverative patterns of self-depreciating and nonrewarding thought and emotion or to inhibit defensive behaviors and visceral responses to stressors (Drevets 1999; Drevets and Raichle 1998). These behaviors may be driven by pathological activity in the amygdala, where abnormally increased CBF and metabolism correlate positively with ratings of depression severity in MDD (Drevets 1999; Drevets et al. 1992, 1995a, 1997a). Given evidence that somatic antidepressant treatments may directly modulate neuronal activity in the amygdala (Broekkamp and Lloyd 1981; Duncan et al. 1986; Ordway et al. 1991; Wang and Aghajanian 1980), the reduction in orbital cortex CBF and metabolism after successful treatment may indicate that the orbital cortex "relaxes" as such treatments inhibit the pathological limbic activity to which they respond (Table 11–1).

If the posterior orbital cortex is activated in MDD to correct emotional or behavioral responses that become inappropriate as reinforcement contingencies change and to modulate emotional expression, dysfunction of this region may yield a state in which the ability to interrupt perseverative melancholic thoughts and anxious responses to ordinarily nonthreatening stimuli is impaired. The postmortem studies of MDD and bipolar disorder that found abnormally reduced gray matter and reduced glia in the posterior orbital cortex suggest that orbital dysfunction may exist in mood disorders (Bowen et al. 1989; Rajkowska et al. 1999). As reviewed earlier in this chapter, glial dysfunction may disturb reciprocal synaptic interactions between orbital cortex neurons and their projections to the amygdala, striatum, cingulate, hypothalamus, or PAG and thereby interfere with the modulation of stress or emotional responses driven by the amygdala or the right subgenual prefrontal cortex (Araque 1999; Carmichael and Price 1995; Magistretti et al. 1995; Price, in press). Furthermore, acquired lesions of the orbital cortex or the striatum—where converging efferent projections from the orbital cortex and amygdala interact to modulate emotional behavior—may similarly produce depressive syndromes that arise later in life. Cerebrovascular lesions of the left prefrontal cortex and striatum (Starkstein and Robinson 1989) and degenerative disorders that affect striatal function (Folstein et al. 1991; Mayeux 1982; Santamaria et al. 1986) increase the risk of major depressive episodes.

Dorsomedial or Dorsal Anterolateral Prefrontal Cortex

Resting CBF and glucose metabolism are abnormal in the dorsomedial dorsal anterolateral prefrontal cortex as well in MDD and bipolar disorder, and it remains unclear whether structural abnormalities underlie physiological disturbances in these regions as well. For example, a large number of studies have found reduced metabolism in multiple sites of the dorsolateral and dorsomedial prefrontal cortex in MDD (Baxter et al. 1989; Bench et al. 1992; Drevets et al. [1999a]). One dorsomedial or dorsal anterolateral prefrontal cortex area lying anterior to the anterior cingulate gyrus (Brodmann's area 9) in which there was abnormal reduction (Bell et al. 1999) was recently shown to be a site where both neurons and glia are abnormally reduced in brain tissue acquired post-mortem from subjects with MDD, although cortical thickness was not abnormal in this region (Rajkowska et al. 1999). This cellular abnormality may account for the persistence of the metabolic abnormality in spite of effective treatment in this area in PET studies of MDD (Bell et al. 1999).

In brain mapping studies performed in healthy humans, CBF increases in these areas of Brodmann's area 9 during performance of some tasks that elicit emotional responses or require emotional evaluations (Dolan et al. 1996; Drevets et al. 1995a; Reiman et al. 1997). The relationships between hemodynamic responses and emotion ratings in these studies suggest that this region is activated to modulate emotional responses. For example, during anticipation of a painful electrical shock, CBF increases in this region relative to resting or teeth-clenching control conditions, but within each condition the change in anxiety ratings and heart rate correlate inversely with CBF (Drevets et al. 1994). The dorsomedial prefrontal cortex (Brodmann's area 9) receives and sends extensive projections to the PAG, through which it may modulate emotional behavior and cardiovascular responses (Price, in press). Lesions placed in the dorsomedial prefrontal cortex in experimental animals increase heart rate responses to fear-conditioned stimuli, and electrical and chemical stimulation of sites within this cortex attenuate or inhibit the defensive behavior and associated cardiovascular responses evoked by amygdala stimulation (Frysztak and Neafsey 1994). It is thus hypothesized that these areas of the medial prefrontal cortex normally act to decrease heart rate during stress.

If the dorsomedial prefrontal cortex plays a role in modulating behavioral and cardiovascular responses to stress, the reduction in neurons and glia identified in this region by Rajkowska et al. (1999) suggests that dorsomedial prefrontal cortex dysfunction may contribute to the exaggerated stress responses seen in MDD. Dorsomedial prefrontal cortex dysfunction having other causes may similarly alter stress or emotional responses. For example, this region was shown to have reduced CBF in depressed relative to nondepressed Parkinson's disease patients, possibly related to the dense dopamine innervation this region receives from the VTA (Ring et al. 1994).

Subcortical Structures

Other neuromorphometric MRI abnormalities reported in MDD and bipolar disorder implicate the striatal, thalamic, and mesiotemporal cortex areas that share extensive anatomical connections with the orbital and medial prefrontal cortex. For example, enlargement of the third ventricle has been found in studies of adult and adolescent subjects with bipolar disorder, although the specific tissue in which volume loss results in ex vacuo changes in third ventricle size remains unclear (Botteron and Figiel 1997; Pearlson et al. 1997). The subgenual and orbital prefrontal cortices share extensive, reciprocal, anatomical projections with the periventricular and mediodorsal thalamic nuclei that line the third ventricle, so it is conceivable that the volumetric reductions in these prefrontal cortex areas and third ventricle enlargement are related (Carmichael and Price 1995).

Striatum

The striatum receives major projections from the orbital and medial prefrontal cortex that terminate in the ventromedial caudate and nucleus accumbens (Carmichael and Price 1995; Nauta and Domesick 1984). Krishnan et al. (1992) reported that the volume of the caudate head was abnormally decreased in a combined sample of elderly and middle-aged subjects. Post hoc assessments of these data suggested that this abnormality applied to both the elderly subjects and the young subjects with early-onset disease within this sample. Establishing this conclusion will prove critical for determining whether the PET findings of abnormally decreased resting CBF and metabolism in the caudate in middle-aged MDD subjects reflect partial volume effects (Baxter et al. 1985; Drevets et al. 1992) (Figure 11–5). Understanding the nature of these striatal abnormalities is also likely to be an important key to elucidating the pathophysiology of mood disorders, given that, as reviewed earlier, the synaptic interactions between the striatal targets of converging fibers from the orbital and medial prefrontal cortex and the amygdala appear critical for mod-

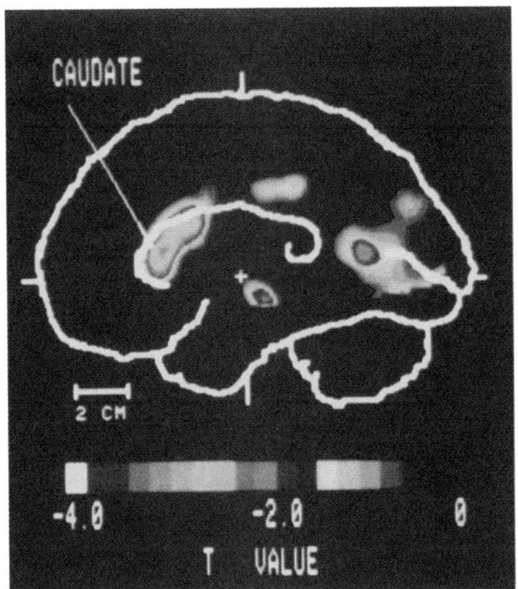

FIGURE 11–5. Areas of decreased activity in depressed subjects with major depressive disorder (MDD), relative to control subjects, in the left medial caudate. This *t* image is a sagittal projection of the greatest voxel *t* values in all planes between the midline and 10 mm left of midline. This observation may be accounted for by a reduction in caudate volume in MDD (Krishnan et al. 1992). Anterior is to the left.
Source. Reprinted from Drevets WC, Videen TO, Price JL, et al.: "A Functional Anatomical Study of Unipolar Depression." *Journal of Neuroscience* 12:3628–3641, 1992. Used with permission.

ulating emotional behavior (Nauta and Domesick 1984) and that neurological disorders that disturb striatal function are associated with an increased risk of major depression (Folstein et al. 1991; Mayeux 1982; Santamaria et al. 1986; Starkstein and Robinson 1989).

Mesiotemporal Cortex

The volume of some mesiotemporal cortex structures may also differ between depressed patients and control subjects. In tissue acquired post-mortem, Bowen et al. (1989) found that the gray matter wet weight of the parahippocampal gyrus was reduced by 34% in MDD and bipolar disorder subjects dying from natural causes, compared with control subjects, although this finding awaits replication. Subtle reductions in hippocampal volume in mood disorder patients relative to control subjects have been found in some (Sheline et al.

1996; Swayze et al. 1992) but not other (Altshuler et al. 1998; Axelson et al. 1993; Hauser et al. 1989; Pearlson et al. 1997) neuromorphometric MRI studies. Published studies are also in disagreement regarding amygdala volume, which Pearlson et al. (1997) found to be abnormally decreased in bipolar disorder but which Altshuler et al. (1998) found to be abnormally increased in the same disorder. Tebartz and colleagues (1999) recently reported that subjects with temporal lobe epilepsy who have increased Beck Depression Inventory scores have a larger mean amygdala volume than do both temporal lobe epilepsy subjects with low scores and healthy control subjects.

Resolving whether amygdala volume is abnormal in mood disorders may be particularly relevant to understanding the pathophysiology of these conditions, given that functional imaging studies have shown that resting CBF and glucose metabolism are abnormally increased in the amygdala in depressed patients compared with control subjects and correlate positively with depression severity (Abercrombie et al. 1996; Drevets 1999; Drevets et al. 1992, 1995a, 1997a; Wu et al. 1992). In addition to being increased in the depressed state, CBF and metabolism in the left amygdala appear abnormally increased (though to a lesser extent) in patients with remitted depression who are not taking antidepressant drugs (Drevets et al. 1992). Conversely, antidepressant drug treatment that both induces and maintains remission is associated with normalization of amygdala metabolism (Drevets et al. 1996). Consistent with these observations, antidepressant drug–treated subjects with remitted MDD who relapse when on a tryptophan-free diet (which putatively reduces 5-HT levels in the central nervous system) have higher baseline amygdala metabolism (i.e., before depletion) than do similar subjects who do not relapse (Bremner et al. 1997). Abnormal activity in the amygdala may thus be associated with an increased susceptibility to recurrence of major depression. However, the magnitude of the increase in amygdala activity corresponds to the level expected for physiological activation rather than seizure activity (Drevets 1999; Drevets et al. 1992; LeDoux et al. 1983; Links et al. 1996).

■ NEURORECEPTOR RADIOLIGANDS AS HISTOLOGICAL MARKERS IN DEPRESSION

Some neuroreceptor ligands for PET and SPECT may prove useful as histological markers through labeling cells on which their target receptors are expressed. The extent to which radiolabeled receptor antagonist binding may reflect the density of the cells the receptors label is limited by the numerous dynamic regulatory mechanisms influencing receptor availability that are unrelated to cell number or density. Receptor sites may be upregulated or downregulated or internalized by exposure to altered neurotransmitter concentrations or other factors associated with disease or its treatment. Interpretation of differences in neuroreceptor radioligand binding between depressed patients and control subjects identified using PET will therefore depend on histopathological correlation in clinically similar subjects post-mortem.

Nevertheless, the use of neuroimaging markers ante-mortem in clinically well-characterized cases of MDD or bipolar disorder holds potential for facilitating and complementing postmortem studies involving clinically similar subjects. Because of the limited availability of brain tissue suitable for modern immunohistochemical staining from subjects with primary mood disorders, the determination of whether abnormalities are specific to particular clinical subtypes may be most effectively accomplished using the larger sample sizes that can be studied with PET. With in vivo receptor imaging, the entire brain can also be surveyed more quickly than with relatively tedious microscopic analyses to delimit areas where postmortem immunohistochemical assessments in brain tissue are likely to identify differences between mood disorder patients and control subjects (Drevets et al. 1998; Öngür et al. 1998). Finally, because PET permits repeated measures across clinical conditions, the effects of mood state, treatment, illness duration, comorbid disorders, and prolonged remission on receptor BP can be more easily characterized using in vivo neuroimaging.

Serotonin$_{1A}$ Receptor Imaging in Mood Disorders

5-HT$_{1A}$ receptor antagonists were previously proposed by neuropathologists as potential histological markers for some cell types within the cerebral cortex (Bowen et al. 1989; Middlemiss et al. 1986). Cortical 5-HT$_{1A}$ receptors are abundantly expressed on pyramidal neurons, some GABAergic interneurons, astrocytes, and some other glia located in cerebral cortex and limbic structures (Azmitia et al. 1996). The 5-HT$_{1A}$ receptor density and messenger RNA expression appear remarkably insensitive to reductions in 5-HT transmission associated with lesioning of the raphe or administration of parachloroamphetamine (PCPA) (Frazer and Hensler 1990; Hensler et al. 1991; Pranzatelli 1994; Verge et al. 1986). Similarly, increases in 5-HT transmission resulting from chronic administration of selective serotonin reuptake inhibitors (SSRIs) or monoamine oxidase inhibitors (MAOIs) does not consistently alter 5-HT$_{1A}$ receptor density or messenger RNA in the cortex, hippocampus, amygdala, or hypothalamus (Carli et al. 1996; Hensler et al. 1991; Spurlock et al. 1994; Welner et al. 1989). In the raphe, chronic SSRI or MAOI administration desensitizes presynaptic somatodendritic 5-HT$_{1A}$ receptors (Chaput et al. 1991), but this effect may not be evident in 5-HT$_{1A}$ receptor images, given that [^{3}H]8-OH-DPAT binding in the raphe is not consistently altered by chronic SSRI administration in rats (Frazer and Hensler 1990; Welner et al. 1989). The most clearly established dynamic influence on 5-HT$_{1A}$ receptor density is that postsynaptic 5-HT$_{1A}$ receptor gene expression in the hippocampus (but not in other structures examined) is under tonic inhibition by adrenal steroids (reviewed by López et al. [1998]). Hippocampal 5-HT$_{1A}$ receptor binding may thus be altered in depressed patients with limbic-hypothalamic-pituitary-adrenal–axis dysregulation (López et al. 1998).

Although 5-HT$_{1A}$ receptor binding is not specific for a single cell type, in regions where the pyramidal neurons, interneurons, or astrocytes expressing these receptors are specifically affected by disease, neuroimaging measures of 5-HT$_{1A}$ receptor binding may prove more sensitive than MRI-based measures of gray matter volume for guiding postmortem studies (Azmitia et al. 1996; Bowen et al. 1989). For example, Bowen et al. (1989) demonstrated that in tissue acquired post-mortem from subjects with MDD or bipolar disorder, 29% and 38% mean reductions in gray matter wet weight in the lateral orbital cortex and temporal polar cortex, respectively, were associated with proportionately greater reductions in 5-HT$_{1A}$ receptor binding of 45% and 59%, respectively. In accordance with these data, our preliminary PET measures of [^{11}C]WAY-100635 binding in these cases have shown 30%–40% reductions in mean 5-HT$_{1A}$ receptor BP in areas where we and others identified proportionately smaller decreases in gray matter volume in MDD subjects relative to control subjects (Drevets et al. 1999c; Rajkowska et al. 1999). These observations may reflect decreased 5-HT$_{1A}$ receptor binding to astroglia, given that the magnitude of reductions of glia also exceeds that of the corresponding gray matter volume reduction (Drevets et al. 1998; Öngür et al. 1998). Moreover, in the posterior orbital cortex and subgenual prefrontal cortex where postmortem studies of MDD demonstrated reductions of glia with no equivalent loss of neurons, PET measures of 5-HT$_{1A}$ receptor density may reflect more specific markers for glial pathology.

Using PET and the selective 5-HT$_{1A}$ receptor radioligand carbonyl [^{11}C]WAY-100635, we also demonstrated abnormal 5-HT$_{1A}$ receptor binding in the mesiotemporal cortex (hippocampus, amygdala, and parahippocampal cortex) and the midbrain raphe in unmedicated, depressed subjects (Drevets et al. 1999b). Histological abnormalities may contribute to this reduction in mesiotemporal 5-HT$_{1A}$ receptor BP in mood disorders, given that seven MDD and bipolar disorder subjects dying from natural causes were found to have a 34% reduction in gray matter wet weight of the parahippocampal gyrus, compared with control subjects (Bowen et al. 1989), and that four patients with bipolar disorder were found to have abnormally decreased non-pyramidal neuron counts in hippocampal sector CA2 (Benes et al. 1998). Additionally or alternatively, the effects of cortisol hypersecretion on hippocampal 5-HT_{1A} receptor gene expression may contribute to the reduced 5-HT_{1A} receptor BP in the mesiotemporal cortex (López et al. 1998).

Finally, the abnormal 5-HT_{1A} receptor BP in the midbrain raphe may reflect morphological abnormalities in the DRN. Baumann and Bogerts (1998) found reduced numbers of Nissl staining neurons in the DRN in bipolar disorder and MDD subjects relative to control subjects post-mortem. Kassir et al. (1998) showed that both the 5-HT_{1A} receptor density and the DRN size are abnormally decreased in individuals who commit suicide. If the DRN is abnormally small in MDD and bipolar disorder, this abnormality may appear as decreased 5-HT_{1A} receptor BP in PET images.

It is noteworthy that during neural development the astroglia play a critical role in 5-HT system growth, because stimulation of astroglial 5-HT_{1A} receptors causes astrocytes to secrete S-100, a neurotrophic factor that promotes growth and arborization of serotonergic axons (Azmitia and Whitaker-Azmitia 1991; Whitaker-Azmitia and Azmitia 1989). In the rat, cells that double-label 5-HT_{1A} receptors and glial fibrillary acidic protein (which labels astrocytes) predominate in the hippocampus, cingulate gyrus, amygdala, temporal cortex, and lateral septal nuclei (Whitaker-Azmitia et al. 1993). It is conceivable that a regional reduction of astroglia during development may result in local deficits of serotonergic innervation in regions where such double-labeled cells predominate. A reduction in serotonergic innervation of these structures may also be associated with reduced DRN volume. The reductions in astroglia in the limbic prefrontal cortex (Drevets et al. 1998; Öngür et al. 1998; Rajkowska et al. 1999) and the decrements in 5-HT_{1A} receptor BP and neuronal counts in the midbrain raphe (Baumann and Bogerts 1998; Drevets et al. 1999b; Kassir et al. 1998) may thus reflect related processes in MDD and bipolar disorder. Taken together, these data suggest mechanisms by which serotonergic function becomes blunted in MDD and why drugs that enhance 5-HT transmission have antidepressant efficacy in MDD (Chaput et al. 1991; Haddjeri et al. 1998).

Finally, neuroimaging measures of 5-HT_{1A} receptor binding may prove useful for investigating the histopathological heterogeneity within samples of subjects prone to suicide or depression. For example, Arango et al. (1997) found decreased 5-HT_{1A} receptor binding in the ventrolateral prefrontal cortex in alcoholic individuals who committed suicide but increased binding in nonalcoholic individuals who committed suicide, relative to control subjects. Furthermore, whereas persons who committed suicide had abnormally reduced 5-HT_{1A} receptor density and area in the DRN (Kassir et al. 1998), individuals with chronic alcoholism had an abnormally (2.2-fold) increased density of serotonergic neuronal processes in the DRN (Underwood et al. 1998). Potentially compatible with these data is our preliminary evidence that subjects with depression spectrum disease or depression secondary to alcohol dependence show a tendency toward having abnormally increased 5-HT_{1A} receptor BP in the raphe.

■ SUMMARY

Neuroimaging studies have identified abnormalities of brain function and structure in mood disorders. These findings confirm results of previous neuropathological studies and have begun to guide postmortem studies aimed at discovering new histopathological abnormalities in mood disorders. The brain structures implicated by these studies have been shown by other types of research to play central roles in the expression and modulation of emotional behavior (Drevets et al. 1999a). These data thus converge with results of lesion analysis studies to support neural models of depression in which dysfunction of modulatory systems within the prefrontal cortex, striatum, and brain stem disinhibits emotional and stress responses generated through the amygdala and its projections to the hypothalamus, PAG, and other limbic structures.

■ REFERENCES

Abercrombie HC, Larson CL, Ward, RT, et al: Metabolic rate in the amygdala predicts negative affect and depression severity in depressed patients: an FDG-PET study (abstract). Neuroimage 3:S217, 1996

Altshuler LL, Bartzokis, G, Grieder T, et al: Amygdala enlargement in bipolar disorder and hippocampal reduction in schizophrenia: an MRI study demonstrating neuroanatomic specificity. Arch Gen Psychiatry 55:663–664, 1998

Arana GW, Baldessarini RJ, Ornsteen M: The dexamethasone suppression test for diagnosis and prognosis in psychiatry: commentary and review. Arch Gen Psychiatry 42:1193–1204, 1985

Arango V, Underwood MD, Kassir SA, et al: 5HT_{1A} binding alterations are more pronounced in young suicide victims and alcoholics (abstract). Society of Neuroscience Abstracts 23:1676, 1997

Araque A: Tripartite synapses: glia, the unacknowledged partner. Trends Neurosci 22:208–215, 1999

Awad IA, Spetzler RF, Hodak JA, et al: Incidental subcortical lesions identified on magnetic resonance imaging in the elderly, I: correlation with age and cerebrovascular risk factors. Stroke 17:1084–1089, 1986a

Awad IA, Johnson PC, Spetzler RF, et al: Incidental subcortical lesions identified on magnetic resonance imaging in the elderly, II: postmortem pathological correlations. Stroke 17:1090–1097, 1986b

Axelson DA, Doraiswamy PM, McDonald WM, et al: Hypercortisolemia and hippocampal changes in depression. Psychiatry Res 47:167–173, 1993

Azmitia EC, Whitaker-Azmitia PM: Awakening the sleeping giant: anatomy and plasticity of the brain serotonergic system. J Clin Psychiatry 52:4–16, 1991

Azmitia EC, Gannon PJ, Kheck NM, et al: Cellular localization of the $5HT_{1A}$ receptor in primate brain neurons and glial cells. Neuropsychopharmacology 14:35–46, 1996

Barden N, Reul J, Holsboer F: Do antidepressants stabilize mood through actions on the hypothalamic-pituitary-adrenocortical system? Trends Neurosci 18:6–11, 1995

Baumann BG, Bogerts B: Post mortem studies of bipolar disorder. Paper presented at the Stanley Foundation European Bipolar Symposium, Royal Society, London, September 24, 1998

Baxter LR, Phelps ME, Mazziotta JC, et al: Cerebral metabolic rates for glucose in mood disorders. Arch Gen Psychiatry 42:441–447, 1985

Baxter LR, Phelps ME, Mazziotta JC, et al: Local cerebral glucose metabolic rates in obsessive-compulsive disorder—a comparison with rates in unipolar depression and in normal controls. Arch Gen Psychiatry 44:211–218, 1987

Baxter LR, Schwartz JM, Phelps ME, et al: Reduction of prefrontal cortex glucose metabolism common to three types of depression. Arch Gen Psychiatry 46:243–250, 1989

Bell KA, Kupfer DJ, Drevets WC: Decreased glucose metabolism in the dorsomedial prefrontal cortex in depression (abstract). Biol Psychiatry 45:118S, 1999

Bench CJ, Friston KJ, Brown RG, et al: The anatomy of melancholia—focal abnormalities of cerebral blood flow in major depression. Psychol Med 22:607–615, 1992

Benes FM, Kwok EW, Vincent SL, et al: A reduction of nonpyramidal cells in sector CA2 of schizophrenics and manic depressives. Biol Psychiatry 44:88–97, 1998

Biver F, Goldman S, Delvenne V, et al: Frontal and parietal metabolic disturbances in unipolar depression. Biol Psychiatry 36:381–388, 1994

Bonne O, Krausz Y, Shapira B, et al: Increased cerebral blood flow in depressed patients responding to electroconvulsive therapy. J Nucl Med 37:1075–1080, 1996

Botteron KN, Figiel GS: The neuromorphometry of affective disorders, in Brain Imaging in Clinical Psychiatry. Edited by Krishnan KRR, Doraiswamy PM. New York, Marcel Dekker, 1997, pp 145–184

Botteron KN, Raichle ME, Heath AC, et al: An epidemiological twin study of prefrontal neuromorphometry in early onset depression (abstract). Biol Psychiatry 45:59S, 1999

Bowen DM, Najlerahim A, Procter AW, et al: Circumscribed changes of the cerebral cortex in neuropsychiatric disorders of later life. Proc Natl Acad Sci U S A 86:9504–9508, 1989

Bremner JD, Innis RB, Salomon RM, et al: Positron emission tomography measurement of cerebral metabolic correlates of tryptophan depletion-induced depressive relapse. Arch Gen Psychiatry 54:346–374, 1997

Broekkamp CL, Lloyd KG: The role of the amygdala on the action of psychotropic drugs, in The Amygdaloid Complex. Edited by Ben-Ari Y. Amsterdam, Elsevier North-Holland Biomedical, 1981, pp 219–225

Buchsbaum MS, Wu J, Siegel BV, et al: Effect of sertraline on regional metabolic rate in patients with affective disorder. Biol Psychiatry 41:15–22, 1997

Carli M, Afkhami-Dastjerdian S, Reader TA: [^{3}H]8-OH-DPAT binding and serotonin content in rat cerebral cortex after acute fluoxetine, desipramine, or pargyline. J Psychiatry Neurosci 21:114–122, 1996

Carmichael ST, Price JL: Limbic connections of the orbital and medial prefrontal cortex in macaque monkeys. J Comp Neurol 363:615–641, 1995

Carney RM, Rich MW, Freedland KE, et al: Major depressive disorder predicts cardiac events in patients with coronary artery disease. Psychosom Med 50:627–633, 1988

Carney RM, Freedland KE, Rich MW, et al: Ventricular tachycardia and psychiatric depression in patients with coronary artery disease. Am J Med 95:23–28, 1993

Carroll BJ: Brain mechanisms in manic depression. Clin Chem 40:303–308, 1994

Chaput Y, de Montigny C, Blier P: Presynaptic and postsynaptic modifications of the serotonin system by long-term administration of antidepressant treatments: an in vivo electrophysiologic study in the rat. Neuropsychopharmacology 5:219–229, 1991

Chen G, Zeng WZ, Yuan PX, et al: The mood-stabilizing agents lithium and valproate robustly increase the levels of the neuroprotective protein bcl-2 in the CNS. J Neurochem 72:879–882, 1999

Chergui K, Nomikos GG, Mathe JM, et al: Tonic activation of NMDA receptors causes spontaneous burst discharge of rat midbrain dopamine neurons in vivo. Eur J Neurosci 5:137–144, 1993

Chimowitz MI, Estes ML, Furlan AJ, et al: Further observations on the pathology of subcortical lesions identified on magnetic resonance imaging. Arch Neurol 49:747–752, 1992

Coffey CE, Wilkinson WE, Weiner RD, et al: Quantitative cerebral anatomy in depression: a controlled magnetic resonance imaging study. Arch Gen Psychiatry 50:7–16, 1993

Cohen RM, Gross M, Nordahl TE, et al: Preliminary data on the metabolic brain pattern of patients with winter seasonal affective disorder. Arch Gen Psychiatry 49:545–552, 1992

Coryell W, Zimmerman M: Outcome following ECT for primary unipolar depression: a test of newly proposed response predictors. Am J Psychiatry 141:862–867, 1984

Crino PB, Morrison JH, Hof PR: Monoaminergic innervation of cingulate cortex, in Neurobiology of Cingulate Cortex and Limbic Thalamus. Edited by Vogt BA, Gabriel M. Boston, Birkhauser, 1993, pp 285–312

Damasio AR, Tranel D, Damasio H: Individuals with sociopathic behavior caused by frontal damage fail to respond autonomically to social stimuli. Behav Brain Res 41:81–94, 1990

Damasio AR, Grabowski TJ, Bechara A, et al: Neural correlates of the experience of emotions (abstract). Soc Neurosci Abstr 24:258, 1998

Derdeyn CP, Yundt KD, Videen TO, et al: Increased oxygen extraction fraction is associated with prior ischemic events in patients with carotid occlusion. Stroke 29:754–758, 1998

Diorio D, Viau V, Meaney MJ: The role of the medial prefrontal cortex (cingulate gyrus) in the regulation of hypothalamic-pituitary-adrenal responses to stress. J Neurosci 13:3839–3847, 1993

Dolan RJ, Fletcher P, Morris J, et al: Neural activation during covert processing of positive emotional expressions. Neuroimage 4:194–200, 1996

Drevets WC: Geriatric depression: brain imaging correlates and pharmacologic considerations. J Clin Psychiatry 55:71–81, 1994

Drevets WC: Neuroimaging in depression: implications for studies of histopathology and antidepressant treatment mechanisms. Paper presented at the annual meeting of the American College of Neuropsychopharmacology, Hawaii, December 11, 1997

Drevets WC: Prefrontal cortical-amygdalar metabolism in major depression. Ann N Y Acad Sci 877:614–637, 1999

Drevets WC, Raichle ME: Neuroanatomical circuits in depression: implications for treatment mechanisms. Psychopharmacol Bull 28:261-274, 1992

Drevets WC, Raichle ME: Reciprocal suppression of regional cerebral blood flow during emotional versus higher cognitive processes: implications for interactions between emotion and cognition. Cognition and Emotion 12:353–385, 1998

Drevets WC, Todd RD: Depression, mania and related disorders, in Adult Psychiatry. Edited by Guze SB. St. Louis, MO, CV Mosby, 1997, pp 99–141

Drevets WC, Videen TO, Price JL, et al: A functional anatomical study of unipolar depression. J Neurosci 12:3628–3641, 1992

Drevets WC, Videen TO, Snyder AZ, et al: Regional cerebral blood flow changes during anticipatory anxiety (abstract). Society of Neuroscience Abstracts 20:368, 1994

Drevets WC, Spitznagel E, Raichle ME: Functional anatomical differences between major depressive subtypes (abstract). J Cereb Blood Flow Metab 15:S93, 1995a

Drevets WC, Simpson JR, Raichle ME: Regional blood flow changes in response to phobic anxiety and habituation. J Cereb Blood Flow Metab 15:S856, 1995b

Drevets WC, Price JL, Simpson JS, et al: State- and trait-like neuroimaging abnormalities in depression: effects of antidepressant treatment (abstract). Soc Neurosci Abstr 22:266, 1996

Drevets WC, Price JL, Todd RD, et al: PET measures of amygdala metabolism in bipolar and unipolar depression: correlation with plasma cortisol (abstract). Soc Neurosci 23:1407, 1997a

Drevets WC, Price JL, Simpson JR, et al: Subgenual prefrontal cortex abnormalities in mood disorders. Nature 386:824–827, 1997b

Drevets WC, Öngür D, Price JL: Neuroimaging abnormalities in the subgenual prefrontal cortex: implications for pathophysiology of familial mood disorders. Mol Psychiatry 3:220–226, 1998

Drevets WC, Gadde K, Krishnan KRR: Neuroimaging studies of depression, in The Neurobiological Foundation of Mental Illness. Edited by Charney DS, Nestler EJ, Bunney BJ. New York, Oxford University Press, 1999a, pp 394–418

Drevets WC, Frank E, Price JC, et al: PET imaging of serotonin 1A receptor binding in depression. Biol Psychiatry 46:1375–1387, 1999b

Duncan GE, Breese GR, Criswell H, et al: Effects of antidepressant drugs injected into the amygdala on behavioral responses of rats in the forced swim test. J Pharmacol Exp Ther 238:758–762, 1986

Ebert D, Feistel H, Barocka A: Effects of sleep deprivation on the limbic system and the frontal lobes in affective disorders: a study with Tc-99m-HMPAO SPECT. Psychiatry Res 40:247–251, 1991

Fazekas F: Magnetic resonance signal abnormalities in asymptomatic individuals: their incidence and functional correlates. Eur Neurol 29:164–168, 1989

Folstein SE, Peyser CE, Starkstein SE, et al: Subcortical triad of Huntington's disease: a model for a neuropathology of depression, dementia, and dyskinesia, in Psychopathology and the Brain. Edited by Carroll BJ, Barrett JE. New York, Raven, 1991, pp 65–75

Frackowiak R, Friston KJ, Frith CD, et al: Human Brain Function. San Diego, CA, Academic Press, 1997

Frasure-Smith N, Lespérance F, Talajic M: Depression and 18-month prognosis after myocardial infarction. Circulation 91:999–1005, 1995

Frazer A, Hensler JG: 5-HT_{1A} receptors and 5-HT_{1A}-mediated responses: effect of treatments that modify serotonergic neurotransmission. Ann N Y Acad Sci 600:460–475, 1990

Frysztak RJ, Neafsey EJ: The effect of medial frontal cortex lesions on cardiovascular conditioned emotional responses in the rat. Brain Res 643:181–193, 1994

Fujikawa T, Yamawaki S, Touhouda Y: Background factors and clinical symptoms of major depression with silent cerebral infarction. Stroke 25:798–801, 1994

Fujikawa T, Yokota N, Muraoka M, et al: Response of patients with major depression and silent cerebral infarction to antidepressant drug therapy, with emphasis on central nervous system adverse effects. Stroke 27:2040–2042, 1996

Fuster JM: The Prefrontal Cortex: Anatomy, Physiology, and Neuropsychology of the Frontal Lobe. New York, Raven, 1989

George MS, Ketter TA, Parekh PI, et al: Brain activity during transient sadness and happiness in healthy women. Am J Psychiatry 152:341–351, 1995

Goodwin GM, Austin MP, Dougall N, et al: State changes in brain activity shown by the uptake of ^{99m}Tc-exametazine with SPET in major depression before and after treatment. J Affect Disord 29:243–253, 1993

Greenwald BS, Kramerginsberg E, Krishnan KRR, et al: MRI signal hyperintensities in geriatric depression. Am J Psychiatry 153:1212–1215, 1996

Greenwald BS, Kramerginsberg E, Krishnan KRR, et al: Localization of magnetic resonance imaging signal hyperintensities in geriatric depression. Stroke 29:613–617, 1998

Haddjeri N, Blier P, de Montigny C: Long-term antidepressant treatments result in a tonic activation of forebrain 5-HT_{1A} receptors. J Neurosci 18:10150–10156, 1998

Hauser P, Altshuler LL, Berrettini W, et al: Temporal lobe measurement in primary affective disorder by magnetic resonance imaging. J Neuropsychiatry Clin Neurosci 1:128–134, 1989

Hensler J, Kovachich G, Frazer A: A quantitative autoradiographic study of $serotonin_{1A}$ receptor regulation. Neuropsychopharmacology 4:131–144, 1991

Hirayasu Y, Shenton ME, Salisbury DF, et al: Subgenual cingulate cortex volume in first-episode psychosis. Am J Psychiatry 156:1091–1093, 1999

Iversen SD, Mishkin M: Perseverative interference in monkeys following selective lesions of the inferior prefrontal convexity. Exp Brain Res 11:376–386, 1970

Kassir SA, Underwood MD, Bakalian MJ, et al: $5HT_{1A}$ binding in dorsal and median raphe nuclei of suicide victims (abstract). Soc Neurosci Abstr 24:1274, 1998

Kegeles LS, Malone KM, Slifstein M, et al: Response of cortical metabolic deficits to serotonergic challenges in mood disorders (abstract). Biol Psychiatry 45:76S, 1999

Krishnan KRR, McDonald WM, Escalona PR, et al: Magnetic resonance imaging of the caudate nuclei in depression: preliminary observations. Arch Gen Psychiatry 49:553–557, 1992

Krishnan KRR, McDonald WM, Doraiswamy PM, et al: Neuroanatomical substrates of depression in the elderly. Eur Arch Psychiatry Clin Neurosci 243:41–46, 1993

Kupfer DJ, Targ E, Stack J: Electroencephalographic sleep in unipolar depressive subtypes: support for a biological and familial classification. J Nerv Ment Dis 170:494–498, 1992

LeDoux JE: Emotion, in Handbook of Physiology: The Nervous System/V, 5th Edition. Edited by Mills J, Mountcastle VB, Plum F, et al. Baltimore, MD, Williams & Wilkins, 1987, pp 373–417

LeDoux JE, Thompson ME, Iadecola C, et al: Local cerebral blood flow increases during auditory and emotional processing in the conscious rat. Science 221:576–578, 1983

Leichnetz GR, Astruc J: The efferent projections of the medial prefrontal cortex in the squirrel monkey *(Saimiri sciureus)*. Brain Res 109:455–472, 1976

Lesser IM, Mena I, Boone KB, et al: Reduction of cerebral blood flow in older depressed patients. Arch Gen Psychiatry 51:677–686, 1994

Lesser IM, Boone KB, Mehringer CM, et al: Cognition and white matter hyperintensities in older depressed patients. Am J Psychiatry 153:1280–1287, 1996

Lewis DA, McChesney C: Tritiated imipramine binding distinguishes among subtypes of depression. Arch Gen Psychiatry 42:485–488, 1985

Lewis DA, Kathol RG, Sherman BM, et al: Differentiation of depressive subtypes by insulin insensitivity in the recovered phase. Arch Gen Psychiatry 40:167–170, 1983

Links JM, Zubieta JK, Meltzer CC, et al: Influence of spatially heterogeneous background activity on "hot object" quantitation in brain emission computed tomography. J Comput Assist Tomogr 20:680–687, 1996

López JF, Chalmers DT, Little KY, et al: A.E. Bennett Research Award. Regulation of serotonin$_{1A}$, glucocorticoid, and mineralocorticoid receptor in rat and human hippocampus: implications for the neurobiology of depression. Biol Psychiatry 43:547–573, 1998

Maes M, Dierckx R, Meltzer HY, et al: Regional cerebral blood flow in unipolar depression measured with Tc-99m-HMPAO single photon emission computed tomography: negative findings. Psychiatry Res 50:77–88, 1993

Magistretti PJ, Pellerin L, Martin JL. Brain energy metabolism: an integrated cellular perspective, in Psychopharmacology: The Fourth Generation of Progress. Edited by Bloom FE, Kupfer DJ. New York, Raven, 1995, pp 921–932

Makkos Z, Miguel-Hidalgo JJ, Dilley G, et al: GFAP-immunoreactive glia in the prefrontal cortex in schizophrenia and major depression (abstract). Society of Neuroscience Abstracts 581:16, 2000

Mayberg HS, Brannan SK, Mahurin RK, et al: Cingulate function in depression: a potential predictor of treatment response. Neuroreport 8:1057–1061, 1997

Mayberg HS, Liotti M, Brannan SK, et al: Reciprocal limbic-cortical function and negative mood: converging PET findings in depression and normal sadness. Am J Psychiatry 156:675–682, 1999

Mayeux R: Depression and dementia in Parkinson's disease, in Movement Disorders. Edited by Marsden CO, Fahn S. London, Butterworth, 1982, pp 75–95

Mazziotta JC, Phelps ME, Plummer D, et al: Quantitation in positron emission computed tomography, 5: physical-anatomical effects. J Comput Assist Tomogr 5:734–743, 1981

Meltzer CC, Kinahan PE, Greer PJ, et al: Comparative evaluation of MR-based partial-volume correction schemes for PET. J Nucl Med 40:2053–2065, 1999

Middlemiss DN, Palmer AM, Edel N, et al: Binding of the novel serotonin agonist 8-hydroxy-2-(di-n-propylamino) tetralin in normal and Alzheimer brain. J Neurochem 46:993–996, 1986

Morgan MA, LeDoux JE: Differential contribution of dorsal and ventral medial prefrontal cortex to the aquisition and extinction of conditioned fear in rats. Behav Neurosci 109:681–688, 1995

Murase S, Grenhoff J, Chouvet G, et al: Prefrontal cortex regulates burst firing and transmitter release in rat mesolimbic dopamine neurons. Neurosci Lett 157:53–56, 1993

Nauta WJ, Domesick V: Afferent and efferent relationships of the basal ganglia, in Function of the Basal Ganglia (CIBA Foundation Symposium 107). London, Pitman, 1984, pp 3–29

Neafsey EJ, Hurley-Gius KM, Arvanitis D: The topographical organization of neurons in the rat medial frontal, insular and olfactory cortex projecting to the solitary nucleus, olfactory bulb, periaqueductal gray and superior colliculus. Brain Res 377:561–570, 1986

Neafsey EJ, Terreberry RR, Hurley KM, et al: Anterior cingulate cortex in rodents: connections, visceral control functions, and implications for emotion, in Neurobiology of Cingulate Cortex and Limbic Thalamus. Edited by Vogt BA, Gabriel M. Boston, MA, Birkhauser, 1993, pp 206–223

Nibuya M, Morinobu S, Duman RS: Regulation of BDNF and trkB mRNA in rat brain by chronic electroconvulsive seizure and antidepressant drug treatments. J Neurosci 15:7539–7547, 1995

Nobler MS, Sackeim HA, Prohovnik I, et al: Regional cerebral blood flow in mood disorders, III: treatment and clinical response. Arch Gen Psychiatry 51:884–897, 1994

Nowak G, Trullas R, Layer RT, et al: Adaptive changes in the *N*-methyl-D-aspartate receptor complex after chronic treatment with imipramine and 1-aminocyclopropanecarboxylic acid. J Pharmacol Exp Ther 265:1380–1386, 1993

Nowak G, Ordway GA, Paul IA: Alterations in the *N*-methyl-D-aspartate (NMDA) receptor complex in the frontal cortex of suicide victims. Brain Res 675:157–164, 1995

Öngür D, Drevets WC, Price JL: Glial reduction in the subgenual prefrontal cortex in mood disorders. Proc Natl Acad Sci U S A 95:13290–13295, 1998

Ordway GA, Gambarana C, Tejani-Butt SM, et al: Preferential reduction of binding of ^{125}I-iodopindolol to beta-1 adrenoreceptors in the amygdala of rat after antidepressant treatments. J Pharmacol Exp Ther 257:681–690, 1991

Pagani M, Lombardi F, Guzzetti S, et al: Power spectral analysis of heart rate and arterial pressure variabilities as a marker for sympathovagal interaction in man and conscious dog. Circ Res 59:178–193, 1986

Pardo JV, Pardo PJ, Raichle ME: Neural correlates of self-induced dysphoria. Am J Psychiatry 150:713–719, 1993

Paul IA, Nowak G, Layer RT, et al: Adaptation of the *N*-methyl-D-aspartate receptor complex following chronic antidepressant treatments. J Pharmacol Exp Ther 269:95–102, 1994

Pearlson GD, Barta PE, Powers RE, et al: Medial and superior temporal gyral volumes and cerebral asymmetry in schizophrenia versus bipolar disorder. Biol Psychiatry 41:1–14, 1997

Poline JB, Worsley KJ, Evans AC, et al: Combining spatial extent and peak intensity to test for activations in functional imaging. Neuroimage 5:83–96, 1997

Post RM: Transduction of psychosocial stress into the neurobiology of recurrent affective disorder. Am J Psychiatry 149:999–1010, 1992

Pranzatelli MR: Dissociation of the plasticity of $5HT_{1A}$ sites and 5HT transporter sites. Neurochem Res 19:311–315, 1994

Price JL: Networks within the orbital and medial prefrontal cortex. Neurocase 5:231–241, 1999

Price JL, Carmichael ST, Drevets WC: Networks related to the orbital and medial prefrontal cortex: a substrate for emotional behavior? Prog Brain Res 107:523–536, 1996

Raichle ME: Circulatory and metabolic correlates of brain function in normal humans, in Handbook of Physiology: The Nervous System/V, 5th Edition. Edited by Brookhart JM, Mountcastle VB. Baltimore, MD, Williams & Wilkins, 1987, pp 643–674

Rajkowska G, Selemon LD, Goldman-Rakic PS: Marked glial neuropathology in prefrontal cortex distinguishes bipolar disorder from schizophrenia (abstract). Schizophr Res 24:41, 1997

Rajkowska G, Miguel-Hidalgo JJ, Wei J, et al: Morphometric evidence for neuronal and glial prefrontal cell pathology in major depression. Biol Psychiatry 45:1085–1098, 1999

Rauch SL, Jenike MA, Alpert NM, et al: Regional cerebral blood flow measured during symptom provocation in obsessive-compulsive disorder using oxygen 15-labeled carbon dioxide and positron emission tomography. Arch Gen Psychiatry 51:62–70, 1994

Rauch SL, Savage CR, Alpert NM, et al: A positron emission tomographic study of simple phobic symptom provocation. Arch Gen Psychiatry 52:20–28, 1995

Rauch SL, van der Kolk BA, Evans AC, et al: A symptom provocation study of post-traumatic stress disorder using positron emission tomography and script driven imagery. Arch Gen Psychiatry 53:380–387, 1996

Reiman EM, Lane RD, Ahern GL, et al: Neuroanatomical correlates of externally and internally generated human emotion. Am J Psychiatry 154:918–925, 1997

Ring HA, Bench CJ, Trimble MR, et al: Depression in Parkinson's disease: a positron emission study. Br J Psychiatry 165:333–339, 1994

Rolls ET: A theory of emotion and consciousness, and its application to understanding the neural basis of emotion, in The Cognitive Neurosciences. Edited by Gazzaniga M. Cambridge, MA, MIT Press, 1995, pp 1091–1106

Rosenkilde CE, Bauer RH, Fuster JM: Single cell activity in ventral prefrontal cortex of behaving monkeys. Brain Res 209:375–394, 1981

Roth RH, Elsworth JD: Biochemical pharmacology of midbrain dopamine neurons, in Psychopharmacology: The Fourth Generation of Progress. Edited by Bloom FE, Kupfer DJ. New York, Raven, 1995, pp 227–243

Rubin E, Sackeim HA, Nobler MS, et al: Brain imaging studies of antidepressant treatments. Psychiatric Annals 24:653–658, 1994

Santamaria J, Tolosa E, Valles A: Parkinson's disease with depression: a possible subgroup of idiopathic parkinsonism. Neurology 36:1130–1133, 1986

Schneider F, Gur RE, Alav A, et al: Mood effects on limbic blood flow correlate with emotion self-rating: a PET study with oxygen-15 labeled water. Psychiatry Res 61:265–283, 1995

Schultz W: Dopamine neurons and their role in reward mechanisms. Curr Opin Neurobiol 7:191–197, 1997

Sesack SR, Pickel VM: Prefrontal cortical efferents in the rat synapse on unlabeled neuronal targets of catecholamine terminals in the nucleus accumbens septi and on dopamine neurons in the ventral tegmental area. J Comp Neurol 320:145–160, 1992

Sesack SR, Deutch AY, Roth RH, et al: Topographical organization of the efferent projections of the medial prefrontal cortex in the rat: an anterograde tract-tracing study using *Phaseolus vulgaris* leucoagglutinin. J Comp Neurol 290:213–242, 1989

Sheline YI, Wang PW, Gado MH, et al: Hippocampal atrophy in recurrent major depression. Proc Natl Acad Sci U S A 93:3908–3913, 1996

Silfverskiöld P, Risberg J: Regional blood flow in depression and mania. Arch Gen Psychiatry 46:253–259, 1989

Sporn J, Sachs G: The anticonvulsant lamotrigine in treatment-resistant manic-depressive illness. J Clin Psychopharmacol 17:185–189, 1997

Spurlock G, Buckland P, O'Donovan M, et al: Lack of effect of antidepressant drugs on the levels of mRNAs encoding serotonergic receptors, synthetic enzymes and 5HT transporter. Neuropharmacology 33:433–440, 1994

Starkstein SE, Robinson RG: Affective disorders and cerebral vascular disease. Br J Psychiatry 154:170–182, 1989

Sullivan RM, Gratton A: Lateralized effects of medial prefrontal cortex lesions on neuroendocrine and autonomic stress responses in rats. J Neurosci 19:2834–2840, 1999

Swayze SM, Andreasen NC, Alliger RJ, et al: Subcortical and temporal lobe structures in affective disorder and schizophrenia: a magnetic resonance imaging study. Biol Psychiatry 31:221–240, 1992

Taber MT, Fibiger HC: Electrical stimulation of the medial prefrontal cortex increases dopamine release in the striatum. Neuropsychopharmacology 9:271–275, 1993

Tebartz van Elst L, Woermann FG, Lemieux L, et al: Amygdala enlargement in dysthymia: a volumetric study of patients with temporal lobe epilepsy. Biol Psychiatry 46:1614–1623, 1999

Thorpe SJ, Rolls ET, Maddison S: Neuronal activity in the orbitofrontal cortex of the behaving monkey. Exp Brain Res 49:93–115, 1983

Timms RJ: Cortical inhibition and facilitation of the defense reaction. J Physiol (Lond) 266:98–99, 1977

Underwood MD, Johnson VL, Bakalian MJ, et al: Morphometry of dorsal raphe nucleus serotonergic neurons in alcoholics (abstract). Soc Neurosci Abstr 24:1273, 1998

Veith RC, Lewis N, Linares OA, et al: Sympathetic nervous system activity in major depression. Arch Gen Psychiatry 51:411–422, 1994

Verge D, Davel G, Marcinkiewicz M, et al: Quantitative autoradiography of multiple $5HT_1$ receptor subtypes in the brain of control and 5,7 dihydroxytryptamine treated rats. J Neurosci 6:3474–3482, 1986

Wang RY, Aghajanian GK: Enhanced sensitivity of amygdaloid neurons to serotonin and norepinephrine after chronic antidepressant treatment. Commun Psychopharmacol 4:83–90, 1980

Welner SA, de Montigny C, Desroches J, et al: Autoradiographic quantification of $serotonin_{1A}$ receptors in rat brain following antidepressant drug treatment. Synapse 4:347–352, 1989

Whitaker-Azmitia PM, Azmitia EC: Stimulation of astroglial serotonin receptors produces culture media which regulates growth of serotonergic neurons. Brain Res 497:80–85, 1989

Whitaker-Azmitia PM, Clarke C, Azmitia EC: Localization of $5\text{-}HT_{1A}$ receptors to astroglial cells in adult rats: implications for neuronal-glial interactions and psychoactive drug mechanism of action. Synapse 14:201–205, 1993

Winokur G: The development and validity of familial subtypes in primary unipolar depression. Pharmacopsychiatry 15:142–146, 1982

Wu JC, Gillin JC, Buchsbaum MS, et al: Effect of sleep deprivation on brain metabolism of depressed patients. Am J Psychiatry 149:538–543, 1992

12

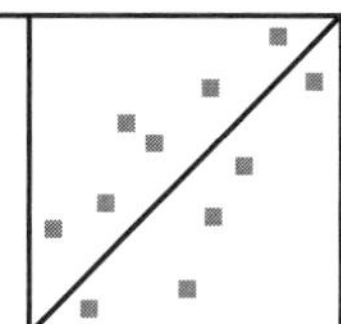

MAGNETIC RESONANCE SPECTROSCOPY IN PSYCHIATRIC ILLNESS

Michael E. Henry, M.D.
Blaise deB. Frederick, Ph.D.
Constance M. Moore, Ph.D.
Eve Stoddard
Perry F. Renshaw, M.D., Ph.D.

In vivo magnetic resonance spectroscopy (MRS), an extension of nuclear MRS methods used in analytic chemistry, is a brain imaging technique that permits the study of a limited number of endogenous brain chemicals without the introduction of exogenous tracers or exposure to ionizing radiation. Given that MRS can be performed with a standard clinical magnetic resonance scanner with some modification of head coils and software, the technology to carry out these studies is available at many academic and clinical research centers. In this chapter, we review the MRS literature on affective disorders, schizophrenia, and dementia to illustrate the applications of this technology to date. We then outline potential areas for the use of this technology in future psychiatric research.

■ Magnetic Resonance Spectroscopy

MRS is based on the fact that every nucleus has angular momentum, or spin, which can be described by a spin angular momentum quantum number. This number, I, can take on half integer values (e.g., 0, $\frac{1}{2}$, 1, $\frac{3}{2}$) (Bovey 1988), and, within a magnetic field (B_o), nuclei with nonzero quantum numbers will have 2I + 1 equally spaced energy levels. The energy separating these levels (ΔE) is described by the relationship $\Delta E = \mu B_o / I$, where μ is the nuclear magnetic moment. In MRS, energy at an appropriate frequency is applied to the nucleus to cause a transition between energy levels. The frequency of energy needed to induce this transition, called the *resonance frequency* (ν_o), is described by the relationship $\nu_o = \Delta E/h$, where h is Planck's constant. Combining these two equations, it is possible to calculate the resonance frequency, or Larmor frequency, for each nucleus under study. Energy supplied at the Larmor frequency causes the nuclei to transition between energy levels.

The lowest energy level available to the nucleus occurs when the magnetic moment of the nucleus aligns with the magnetic field. The highest energy level occurs when the magnetic moment aligns against the magnetic field. When groups of nuclei are studied simultaneously, as in brain tissue, the net magnetic moment reflects the sum of the individual magnetic moments.

In MRS, nuclei under study are initially placed in the external magnetic field (B_o), where they align with the magnetic field, which, by convention, is oriented along the Z axis. Because the nuclei still have angular momentum, they spin like a top around this axis. Application of radiofrequency energy at the resonance frequency has the effect of moving the net magnetic moment off the Z axis and into the XY, or transverse, plane. A coordinate system rotating around the Z axis at the Larmor frequency is often considered a reference point, or a "rotating frame" from which observations are made. Therefore, the degree to which the magnetic moment deviates from the Z axis and projects onto the XY plane in this system determines the magnitude of the signal that may be observed. Once the application of energy is stopped, the observable signal within the XY plane disappears with a relaxation time constant, T2. The recovery of the spin along the Z axis occurs according to the spin lattice relaxation time T1. As the system relaxes back to a lower energy state, the energy released can be detected near the Larmor frequency for each chemical species.

The electron clouds from chemical bonds surrounding each nucleus modify the strength of the magnetic field that impinges on the nucleus. This modification results in a change in the resonance (Larmor) frequency for that particular nucleus, known as a *chemical shift*. In general, the stronger the bond, the stronger the influence on the local magnetic field and the greater the chemical shift.

Relaxation parameters become important when excitation and observation strategies are being designed for experiments. Because the signal generated from one cycle of excitation and relaxation is small, the signals obtained from multiple acquisition cycles are averaged to increase the signal-to-noise ratio. The *repetition time* (TR) between excitations determines the effect of T1 on the spectra obtained. When short TRs are used, the spectra obtained are weighted toward the nuclei with short T1 values relative to the nuclei with long T1 relaxation times. In this case, the signals from the long T1 species are considered saturated. The time that passes between excitation and observation of magnetic resonance signals is referred to as the *echo time* (TE). When longer TE values are chosen, the spectra are weighted toward the nuclei with longer T2 values.

For the signal received from the sample to be quantitated, the signal intensity must be calibrated against known standards. However, variables such as tuning of the receiver and regional relaxation times can differ from subject to subject. To compensate, investigators often use estimated relaxation times to correct for relaxation effects and compare resonance signal intensities with those that arise from chemical species whose concentrations are considered constant throughout the brain. For example, the concentration of protons in pure water is approximately 110 M, and the brain is 70%–80% water. Creatine (Cr), another chemical used as an internal reference, is found at a concentration of approximately 11 mM (Barker et al. 1993).

Some of the earliest in vivo MRS assessments of tissue biochemistry involved the evaluation of phosphorus (^{31}P) metabolism using surface coils (Ackerman et al. 1980). The geometry and size of the surface coil define the sensitive volume from which the spectral signals arise. Depth-resolved surface coil spectroscopy (Bottomley et al. 1984) allows for localized signal detection from slices at different distances from the surface coil.

It is now possible to use ^{31}P coils that entirely surround the head for MRS studies of human brain. These volume coils provide more homogeneous radiofrequency excitation and are commonly used in conjunction with a localizing pulse sequence. One of the earliest localization methods proposed was image-selected in vivo spectroscopy (ISIS) (Ordidge et al. 1986). With ISIS, signals arising from a cubic volume may be selected as a result of the addition and subtraction of eight separate acquisitions. ISIS allows for the volume of interest (VOI) to be selected from a standard magnetic resonance proton image. Both ISIS and depth-resolved surface coil spectroscopy are well suited for ^{31}P spectroscopy, because the delay between excitation of the nuclei and signal detection for these sequences is quite short. This short delay allows for detection of nuclei with short T2 relaxation times, such as the phosphorus in nucleoside 5′-triphosphate (NTP). Spectra can also be acquired by chemical shift imaging, which produces a two- or three-dimensional map of metabolite distribution as a matrix of spectra acquired over the voxel of interest (Brown et al. 1982; Podo et al. 1998). Chemical shift imaging may be time-consuming, and the signal-to-noise ratio of the individual spectra may be too low for quantitation.

^{1}H or proton spectroscopy is complicated by the fact that the signals from most metabolites of interest are 10^5 times smaller than the signals arising from tissue water and lipid. However, using specially developed sequences, it has become possible in recent years to suppress the water signal. Using water-suppressed localized ^{1}H spectroscopy, it is therefore possible to acquire ^{1}H spectra from defined brain regions.

Techniques commonly used for water-suppressed localized proton spectroscopy include stimulated-echo acquisition mode (STEAM) spectroscopy (Frahm et al. 1989) and point-resolved spectroscopy (PRESS) (Bottomley et al. 1984). STEAM spectroscopy produces a stimulated echo from a cubic VOI within a single experiment. As with ISIS, the location of the VOI may be selected from a magnetic resonance image. A major advantage of this sequence is that it permits variation of the TE, so the sequence may be optimized to investigate metabolites with short T2 values. PRESS is similar to STEAM spectroscopy; however, the PRESS sequence samples the entire signal, whereas STEAM spectroscopy, as a stimulated-echo technique, samples only half the signal originating from within the VOI. PRESS is also less sensitive to motion artifacts. However, STEAM spectroscopy allows for shorter TEs to be used (Moonen et al. 1989). Chemical shift imaging may also be used to acquire a map of metabolite distribution in conjunction with either STEAM or PRESS spectroscopy.

In the majority of studies of psychiatric illnesses, phosphorus and proton spectroscopy have been most commonly employed. ^{31}P is present in significant quantities in phospholipid membranes, their precursors, and high-energy nucleoside phosphates. ^{31}P spectroscopy can provide important information about membrane metabolism, cellular energetics, and pH. In particular, ^{31}P spectra typically contain resonances from phosphomonoesters (PMEs) and phosphodiesters (PDEs); the high-energy phosphates phosphocreatine (PCr) and α-, β-, and γ-NTP; and inorganic phosphate (Pi).

The primary precursors and metabolites of phospholipids are PMEs and PDEs, respectively (Buchli et al. 1994). ^{31}P PME resonance arises from phosphoethanolamine, phosphocholine, and sugar phosphates. Phosphoethanolamine is a precursor of the membrane phospholipid phosphatidylethanolamine (Gyulai et al. 1984). The principal components of the PDE resonance are more mobile phospholipids and the freely soluble molecules glycerophosphocholine and glycerophosphoethanolamine (Kilby et al. 1991). ^{31}P-MRS brain spectra are dominated by a broad baseline resonance arising from the bilayer phospholipids; this "hump" is generally removed by postprocessing before data analysis (Kilby et al. 1991). As a result, a large fraction of the phospholipid content of spectra is essentially "invisible" in analysis, a fact that must be considered in interpreting spectral results.

Information on alterations in high-energy phosphate metabolism may be gained by measuring the relative levels of PCr, NTP, and Pi (Buchli et al.

1994). The brain NTP resonance is primarily derived from adenosine triphosphate (ATP), which is found universally in living systems and is the "currency" by which energy is transferred within the cell. The energy supplied by ATP is constantly being used to support a number of critical functions. Because the supply of ATP at any given time is limited, a mechanism exists to replenish it: specifically, a phosphate group is transferred by creatine kinase from PCr to adenosine diphosphate to produce ATP. Creatinine kinase is present only in muscle and in brain, where states of rapidly increased metabolism are common.

In proton spectroscopy, a number of chemical species are measured, including cytosolic choline (Cho), *myo*-inositol (Ino), and *N*-acetylaspartate (NAA), as well as Cr/PCr resonance. Most Cho in the brain is in the form of membrane phospholipids. However, because Cho is tightly bound in these molecules, its relaxation time is very short and it is not detectable by MRS. The major contributors to the Cho peak are phosphocholine and glycerophosphocholine (Barker et al. 1994; Miller et al. 1996), in addition to smaller contributions from Cho and acetylcholine (Charles et al. 1994; Stoll et al. 1995). Ino is a sugar that is involved in second messenger systems through the phosphatidylinositol cycle (Berridge et al. 1989). PCr is a high-energy phosphate, and the Cr/PCr resonance is often used as a reference standard, because the total concentration of Cr and PCr remains approximately the same throughout the brain (Petroff et al. 1989). NAA is a cell marker that is specific for neurons. Although its function is unclear, NAA is found almost exclusively in neurons, and its concentration correlates with neuronal density.

■ Affective Disorders

MRS studies of affective disorders are listed in Table 12–1. These studies have generally focused on the frontal lobes, the basal ganglia, and temporal lobes, regions that have been implicated in the pathophysiology of mood disorders. ^{31}phosphorous and proton spectroscopy have been used to assess metabolites involved in membrane metabolism (PME, PDE, Cho), cellular energetics (NTP, Cr/PCr), and neuronal integrity (NAA).

Bipolar Disorder

Because bipolar patients can alternate between manic, depressed, mixed, and euthymic states, the potential for misdiagnosis and subsequent patient misclassification is substantial. Furthermore, defining trait markers requires that

TABLE 12–1. Magnetic resonance spectroscopy and affective disorders

Reference	Subjects	Brain region(s) studied	Type(s) of spectroscopy	Finding(s)
Kato et al. 1995	11 bipolar depressed pts 12 manic bipolar pts 21 euthymic bipolar pts 21 control subjects	Frontal lobe	^{31}P	PCr level decr in left frontal cortex in depressed state PCr level decr in right frontal cortex in manic and euthymic states
Kato et al. 1998	7 drug-free, euthymic bipolar pts 60 control subjects	Frontal lobe	^{31}P	Intracellular pH level decr in pts
Deicken et al. 1995a	12 unmedicated, euthymic bipolar pts 16 control subjects	Frontal lobes	^{31}P	PME level decr and PDE level incr in both frontal lobes in pts PCr level incr in right vs. left frontal lobe in pts
Deicken et al. 1995b	12 unmedicated, euthymic bipolar pts 14 control subjects	Temporal lobes	^{31}P	PME level decr in left and right temporal lobes
Kato et al. 1994a	14 pts with BD I 15 pts with BD II 59 psychiatrically healthy control subjects	Frontal lobe	^{31}P	PCr level decr in all phases of BD II pH level decr in euthymic state in pts with BD I PME level incr in hypomanic and depressive states in pts with BD II
Kato et al. 1993	17 bipolar pts	Frontal lobe	^{31}P	PME and pH levels incr in mania PME and pH levels decr in euthymic state relative to control subjects

TABLE 12–1. Magnetic resonance spectroscopy and affective disorders *(continued)*

Reference	Subjects	Brain region(s) studied	Type(s) of spectroscopy	Finding(s)
Kato et al. 1991	11 manic pts with BD I 11 euthymic pts with BD I 9 drug-free control subjects	Frontal lobe	^{31}P	PME level incr in manic state
Kato et al. 1992	10 bipolar depressed pts 12 unipolar depressed pts	Frontal lobe	^{31}P	PME and pH levels incr in bipolar depressed pts relative to euthymic state PME and pH levels decr in bipolar pts relative to control subjects PCr level decr in severely depressed (?bipolar vs. combined) pts
Kato et al. 1994b	40 bipolar pts 60 control subjects	Frontal lobe	^{31}P, ^{1}H	PME level negatively correlated with age in pts PME level decr in pts with BD I Duration of lithium effect correlated with pH level
Volz et al. 1998	14 unipolar depressed pts 8 matched control subjects	Frontal lobe	^{31}P	PME level incr ATP level decr
Moore et al. 1997	35 unmedicated depressed pts 18 comparison subjects	Basal ganglia	^{31}P	ATP level 16% lower in pts
Stoll et al. 1996	6 pts with rapid-cycling BD treated with lithium and Cho	Basal ganglia	^{1}H	Cho level incr in responders to Cho augmentation
Kato et al. 1996	19 euthymic bipolar pts 19 age-matched control subjects	Basal ganglia	^{1}H	Cho/Cr ratio incr in pts

TABLE 12–1. Magnetic resonance spectroscopy and affective disorders *(continued)*

Reference	Subjects	Brain region(s) studied	Type(s) of spectroscopy	Finding(s)
Hamakawa et al. 1998	18 bipolar pts 22 unipolar depressed pts 20 control subjects	Basal ganglia	^{1}H	Cho level incr in bipolar depressed pts Cho/Cr and Cho/NAA ratios incr in bipolar depressed pts and euthymic bipolar pts Cho/NAA ratio incr in unipolar depressed pts
Sharma et al. 1992	Bipolar pts treated with lithium	Basal ganglia, occipital cortex	^{1}H	NAA/PCr, Cho/PCr, and Ino/PCr ratios incr in basal ganglia in pts
Frey et al. 1998	22 depressed pts 22 control subjects	Frontal lobe	^{1}H	MI/Cr ratio in right frontal lobe positively correlated with age MI/Cr ratio decr in treated pts relative to control subjects
Charles et al. 1994	7 depressed pts 7 matched control subjects	Subcortical region	^{1}H	Cho level incr in depressed state

Note. ATP = adenosine triphosphate; BD = bipolar disorder; Cho = choline; Cr = creatine; decr = decreased; incr = increased; Ino = *myo*-inositol; MI = myo-inositol; NAA = *N*-acetylaspartate; PCr = phosphocreatine; PDE = phosphodiester; PME = phosphomonoester; pts = patients.

these markers be present in all phases of the illness. Nonetheless, some interesting trends have emerged from MRS studies.

Phosphorus MRS Studies

Euthymic and depressed patients with bipolar disorder have decreased PME and increased PDE levels relative to euthymic control subjects. Deicken et al. (1995a, 1995b) reported these findings in both the frontal and temporal lobes, and Kato et al. (1994b) reported similar findings in the frontal lobe. Because the PME signal is generally composed of membrane precursors and the PDE signal of membrane breakdown products and mobile phospholipids, these findings suggest that, in the depressed and euthymic states, membrane turnover may be increased, or that phospholipid synthesis may be decreased in bipolar subjects more than in control subjects. Conversely, manic subjects studied by Kato et al. in 1991 and 1993 showed increased frontal lobe PME levels. However, these patients were treated with lithium, which may increase PME levels transiently when first administered (Renshaw et al. 1985). Kato et al. (1994a) suggested that the increase in PME levels observed in these patients reflects the combined effects of lithium and catecholaminergic activation associated with the manic state.

In terms of cellular energetics, Kato and colleagues (1995), reported decreased PCr levels in the left prefrontal cortex in the depressed state and in the right prefrontal cortex in the manic and euthymic states. In bipolar II disorder, which is characterized by deep depression and occasional hypomanias, this same group reported decreased frontal lobe PCr levels in all phases. In contrast, Deicken et al. (1995a), studying 12 euthymic bipolar patients and 16 control subjects, found that PCr levels in patients were increased in the right frontal lobe compared with the left frontal lobe but that PCr levels in patients were not increased compared with those in control subjects. The patients studied by Kato et al. (1995) were receiving medication, whereas the patients studied by Deicken and colleagues (1995a) were medication free for 1 week before the study.

Because it has been postulated that acute increases in cerebral metabolism are associated with decrements in PCr concentrations, it is difficult to reconcile these data with findings, obtained in other functional imaging studies of depression, of decreased metabolic activity in the left prefrontal cortex in depressed patients. However, given that relatively little is known about brain disorders associated with chronic decreases in metabolic activity, one possibility is that the decreased PCr level reflects a resetting of the system at a lower energy state. It should also be noted that both Mayberg et al. (1997) and Wu et al. (1992), using positron emission tomography (PET), found increased metabolic activity in the cingulate gyrus in depressed subjects. It is also important to consider that decreased PCr levels may reflect medication effects rather than metabolic demands.

Proton MRS Studies

In two proton MRS studies in which the temporal lobes were examined, no differences were found between bipolar patients and control subjects. Kato et al. (1996), Lafer et al. (1994), and Sharma et al. (1992) reported an increased Cho/Cr ratio in the basal ganglia of bipolar patients compared with control subjects. Stoll et al. (1996) reported on four of six patients with bipolar mixed states who responded to augmentation of their lithium with Cho. In this small group, responders had increased basal ganglia Cho levels after augmentation, whereas nonresponders did not.

One possible explanation for the increase in Cho levels observed in these studies is drug effect. Lithium is known to increase intracellular levels of Cho by inhibition of Cho transport (Stoll et al. 1991). Alternatively, because the Cho peak measured by spectroscopy largely reflects membrane precursors and metabolites, these data also appear to be consistent with the ^{31}P-MRS results that indicate differences in membrane dynamics between bipolar patients and control subjects.

One leading theory is that depression and mania result from dysfunctional regulation of the catecholaminergic neurotransmitter circuits in brain regions such as the frontal lobes and the basal ganglia (Siever and Davis 1985). If this theory is correct, then it is easy to hypothesize that the dysfunctional regulation increases membrane turnover, by overloading the postsynaptic neuron with increased use of ion channels or need for precursors of second messenger systems. Janowsky et al. (1972) proposed an "adrenergic-cholinergic balance" hypothesis, suggesting that mania is associated with cholinergic underactivity and adrenergic overactivity. Consistent with this hypothesis, lithium exerts a potent and specific inhibitory effect on human Cho transport (Stoll et al. 1991), and treatment with phosphatidylcholine has been shown to have a moderate antimanic effect (Cohen et al. 1980, 1984; Leiva 1990; Schreier 1982).

Unipolar Depression

Unipolar depression has been the focus of fewer MRS studies than has bipolar disorder.

Phosphorus MRS Studies

Christensen et al. (1994) reported increased PDE levels in the basal ganglia of 9 depressed patients relative to control subjects. Volz et al. (1998a) reported increased PME levels in the frontal lobe in 14 unipolar depressed patients compared with control subjects. This same group also reported decreased ATP levels in the depressed patients. Moore et al. (1997) expanded on the preliminary data of Christensen et al. (1994) and reported decreased ATP levels in the basal ganglia of depressed patients. The finding of decreased ATP levels in the basal ganglia and frontal lobes of unipolar depressed patients is consistent with the finding of decreased metabolism in these two areas by other functional imaging modalities. However, because ATP is usually replenished rapidly after a response to an acute metabolic need, the decrease in levels suggests that, under chronic conditions of decreased metabolism, there may be a resetting of the system to lower concentrations of key molecules involved in neuronal energetics. The similarity of findings in the frontal lobes and the basal ganglia is consistent with [^{18}F]fluorodeoxyglucose–PET findings of a linkage between the metabolic activity of the caudate nucleus and the ipsilateral frontal lobe (Mayberg et al. 1992).

Proton MRS Studies

In two proton MRS studies, Cho/Cr ratios were examined in depressed versus euthymic patients and control subjects. Charles and colleagues (1994) examined Cho/Cr ratios in 7 geriatric depressed patients, using a relatively large voxel (27 cm^3) that included the basal ganglia, thalamus, and third ventricle. In this population, the researchers reported an increased Cho/Cr ratio in depressed subjects. Renshaw and colleagues (1997) used an 8-cm^3 voxel that was centered on the head of the caudate and putamen in 41 nongeriatric depressed patients. These investigators reported *decreased* Cho/Cr ratios in the depressed group. When grouped by treatment response, responders to fluoxetine therapy had nonsignificantly lower Cho/Cr ratios than did nonresponders. The seemingly contradictory results of these two studies may reflect the differences in voxel size and subcortical structures and/or the age differences between the two populations. Clearly, further work is necessary to interpret the results of these two studies.

Discussion

Overall, the limited number of studies makes it impossible to draw definitive conclusions, but the available data are consistent with altered membrane dynamics and abnormal cellular energetics in patients with mood disorders. Larger samples of bipolar and unipolar patients, stratified according to mood state, medication status, and age, are needed to understand the significance of the data summarized here. In addition, studies in which subjects undergo more than one type of imaging, under similar conditions, may help clarify the interpretation of these results.

■ SCHIZOPHRENIA

Schizophrenia is currently thought to be a neurodevelopmental disorder that arises from a combination of genetic vulnerability, environmental insult or insults in utero, and psychosocial factors (McCarley et al. 1999). Structural studies have demonstrated decreases in volume of brain regions such as the prefrontal cortex, temporal lobes, and thalamus (see McCarley et al. 1999 for a comprehensive review). MRS studies have in turn characterized differences in brain chemistry (Table 12–2). Although the results are not always consistent, the general themes are. Reported findings include disturbances in phospholipid membrane breakdown products and precursors, altered levels of high-energy phosphates, and decreased NAA levels in the frontal cortex, hippocampus, and basal ganglia in schizophrenic patients and cohorts at risk for schizophrenia. These spectroscopy findings are consistent with the findings of the structural studies and with the neuropsychological deficits that have been described in schizophrenic patients (Elliott et al. 1995). The findings suggest that decreased neuronal networking and dysfunctional membrane dynamics and cellular metabolism are important in the pathophysiology and expression of the illness.

Phosphorus MRS Studies

Pettegrew et al. (1991a) reported increased PDE and decreased PME levels in the left prefrontal cortex in a series of 11 neuroleptic-naive patients with first-episode schizophrenia compared with 10 matched control subjects. Subsequently, they reported a case in which measurements were taken 2 years before the onset of overt psychotic symptoms; a similar pattern was found (Pettegrew et al. 1991b). In contrast, Volz et al. (1998) subsequently reported decreased PDE levels in 50 medicated schizophrenic patients, and Shioiri et al. (1994) reported increased PME levels in patients with prominent negative symptoms. One important difference between the study by Pettegrew and colleagues (1991a) and those by Volz and colleagues (1998) and Shioiri and colleagues

TABLE 12–2. Magnetic resonance spectroscopy and schizophrenia

Reference	Subjects	Brain region(s) studied	Type(s) of spectroscopy	Finding(s)
Volz et al. 1998	26 schizophrenic pts 23 control subjects	Frontal lobe	Phosphorus	PCr level and PCr/ATP ratio negatively correlated with WCST score in control subjects only
Shioiri et al. 1997	4 catatonic pts 8 pts with disorganized type of schizophrenia 10 paranoid pts 14 pts with undifferentiated type of schizophrenia	Frontal lobe	Phosphorus	PME level decr in pts with disorganized type of schizophrenia Decr PME level correlated with motor retardation Incr PDE level correlated with emotional withdrawal and blunted affect
Shioiri et al. 1994	26 schizophrenic pts 26 matched control subjects	Frontal lobe	Phosphorus	PME level incr in pts with negative symptoms
Bluml et al. 1999	11 treated schizophrenic pts 2 drug-naive schizophrenic pts 15 comparison subjects	Parietal cortex	Phosphorus	GPCho, GPeth, and PCr levels incr in pts No difference in NAA, Cr, and MI levels compared with control subjects
Hinsberger et al. 1997	10 schizophrenic pts 10 control subjects	Left prefrontal cortex	Phosphorus	PME level decr and intracellular Mg level incr in pts
Volz et al. 1998	50 medicated schizophrenic pts 36 control subjects	Dorsolateral prefrontal cortex	Phosphorus	PDE level incr PCr level and PCr/ATP ratio incr ATP level correlated with CPZ PCr/ATP ratio negatively correlated with CPZ

TABLE 12–2. Magnetic resonance spectroscopy and schizophrenia *(continued)*

Reference	Subjects	Brain region(s) studied	Type(s) of spectroscopy	Finding(s)
Pettegrew et al. 1991	11 drug-naive pts with 1st-episode schizophrenia 10 control subjects	Dorsal prefrontal cortex	Phosphorus	PME level decr in pts PDE level incr in pts ATP level incr in pts
Volz et al. 1997	13 schizophrenic inpatients 14 control subjects	Dorsolateral prefrontal cortex	Phosphorus	PDE level decr in pts
Brooks et al. 1998	16 children with schizophrenia spectrum disorder 12 control subjects	Frontal lobe	Proton	NAA/Cr ratio significantly decr in pts
Fukuzako et al. 1995	30 medicated schizophrenic pts 30 control subjects	Frontal lobe (15 pts, 15 control subjects), medial temporal lobe (15 pts, 15 control subjects)	Proton	NAA/Cho and NAA/Cr ratios decr Cho/Cr ratio incr in left temporal lobe NAA/Cho and NAA/Cr ratios corresponded with age at illness onset
Yurgelun-Todd et al. 1996	16 medicated schizophrenic pts 14 control subjects	Temporal lobe	Proton	NAA/Cr ratio decr bilaterally
Keshavan et al. 1997	Offspring of schizophrenic pts control subjects	Ventral prefrontal cortex	Proton	Trend toward decr NAA/Cho ratio in offspring

TABLE 12–2. Magnetic resonance spectroscopy and schizophrenia *(continued)*

Reference	Subjects	Brain region(s) studied	Type(s) of spectroscopy	Finding(s)
Buckley et al. 1994	28 schizophrenic pts 20 control subjects	Left temporal lobe, left frontal lobe	Proton	NAA level decr and Cho level incr in frontal but not temporal lobe in male pts
Shioiri et al. 1996	21 medicated schizophrenic pts 21 matched control subjects	Basal ganglia	Proton	Cho level and Cho/NAA ratio incr in left basal ganglia NAA level correlated with CPZ Cho/NAA ratio negatively correlated with CPZ
Fujimoto et al. 1996	14 medicated schizophrenic pts	Basal ganglia	Proton	NAA/Cho ratio decr bilaterally Cho level incr in left basal ganglia
Cecil et al. 1999	18 drug-naive schizophrenic pts 24 control subjects	Dorsolateral prefrontal cortex (8 pts), midtemporal lobe (10 pts)	Proton	NAA/Cr ratio decr in frontal and temporal lobes Cho/Cr ratio incr in frontal and decr in temporal lobes NAA/Cr ratio incr in temporal lobe
Bertolino et al. 1996	10 schizophrenic inpatients	Dorsolateral prefrontal cortex, hippocampus	Proton	NAA/Cr and NAA/Cho ratios decr bilaterally
Deicken et al. 1998	30 pts with chronic schizophrenia 18 control subjects	Hippocampus	Proton	NAA level decr in right and left hippocampus Cho level not different Trend toward greater Cr level in left hippocampus

TABLE 12–2. Magnetic resonance spectroscopy and schizophrenia *(continued)*

Reference	Subjects	Brain region(s) studied	Type(s) of spectroscopy	Finding(s)
Maier et al. 1995	25 schizophrenic pts 32 control subjects	Hippocampus	Proton	NAA, Cho, and Cr levels decr in left hippocampus
Nasrallah et al. 1994	11 schizophrenic pts 11 control subjects	Hippocampus	Proton	NAA level decr bilaterally, significant only on the right
Eluri et al. 1998	12 schizophrenic pts 8 control subjects	Pons, cerebellum	Proton	NAA/Cr ratio decr in pons

Note. ATP = adenosine triphosphate; Cho = choline; Cr = creatine; decr = decreased; incr = increased; CPZ = chlorpromazine; GPCho = glycerophosphorylcholine; Gpeth = glycerophospylethanolamine; Mg = magnesium; MI = myo-inositol; NAA = *N*-acetylaspartate; PCr = phosphocreatine; PDE = phosphodiester; PME = phosphomonoester; pts = patients; WCST = Wisconsin Card Sorting Test.

(1994) is that the former study involved unmedicated patients. Given the large number of effects that neuroleptic medications have in the central nervous system, it is not surprising that the results obtained differed markedly between medicated and unmedicated patients. In addition, given the data suggesting that typical and atypical neuroleptics cause different metabolic responses in the brain (Chakos et al. 1995), class of antipsychotic medication may need to be taken into account in the interpretation of future studies.

Proton MRS Studies

Decreased NAA levels in various brain regions of schizophrenic patients have been reported by several investigators (Table 12–2), and this finding is consistent with the finding of decreases in volumes of structures within the frontal and temporal lobes (McCarley et al. 1999). In addition, Keshavan et al. (1997) suggested that decreased NAA levels are present in cohorts at risk for the disease. These data support the hypothesis that pathological changes occur in the brain substantially earlier than the onset of symptoms. Whether these decreases and the regions in which they occur can be used to classify patients by disease types requires further study.

Several groups have examined Cho levels in the frontal lobes, temporal lobes, and basal ganglia (Table 12–2). The majority of these researchers studied medicated patients. Among the studies that found differences, the majority found increased levels of Cho and increased Cho/NAA ratios. Exceptions to this trend were the negative findings of Deicken et al. (1998) and the decrease in Cho levels reported by Maier et al. (1995) and Nasrallah and colleagues (1994). These three groups studied the hippocampus, and the cohort studied by Deicken and colleagues (1998) included patients taking antipsychotic medications, both typical and atypical. Given that the hippocampus is involved in memory function, which relies heavily on acetylcholine, these findings might reflect the anticholinergic effects of antipsychotic medications. Alternatively, the irregular shape of the hippocampus increases the risk of partial volume effects, which are important because white matter has a higher concentration of Cho than does gray matter.

■ Dementia

The majority of spectroscopic studies of dementia have focused on Alzheimer's disease. The data point to neuronal loss, alterations in second messenger systems, and changes in cell membrane metabolite levels.

Postmortem studies of brain tissue from individuals with Alzheimer's disease have found decreased levels of the phospholipids phosphatidylcholine, phosphatidylethanolamine, and phosphatidylinositol (Nitsch et al. 1992; Prasad et al. 1998; Stokes and Hawthorne 1987), as well as increased levels of the phospholipid catabolic intermediates glycerophosphocholine and glycerophosphoethanolamine (Blusztajn et al. 1990). The existence of altered membrane metabolism in Alzheimer's disease creates opportunities for both phosphorus and proton MRS investigation of brain chemistry.

Phosphorus MRS

Given that a number of the compounds just listed are visible in MRS studies, one would expect to see an alteration in the spectra from these compounds in Alzheimer's disease. For example, ^{31}P MRS allows simultaneous observation of a number of membrane phospholipid precursors (e.g., phosphatidylcholine and phosphatidylethanolamine) and breakdown products (e.g., glycerophosphocholine and glycerophosphoethanolamine); a loss of membrane integrity would likely change the relative ratio of these compounds compared with the ratio in healthy tissue.

Selective decreases in temporoparietal perfusion have also been associated with the diagnosis of Alzheimer's disease using emission tomography (Bartenstein et al. 1997; Jagust et al. 1997; Masterman et al. 1997). Given that cerebral metabolism is closely coupled with blood flow, one would also expect that these brain regions might demonstrate altered bioenergetic indices, which could be detected with phosphorus MRS. In this regard, ^{31}P MRS permits localized assessments of brain PCr and ATP concentrations. Metabolic disturbances in brain tissue should cause detectable alterations in the relative concentrations of these high-energy phosphate compounds.

Phosphorus MRS Studies

Results of some phosphorus MRS studies conducted in vitro are presented in Table 12–3.

The findings described in reports of in vivo MRS studies are extremely variable for Alzheimer's disease. Of the nine studies surveyed (involving 144 subjects with dementia), four found no significant differences between the spectra of Alzheimer's disease patients and the spectra of control subjects (Table 12–4). Of the remaining five studies, two found an apparent increase in percent PME in mild Alzheimer's disease, but with a significant negative cor-

TABLE 12–3. Phosphorus magnetic resonance spectroscopy and dementia: in vitro studies

Reference	Parameters	Specimens	Brain region(s) studied	Finding(s)
Bárány et al. 1985	360 MHz, PCA extracts	9 AD brains 9 control brains	Cerebral cortex (predominantly gray matter)	GPC/GPE ratio three times higher in AD
Miatto et al. 1986	Aqueous solutions	7 AD brains 9 control brains	Frontal and parietal regions	% PME decr in AD % PDE incr in AD
Pettegrew et al. 1988b	200 MHz, PCA extracts	11 AD pts	Middle frontal and superotemporal gyri	% PME negatively correlated with number of senile plaques % PDE positively correlated with number of senile plaques
Pettegrew et al. 1988a	TR = 1 second, α = 45, TE = minimum	9 AD brains 3 control brains 4 nondiseased AD brains	Whole brain	PME level 23% higher Pi level 13% lower PDE level 58% higher
			Inferior parietal cortex	PME level 32% higher
			Superior and middle frontal cortex	PME level 38% higher Pi level 20% lower
			Occipital cortex	Pi level 16% lower
Smith et al. 1993	300 MHz, PCA extracts	9 AD brains 3 Pick's disease brains 7 control brains	Parietal gray matter	% Sugar phosphates, % PME, and % PDE higher in AD and Pick's disease
			Parietal white matter	% PME and % PDE higher in AD and Pick's disease

Note. AD = Alzheimer's disease; decr = decreased; GPC = glycerophosphocholine; GPE = glycerophosphoethanolamine; incr = increased PCA = perchloric acid; PDE = phosphodiester; Pi = inorganic phosphate; PME = phosphomonoester; pts = patients; TE = echo time; TR = repetition time.

TABLE 12–4. Phosphorus magnetic resonance spectroscopy and dementia: in vivo studies

Reference	Parameters	Subjects	Brain region(s) studied	Findings
Brown et al. 1989	Surface coil localization, TR=1.512 seconds	10 control subjects 7 MSID pts 11 PRAD pts	Temporoparietal region	*In AD pts (compared with MSID pts):* PCr/Pi ratio 44% lower % Pi 63% higher PME/PDE ratio 24 % higher % PME 21% higher
			Frontal region	*In AD pts (compared with MSID pts):* PCr/Pi ratio 27% lower % Pi 35% higher % PCr 10% lower
Bottomley et al. 1992	Slice selective spectroscopy, TR=15 seconds	11 PRAD pts 14 control subjects	Corpus callosum, superior to orbits (3-cm-thick axial slice)	No significant differences between AD pts and control subjects (limited age matching)
Murphy et al. 1993	Slice selective spectroscopy, TR=15 seconds	9 PRAD pts 8 control subjects	Parallel and superior to inferior orbitomeatal line (3-cm-thick axial slice)	No significant differences between AD pts and control subjects

TABLE 12–4. Phosphorus magnetic resonance spectroscopy and dementia: in vivo studies *(continued)*

Reference	Parameters	Subjects	Brain region(s) studied	Findings
Brown et al. 1993	Surface coil localization, TR=1.512 seconds	18 MSID pts 19 PRAD pts 21 control subjects	Frontal cortex and subadjacent white matter	*In MSID pts (compared with AD pts):* % PME 32% lower % PCr 26% higher *In MSID pts (compared with control subjects):* % PME 22% lower % PCr 22% higher % γ-NTP 21% and 24% higher % α-NTP 14% and 20% higher % β-NTP 13% and 15% higher % total NTP 16% and 20% higher PCr/Pi ratio 38% and 70% higher pH level higher
			Temporoparietal cortex and subadjacent white matter	*In MSID pts (compared with AD pts):* % PCr 17% higher PCr/Pi ratio 80% higher *In MSID pts (compared with control subjects):* % Pi 41% lower % PCr 29% higher % α-NTP 18% higher Total NTP 18% higher PCr/Pi ratio 80% higher

TABLE 12–4. Phosphorus magnetic resonance spectroscopy and dementia: in vivo studies *(continued)*

Reference	Parameters	Subjects	Brain region(s) studied	Findings
Pettegrew et al. 1994	Surface coil localization, 180 degrees at scalp	12 PRAD pts 21 control subjects	Dorsal prefrontal cortex (15–20 cm^3)	% PME higher in mildly demented AD pts than in control subjects % PME correlated with Mattis score % PCr lower in mildly demented AD pts than in control subjects, normal in moderate dementia % γ-NTP lower in mildly demented AD pts % γ-NTP correlated with dementia severity Mitochondrial metabolic rate decr with cognitive decline in AD
Pettegrew et al. 1995	Surface coil localization, 180 degrees at scalp	4 control subjects scanned every 6 months for 33 months	Dorsal prefrontal cortex	Subject who later developed dementia had high initial % PME and low initial % PCr. % PCr increased linearly with time, and % PCr correlated negatively with Mattis score.
Smith et al. 1995	Surface coil localization, 180 degrees at scalp, TR = 1.5 seconds	17 PRAD pts 8 elderly control subjects 15 young control subjects	Midline anterior-superior frontal lobe (50 cm^3)	PCr/Pi ratio 12% lower in AD pts than in elderly control subjects PCr/Pi ratio 20% lower in young control subjects than in elderly control subjects PME/PDE ratio lower in female pts with AD than in male pts with AD

TABLE 12–4. Phosphorus magnetic resonance spectroscopy and dementia: in vivo studies *(continued)*

Reference	Parameters	Subjects	Brain region(s) studied	Findings
Cuenod et al. 1995	Surface coil localization, 180 degrees at scalp, TR=2 seconds, TR=8 seconds	15 PRAD pts 6 control subjects	Prefrontal area	% PME 14% lower in AD pts
		9 PRAD pts 9 control subjects	Prefrontal area	% PME 11% lower in AD pts
González et al. 1996	1D ISIS, TR=15 seconds	16 PRAD pts 8 control subjects	Cerebrum (axial slice)	PME/PDE ratio 50% higher in AD pts than in control subjects (attributed to decrease in PDE level); PDE/β-NTP ratio 33% lower in AD pts than in control subjects

Note. 1D=one dimensional; AD=Alzheimer's disease; decr=decreased; incr=increased; ISIS=image-selected in vivo spectroscopy; MSID=multiple subcortical ischemic dementia; NTP=nucleoside 5′-triphosphate; PCr=phosphocreatine; PDE=phosphodiester; Pi=inorganic phosphate; PRAD=probable Alzheimer's disease; pts=patients; TR=repetition time.

relation with disease severity (Pettegrew et al. 1994, 1995); one found an increased PME/PDE ratio, although this finding appeared to be primarily due to a decrease in PDE levels (as evidenced by a decrease in PDE/γ-NTP ratio) (González et al. 1996); one found no change in phospholipid levels (Smith et al. 1995); and one found a decrease in percent PME (Cuenod et al. 1995). Two factors that complicate direct comparison of these studies are the different brain regions from which spectra were obtained and the differing sensitivity of the magnetic resonance techniques to short T2 species.

Only three of the nine studies found any significant changes in the resonances related to cell energetics. One study found a decrease in mitochondrial metabolic rate correlated with cognitive decline in Alzheimer's disease (Pettegrew et al. 1994). Another found a decrease in percent PCr in mild Alzheimer's disease, percent PCr increasing toward control levels with disease progression (Pettegrew 1995). The third study found a decreased PCr/Pi ratio (Smith 1995). These results are somewhat contradictory, because mitochondrial function is closely and positively associated with the PCr/Pi ratio.

Proton MRS Studies

There is good reason to expect that Alzheimer's disease may cause changes in the concentrations of three of the four major metabolites in cerebral proton spectra: NAA, Cho, and Ino. The first, NAA, is known to be a neuronal marker (Koller et al. 1984; Simmons et al. 1991), and the neurodegeneration accompanying Alzheimer's disease would be expected to decrease the concentration of this metabolite. The alterations of membrane biochemistry accompanying Alzheimer's disease have profound effects on the concentration of various Cho-containing compounds; in proton spectra, these compounds are all summed together in the "choline" peak. As the composition of the Cho pool is altered, the size of this resonance may change. Similarly, there have been postmortem findings of an increase in brain Ino levels and a decrease in phosphatidylinositol levels in the brains of patients with Alzheimer's disease (Stokes and Hawthorne 1987). Because Ino is visible in proton MRS studies and phosphatidylinositol is not, an increase in the relative proportion of Ino would be expected to lead to an increase in the size of the inositol resonance.

Given that dementias are fundamentally disruptions of brain function, one would also expect that the concentrations of inhibitory and excitatory neurotransmitters might also be altered in conditions such as Alzheimer's disease. However, these compounds (e.g., glutamate and γ-aminobutyric acid) though technically visible in MRS studies, are extremely difficult to see in vivo without the use of special techniques, because of low concentrations and overlapping resonances (Keltner et al. 1997). As a result, they are not typically measured in standard in vivo spectroscopy, but in vitro studies have suggested the presence of altered levels of these neurotransmitters (Klunk et al. 1992; Mohanakrishnan et al. 1997) (Table 12–5).

We reviewed 20 proton MRS studies involving 407 patients with dementia (Table 12–6). The studies are extremely consistent in their major findings relative to Alzheimer's disease. Of the 17 studies involving patients with Alzheimer's disease, 14 found that NAA levels (or the metabolite ratio NAA/Cr or NAA/Cho) were decreased in patients with Alzheimer's disease, in both gray and white matter and in a wide variety of brain regions. The magnitude of NAA level decrease (5%–40% depending on the brain region) was quite consistent with the reported findings in vitro. However, this decrease in NAA level is not specific to Alzheimer's disease; it shows up in a range of neurodegenerative disorders, including Down's syndrome (two studies), vascular dementia (two studies), age-associated memory impairment (one study), and frontotemporal dementia (two studies).

Eight studies found an increase in Ino levels (or Ino/Cr ratios), and one study found that the magnitude of increase of inositol levels was correlated with dementia severity and duration. Unlike the decrease in NAA level, the increase in inositol level is seen only in Alzheimer's disease and frontotemporal dementia. This finding has led some researchers to propose that an increase in the Ino/NAA ratio may be used diagnostically as a sensitive indicator of Alzheimer's disease (Doraiswamy et al. 1998; Shonk et al. 1995).

The Cho findings point out an important issue. Three of the studies surveyed found an increase in total Cho (either directly or as the ratio Cho/Cr) in the gray matter of patients with Alzheimer's disease, two found a decrease in Cho level in white matter, and the majority of the studies found no significant changes. The composition of the spectroscopic voxel can have a large effect on the metabolite concentration, especially in cases in which different tissue types have concentration changes in opposite directions. It is difficult to select voxels small enough in vivo to isolate gray or white matter; therefore, it may be valuable to assess the tissue composition of the voxel, to control for the effect of different tissue type (Renshaw et al. 1997).

Treatment Response Studies

MRS has also been proposed as a means to monitor the effects of treatment. Although less work has been conducted in this area, we can describe two re-

TABLE 12–5. Proton magnetic resonance spectroscopy: in vitro studies

Reference	Parameters	Specimens	Brain region(s) studied	Findings
Klunk et al. 1992	500 MHz, PCA extracts	12 AD brains 5 control brains	Superior middle frontal cortex, superior temporal cortex	NAA level negatively correlated with NFTs and senile plaques NAA level decr, glutamate level incr, and GABA level decr in AD
Kwo-On-Yuen et al. 1994	300 MHz, PCA extracts	7 AD brains 7 control brains	Visual cortex	GM NAA level 19% lower in AD
			Parahippocampal gyrus	GM NAA level 50% lower and WM NAA level 30% lower in AD
			Superior temporal cortex	GM NAA level 29% lower in AD
Mohanakrishnan et al. 1995	300 MHz, 90% methanol extraction	13 AD brains 4 control brains	Frontal cortex	GM NAA level 25% lower in AD
			Superior temporal cortex	GM NAA level 29% lower in AD
			Parahippocampal gyrus	GM NAA level 50% lower in AD
			Posterior temporoparietal cortex	NAA level decr with NFTs GABA and NAA levels decr in AD

TABLE 12–5. Proton magnetic resonance spectroscopy: in vitro studies *(continued)*

Reference	Parameters	Specimens	Brain region(s) studied	Findings
Mohanakrishnan et al. 1997	300 MHz, 90% methanol extraction	13 AD brains 4 control brains	Hippocampus	NAA level decr in AD brains relative to control brains and in brains from AD pts matched for PMI relative to control brains GABA level decr in brains from AD pts matched for PMI relative to control brains NAA level decr with increasing neuronal loss in AD brains
			Cerebellum	NAA and GABA levels decr in AD brains relative to control brains and in brains from AD pts matched for PMI relative to control brains

Note. AD = Alzheimer's disease; decr = decreased; GABA = γ-aminobutyric acid; GM = gray matter; incr = increased; NAA = *N*-acetylaspartate; NFT = neurofibrillary tangle; PCA = perchloric acid; PMI = postmortem interval; pts = patients; WM = white matter.

TABLE 12–6. Proton magnetic resonance spectroscopy: in vivo studies

Reference	Parameters	Subjects	Brain region(s) studied	Findings
Koshino et al. 1992	STEAM spectroscopy, TR=2 seconds, TE=272 ms	17 Down's syndrome pts	Frontal area (8 cm^3)	NAA/Cho ratio negatively correlated with age
Murata et al. 1993	STEAM spectroscopy, TR=2 seconds, TE=272 ms	18 Down's syndrome pts 15 control subjects	Frontal left WM (8 cm^3)	Cho/Cr ratio positively correlated with age in pts Cho/Cr ratio higher in pts in 40s than in pts in 20s and control subjects in 40s NAA/Cho ratio negatively correlated with age NAA/Cho ratio lower in pts in 40s than in pts in 20s and 30s and control subjects in 40s
Shiino et al. 1993	STEAM spectroscopy, TR=2.5 seconds, TE=19 ms	9 PRAD pts 26 control subjects	Insular cortex (27 cm^3)	NAA/Cr ratio 40% lower in PRAD (limited age matching)
Miller et al. 1993	TR=1.5 and 5 seconds, TE=30 ms	11 PRAD pts 10 control subjects	Parietal WM (10–15 cm^3)	Ino/Cr ratio 11% higher in PRAD NAA/Cr ratio 5% lower in PRAD
			Occipital GM (10–15 cm^3)	Ino/Cr ratio 22% higher in PRAD NAA/Cr ratio 11% lower in PRAD
Meyerhoff et al. 1994	CSI, TE=272 ms	8 PRAD pts 10 control subjects	Centrum semiovale	Cho/Cr ratio 25%–30% higher in GM

TABLE 12–6. Proton magnetic resonance spectroscopy: in vivo studies *(continued)*

Reference	Parameters	Subjects	Brain region(s) studied	Findings
Moats et al. 1994	TR = 1.5 seconds, TE = 30 ms	10 PRAD pts 7 control subjects	Parietal lobe, parietal WM, occipital GM	NAA/Cr ratio 10%–12% lower in WM Ino level 17% higher in WM in PRAD Ino level 33% higher in PRAD NAA level 11% lower in PRAD Cr level 7% lower in PRAD
Christiansen et al. 1995	STEAM spectroscopy, TR = 1.6 and 6.0 seconds, TE = 20, 46, 82, and 272 ms	12 PRAD pts 8 control subjects	Occipital GM, right frontal lobe (8 cm^3)	Ino level 33% higher in PRAD NAA level 11% lower in PRAD Cr level 7% lower in PRAD NAA level 21% lower in PRAD
Shonk et al. 1995	STEAM spectroscopy, TR = 3 seconds, TE = 30 ms	65 PRAD pts 39 pts with other dementia 10 FTD pts 98 pts without dementia 32 control subjects	Occipital GM	NAA level 8% lower in PRAD Ino level 14% higher in PRAD NAA level 6% lower in other dementia
MacKay et al. 1996	CSI, TE = 272 ms	14 PRAD pts 18 control subjects 8 VD pts	Frontal, medial, and posterior WM	NAA/Cr ratio 10% lower in frontal WM in PRAD NAA/Cr ratio 25% lower in frontal WM in VD Cho/Cr ratio 40% higher in GM in PRAD
Tedeschi et al. 1996	CSI, TR = 2.2 seconds, TE = 272 ms	15 PRAD pts 15 control subjects	Frontal, temporal, parietal, occipital, and insular cortices; thalamus; subcortical WM	NAA/Cr ratio lower in frontal, temporal, and parietal cortices in PRAD Cho/Cr ratio lower in WM in PRAD

TABLE 12–6. Proton magnetic resonance spectroscopy: in vivo studies *(continued)*

Reference	Parameters	Subjects	Brain region(s) studied	Findings
Kattapong et al. 1996	PRESS, TR= 2 seconds, TE=136 ms	10 PRAD pts 8 VD pts	Subcortical WM ($8\ cm^3$)	NAA/Cr ratio 29% lower in VD Cho/Cr ratio 35% lower in VD
Parnetti et al. 1996	STEAM spectroscopy, TR=4 seconds, TE=20 ms	6 PRAD pts 6 AAMI pts 6 control subjects	Temporoparietal region ($10\ cm^3$)	NAA/Cr ratio 12% lower in PRAD NAA/Cr ratio 11% lower in AAMI Ino/Cr ratio 22% higher in PRAD
Parnetti et al. 1997	STEAM spectroscopy, TR=2.6 seconds, TE=35 ms	13 PRAD pts 7 control subjects	Temporal GM	NAA level 17% lower in PRAD Ino level 16% higher in PRAD
			Frontal WM	NAA level 9% lower in PRAD Ino level positively correlated with duration of dementia and negatively correlated with dementia severity
Ernst et al. 1997	PRESS, TR=3 seconds	12 PRAD pts 14 FTD pts 11 control subjects	Frontal GM ($3–7\ cm^3$), temporoparietal GM ($3–7\ cm^3$)	NAA level 28% lower in frontal GM in FTD Ino level 19% higher in frontal GM in FTD Ino level 8% higher in temporoparietal GM in PRAD
Frederick et al. 1997	STEAM spectroscopy, TR=2 seconds, TE=272 ms	33 PRAD pts 8 control subjects	Midline parietal lobe ($27\ cm^3$)	NAA/Cr ratio decr 6% NAA/Cho ratio decr 4%

TABLE 12–6. Proton magnetic resonance spectroscopy: in vivo studies *(continued)*

Reference	Parameters	Subjects	Brain region(s) studied	Findings
		14 PRAD pts 8 control subjects	Medial temporal lobe ($3.4\ cm^3$)	NAA/Cr ratio decr 26% NAA/Cho ratio decr 20% Cho/Cr ratio decr 8%
Fukuzako et al. 1997	STEAM spectroscopy, TR=1.5 seconds, TE=135 ms	36 control subjects	Medial temporal lobe ($8\ cm^3$)	Trend toward decr NAA/Cr ratio with age (larger than in frontal lobe)
Schuff et al. 1997	CSI, TR=1.8 seconds, TE=135 ms	12 PRAD pts 17 control subjects	Frontal lobe ($27\ cm^3$)	Trend toward decr NAA/Cr ratio with age
			Right and left hippocampus	NAA level 16% lower in right and left hippocampus in PRAD Right and left hippocampus 20%–22% smaller in PRAD
Lazeyras et al. 1998	STEAM spectroscopy, CSI, TR=1.5 seconds, TE=20 ms	15 PRAD pts 14 control subjects	Cortical GM	Ino/Cr ratio incr 25% NAA/Cho ratio decr 21% Ino/NAA ratio incr 32%
			Subcortical GM	NAA/Cr ratio decr 15%
			WM	Ino/NAA ratio incr 27%

TABLE 12–6. Proton magnetic resonance spectroscopy: in vivo studies *(continued)*

Reference	Parameters	Subjects	Brain region(s) studied	Findings
Pfefferbaum et al. 1999	CSI, TR=2 seconds, TE=144 ms	16 PRAD pts 15 young control subjects 19 elderly control subjects	Slice parallel to antero-posterior commissure line (1.1-cm^3 voxels)	Levels of *N*-acetyl compounds lower in GM in AD pts than in elderly or young control subjects Cr level higher in GM and WM in AD pts and elderly control subjects than in young control subjects Cho level higher in GM in AD pts than in elderly or young control subjects Cho level higher in GM in elderly control subjects than in young control subjects Cho level lower in WM in AD pts than in elderly control subjects
Doraiswamy et al. 1998	STEAM spectroscopy, CSI, TR=1.5 seconds, TE=20 ms	12 PRAD pts at baseline and 12 months after presentation	Axial slice	NAA/Cr ratio at baseline positively correlated with MMSE score at follow-up NAA/Cr ratio at baseline inversely correlated with change in MMSE score between baseline and follow-up Ino/NAA ratio at baseline inversely correlated with MMSE score at follow-up

Note. AAMI=age-associated memory impairment; Cho=choline; Cr=creatine; CSI=chemical shift imaging; decr=decreased; FTD=frontotemporal dementia; GM=gray matter; Ino=*myo*-inositol; incr=increased; ms=milliseconds; MMSE=Mini-Mental State Exam; NAA=*N*-acetylaspartate; PRAD=probable Alzheimer's disease; PRESS=point-resolved spectroscopy; VD=vascular dementia; WM=white matter.

TABLE 12–7. Proton magnetic resonance spectroscopy: treatment effect studies

Reference	Parameters	Intervention	Subjects	Brain region(s) studied	Findings
Satlin et al. 1997	STEAM spectroscopy, TR=2 seconds, TE=272 ms	Treatment with oral xanomeline (25, 50, or 75 mg) or placebo for 6 months	27 PRAD pts	Midline parietal (27 cm^3)	Cho/Cr ratio decr 16%; larger Cho/Cr ratio decrease in responders
Frederick et al. 1998	STEAM spectroscopy, CSI, TR=2 seconds, TE=30 ms	Transdermal xanomeline therapy for 2 months	16 PRAD pts	Periventricular white matter	Cho/Cr ratio decr 38% between baseline and 2 months in pts with no cognitive decline; smaller, nonsignificant decrease in pts with cognitive decline

Note. Cho=choline; Cr=creatine; CSI=chemical shift imaging; ms=milliseconds; PRAD=probable Alzheimer's disease; STEAM=stimulated-echo acquisition mode; TE=echo time; TR=repetition time.

cent studies (Table 12–7). These studies followed patient groups undergoing treatment with xanomeline, a muscarinic cholinergic agonist. In the first investigation, a single midline parietal voxel proton MRS study, researchers found a 16% decrease in Cho/Cr ratios in patients with Alzheimer's disease taking an oral form of xanomeline, relative to patients receiving placebo, with a larger response in patients who responded to the treatment (as measured by a halt in cognitive decline) (Satlin et al. (1997). In the second study, a longitudinal, chemical shift imaging study involving patients treated with a transdermal formulation of the drug, findings were similar (Frederick et al. 1998). In all patients, there was a decrease in Cho/Cr ratios after 2 months of treatment, relative to baseline.

Discussion

The studies reviewed here show that dementia, and in particular Alzheimer's disease, causes some clearly detectable biochemical changes that can be seen by both phosphorus and proton MRS. The most consistent findings are from the proton MRS studies. A decrease in NAA-containing compounds, indicating a loss of neuronal density, was prominent in most of the studies surveyed, in both in vitro and in vivo studies. An increase in inositol resonance in vivo was also a robust finding, and one that appears to be somewhat specific to Alzheimer's disease. Combining these two findings (in the calculated quantity Ino/NAA) may be the basis for an MRS diagnostic assay for Alzheimer's disease (Doraiswamy et al. 1998; Shonk et al. 1995). Further study will be necessary to determine how this quantity is affected by disease progression and therapies. Another consistent (but less common) proton MRS finding was alteration of Cho resonance (increasing in gray matter in Alzheimer's disease and decreasing in white matter), the progression of which may be alterable with therapy.

■ FUTURE DIRECTIONS

As higher-field-strength magnets become more common, and spatial resolution improves, spectroscopy will become an even more powerful tool for understanding and subtyping individuals with psychiatric illnesses. This prediction is important from at least two perspectives—those of genetic studies and drug development. For example, it is likely that the heterogeneity of illnesses such as schizophrenia has led to the development of drugs that act on several receptor systems, rather than agents specific for one or a few types of neural circuitry. The cost to patients is that their lives are often restricted by drug side effects. In the case of mood disorders, the ability to distinguish between unipolar and bipolar depression and to identify patients who have biological, rather than situational or developmental, mood disorders should decrease placebo response rates. This result is important because high placebo response rates have contributed to termination of the development of several candidate antidepressant compounds.

A corollary of the rationale for using spectroscopy in drug development is that spectroscopy may offer insights into which drugs should be used first in patients with a given pattern or patterns of findings. For example, Shioiri et al. (1994) reported that NAA levels correlated with chlorpromazine equivalents. It is relatively easy to imagine that the pattern associated with greater chlorpromazine equivalents would predict a better response to treatment with clozapine or an atypical antipsychotic, whereas the pattern associated with smaller chlorpromazine equivalents might predict a better response to treatment with traditional neuroleptics.

In genetic studies, the ability to subtype patients should allow for the study of more homogeneous populations and increase the likelihood of identifying candidate genes. However, it should be noted that most psychiatric illnesses appear to result from a combination of inherited genetic susceptibility and environmental insult or insults. Given that the human organism is continuously developing, it seems likely that the amount and timing of an environmental insult has significant impact on the pathology and clinical manifestations of an illness. Given too that the brain has a finite number of final common pathways available for expressing pathology, it is possible that categorizing illnesses on the basis of shared spectroscopy findings may result in the grouping of patients with very different genetic profiles. Nonetheless, it is likely that more effective subtyping of patients with psychiatric illnesses, using MRS and other brain imaging techniques, will significantly decrease the amount of work required to identify the genetic loci of these illnesses.

■ References

Ackerman JJ, Grove TH, Wong CG, et al: Mapping of metabolites in whole animals by 31P NMR using surface coils. Nature 283:167–170, 1980

Bárány M, Yen-Chung C, Arils C, et al: Increased glycerol-3-phosphorylcholine in post-mortem Alzheimer's brain. Lancet 1:517, 1985

Barker PB, Soher BJ, Blackband SJ, et al: Quantitation of proton NMR spectra of the human brain using tissue water as an internal concentration reference. NMR Biomed 6:89–94, 1993

Barker PB, Breiter SN, Soher BJ, et al: Quantitative proton spectroscopy of canine brain: in vivo and in vitro correlations. Magn Reson Med 30:157–163, 1994

Bartenstein P, Minoshima S, Hirsch C, et al: Quantitative assessment of cerebral blood flow in patients with Alzheimer's disease by SPECT. J Nucl Med 38:1095–1101, 1997

Berridge M, Downes C, Hanley M: Neural and developmental actions of lithium: a unifying hypothesis. Cell 59:411–419, 1989

Bertolino A, Nawroz S, Mattay VS, et al: Regionally specific pattern of neurochemical pathology in schizophrenia as assesses by multislice proton magnetic resonance spectroscopic imaging. Am J Psychiatry 153:1554–1563, 1996

Bluml S, Zuckerman E, Tan J, et al. Proton-decoupled 31P magnetic resonance spectroscopy reveals osmotic and metabolic disturbances in human hepatic encephalopathy. J Neurochem 71:1564–1576, 1998

Blusztajn J, Gonzalez-Coviella IL, Logue M, et al: Levels of phospholipid catabolic intermediates, glycerophosphocholine and glycerophosphoethanolamine, are elevated in brains of Alzheimer's disease but not of Down's syndrome patients. Brain Res 536:240–244, 1990

Bottomley PA, Foster TB, Darrow RD, et al: Depth-resolved surface coil spectroscopy (DRESS) for in vivo 1H, 31P, and 13C NMR. J Magn Reson 59:338–343, 1984

Bottomley P, Cousins J, Pendrey D, et al: Alzheimer dementia: quantification of energy metabolism and mobile phosphoesters with P-31 NMR spectroscopy. Radiology 183:695–699, 1992

Brooks WM, Hodde-Vargas J, Vargas LA, et al: Frontal lobe of children with schizophrenia spectrum disorders: a proton magnetic resonance spectroscopic study. Biol Psychiatry 43: 263–269, 1998

Brown GG, Levine SR, Gorell JM, et al: In vivo 31P NMR profiles of Alzheimer's disease and multiple subcortical infarct dementia. Neurology 39:1423–1427, 1989

Brown G, Garcia J, Gdowski J, et al: Altered brain energy metabolism in demented patients with multiple subcortical ischemic lesions: working hypotheses. Arch Neurol 50:384–388, 1993

Brown TR, Kincaid BM, Ugurbil K: NMR chemical shift imaging in three dimensions. Proc Natl Acad Sci U S A 79:3523–3526, 1982

Buchli RC, Duc CO, Martin E, et al: Assessment of absolute metabolite concentrations in human tissue by 31P MRS in vivo, part I: cerebrum, cerebellum, cerebral gray and white matter. Magn Reson Med 32:447–452, 1994

Buckley PF, Moore C, Long H, et al: 1H-magnetic resonance spectroscopy of the left temporal and frontal lobes in schizophrenia: clinical, neurodevelopmental, and cognitive correlates. Biol Psychiatry 36:792–800, 1994

Cecil KM, Lenkinski RE, Gur RE, et al: Proton magnetic resonance spectroscopy in the frontal and temporal lobes of neuroleptic naive patients with schizophrenia. Neuropsychopharmacology 20:131–140, 1999

Chakos MH, Lieberman JA, Alvir J, et al: Caudate nuclei volumes in schizophrenic patients treated with typical antipsychotics or clozapine. Lancet 345:456–457, 1995

Charles HC, Lazeyras F, Krishnan KRR, et al: Brain choline in depression: in vivo detection of potential pharmacodynamic effects of antidepressant therapy using hydrogen localized spectroscopy. Prog Neuropsychopharmacol Biol Psychiatry 18: 1121–1127, 1994

Christensen JD, Renshaw PF, Stoll AL, et al.: 31P spectroscopy of the basal ganglia in major depression (abstract), in Proceedings of the 2nd annual meeting of the Society of Magnetic Resonance Medicine, San Francisco, CA, August 6–12, 1994, p 608

Christiansen P, Schlosser A, Henriksen O: Reduced N-acetylaspartate content in the frontal part of the brain in patients with probable Alzheimer's disease. Magn Reson Imaging 13:457–462, 1995

Cohen BM, Miller AL, Lipinski JF, et al: Lecithin in the treatment of mania: a preliminary report. Am J Psychiatry 137:242–243, 1980

Cohen BM, Lipinski JF, Altesman RI: Lecithin in the treatment of mania: double-blind, placebo controlled trials. Am J Psychiatry 139:1162–1164, 1984

Cuenod CA, Kaplan DB, Michot JL, et al: Phospholipid abnormalities in early Alzheimer's disease. Arch Neurol 52:89–94, 1995

Deicken RF, Fein G, Weiner MW: Abnormal frontal lobe phosphorous metabolism in bipolar disorder. Am J Psychiatry 152:915–918, 1995a

Deicken RF, Weiner MW, Fein G: Decreased temporal lobe phosphomonoesters in bipolar disorder. J Affect Disord 33:195–199, 1995b

Deicken RF, Zhou L, Schuff N, et al: Hippocampal neuronal dysfunction in schizophrenia as measured by proton magnetic resonance spectroscopy. Biol Psychiatry 43:483–488, 1998

Doraiswamy P, Charles H, Krishnan K: Prediction of cognitive decline in early Alzheimer's disease (letter). Lancet 352:1678, 1998

Elliott R, McKenna PJ, Robbins TW, et al: Neuropsychological evidence for frontostriatal dysfunction in schizophrenia. Psychol Med 25:619–630, 1995

Eluri R, Paul C, Roemer R, et al: Single-voxel proton magnetic resonance spectroscopy of the pons and cerebellum in patients with schizophrenia: a preliminary study. Psychiatry Res 84:17–26, 1998

Ernst T, Chang L, Melchor R, et al: Frontotemporal dementia and early Alzheimer disease: differentiation with frontal lobe H-1 MR spectroscopy. Radiology 203:829–836, 1997

Frahm J, Bruhn H, Gyngell ML, et al: Localized high-resolution proton NMR spectroscopy using stimulated echoes: initial applications to human brain in vivo. Magn Reson Med 9:79–93, 1989

Frederick BB, Satlin A, Yurgelun-Todd DA, et al: In vivo proton magnetic resonance spectroscopy of Alzheimer's disease in the parietal and temporal lobes. Biol Psychiatry 42:147–150, 1997

Frederick BB, Satlin A, Wald LL, et al: Clinical response in patients with Alzheimer's disease treated with Xanomeline correlates with a decrease in Cho/Cre: a 1H CSI study (abstract), in Proceedings of the 6th annual meeting of the International Society of Magnetic Resonance Medicine, Sydney, Australia, April 18–24, 1998, p 727

Frey R, Metzler D, Fischer P, et al: Myoinositol in depressive and healthy subjects determined by frontal 1H-magnetic resonance spectroscopy at 1.5 tesla. J Psychiatr Res 32: 411–420, 1998

Fujimoto T, Nakano T, Takano T, et al: Proton magnetic resonance spectroscopy of basal ganglia in chronic schizophrenia. Biol Psychiatry 40:14–28, 1996

Fukuzako H, Takeuchi K, Hokazono Y, et al: Proton Magnetic resonance spectroscopy of the left medial temporal and frontal lobes in chronic schizophrenia: a preliminary report. Psychiatry Res 61:193–200, 1995

Fukuzako H, Hashiguchi T, Sakamoto Y, et al: Metabolite changes with age measured by proton magnetic resonance spectroscopy in normal subjects. Psychiatry Clin Neurosci 51:261–263, 1997

González RG, Guimaraes AR, Moore GJ, et al: Quantitative in vivo 31P magnetic resonance spectroscopy of Alzheimer disease. Alzheimer Dis Assoc Disord 10:46–52, 1996

Gyulai L, Bolinger L, Leigh JS Jr, et al: Phosphorylethanolamine—the major constituent of the phosphomonoester peak observed by 31P-NMR on developing dog brain. FEBS Lett 178:137–42, 1984

Hamakawa H, Kato T, Shioiri T, et al: Quantitative proton magnetic resonance spectroscopy of the bilateral frontal lobes on patients with bipolar disorder. Psychol Med 29:639–644, 1999

Hinsberger AD, Williamson PC, Carr TJ, et al: Magnetic resonance imaging volumetric and phosphorus 31 magnetic resonance spectroscopy measurements in schizophrenia. J Psychiatry Neurosci 22:111–117, 1997

Jagust W, Eberling J, Reed B, et al: Clinical studies of cerebral blood flow in Alzheimer's disease. Ann N Y Acad Sci 826:254–262, 1997

Janowsky DS, el-Yousef MK, Davis JM, et al: A cholinergic-adrenergic hypothesis of mania and depression. Lancet 2:632–635, 1972

Kato T, Shioiri T, Takahashi S, et al: Measurement of brain phosphoinositide metabolism in bipolar patients using in vivo 31P-MRS. J Affect Disord 22:185–190, 1991

Kato T, Shioiri T, Inubushi T, et al: Brain lithium concentrations measured with lithium-7 magnetic resonance spectroscopy in patients with affective disorders: relationship to erythrocyte and serum concentrations. Biol Psychiatry 33:147–152, 1993

Kato T, Takahashi S, Inubushi T: Brain lithium concentration by 7Li- and 1H-magnetic resonance spectroscopy in bipolar disorder. Psychiatry Res 45:53–63, 1994a

Kato T, Takahashi S, Shioiri T, et al: Reduction of brain phosphocreatine in bipolar II disorder detected by phosphorus-31 magnetic resonance spectroscopy. J Affect Disord 31:125–133, 1994b

Kato T, Shioiri T, Murashita J, et al: Lateralized abnormality of high energy phosphate metabolism in the frontal lobes of patients with bipolar disorder detected by phase-encoded 31P-MRS. Psychol Med 25:557–566, 1995

Kato T, Hamakawa H, Shioiri T, et al: Choline-containing compounds detected by proton magnetic resonance spectroscopy in the basal ganglia in bipolar disorder. J Psychiatry Neurosci 21:248–254, 1996

Kattapong V, Brooks W, Wesley M, et al: Proton magnetic resonance spectroscopy of vascular- and Alzheimer-type dementia. Arch Neurol 53:678–680, 1996

Keltner JR, Wald LL, Frederick BD, et al: In vivo detection of GABA in human brain using a localized double-quantum filter technique. Magn Reson Med 37:366–371, 1997

Keshavan MS, Montrose DM, Pierri JN, et al: Magnetic resonance imaging and spectroscopy in offspring at risk for schizophrenia: preliminary studies. Prog Neuropsychopharmacol Biol Psychiatry 21:1285–1295, 1997

Kilby PM, Bolas NM, Radda GK: 31P-NMR study of brain phospholipid structures in vivo. Biochim Biophys Acta 1085:257–264, 1991

Klunk WE, Panchalingam K, Moossy J, et al: N-Acetyl-l-aspartate and other amino acid metabolites in Alzheimer's disease brain: a preliminary proton nuclear magnetic resonance study. Neurology 42:1578–1585, 1992

Koller KJ, Zaczek R, Coyle JT: N-Acetyl-aspartyl-glutamate: regional levels in rat brain and the effects of brain lesions as determined by a new HPLC method. J Neurochem 43:1136–1142, 1984

Koshino Y, Murata T, Oomori M, et al: In vivo proton magnetic resonance spectroscopy in adult Down's syndrome. Biol Psychiatry 32:625–627, 1992

Kwo-On-Yuen PF, Newmark RD, Budinger TF, et al: Brain N-acetyl-L-aspartic acid in Alzheimer's disease: a proton magnetic resonance spectroscopy study. Brain Res 667:167–174, 1994

Lafer B, Renshaw PF, Sachs G, et al: Proton MRS of the basal ganglia in bipolar disorder (abstract). Biol Psychiatry 35:685, 1994

Lazeyras F, Charles H, Erickson R, et al: Metabolic brain mapping in Alzheimer's disease using high-resolution proton magnetic resonance spectroscopy. Psychiatry Res 82:95–106, 1998

Leiva DB: The neurochemistry of mania: a hypothesis of etiology and a rationale for treatment. Prog Neuropsychopharmacol Biol Psychiatry 14:423–429, 1990

MacKay S, Meyerhoff DJ, Constans JM, et al: Regional gray and white matter metabolite differences in subjects with AD, with subcortical ischemic vascular dementia, and elderly controls with 1H magnetic resonance spectroscopic imaging. Arch Neurol 53:167–174, 1996

Maier M, Ron MA, Barker GJ, et al: Proton magnetic resonance spectroscopy: an in vivo method of estimating hippocampal neuronal depletion in schizophrenia. Psychol Med 25:1201–1209, 1995

Masterman DL, Mendez MF, Fairbanks LA, et al: Sensitivity, specificity, and positive predictive value of technetium 99-HMPAO SPECT in discriminating Alzheimer's disease from other dementias. J Geriatr Psychiatry Neurol 10:15–21, 1997

Mayberg HS, Starkstein SE, Peyser CE, et al: Paralimbic frontal lobe hypometabolism in depression associated with Huntington's disease. Neurology 42:1791–1797, 1992

Mayberg HS, Brannan SK, Mahurin RK, et al: Cingulate function in depression: a potential predictor of treatment response. Neuroreport 8:1057–1061, 1997

McCarley RW, Wible CG, Frumin M, et al: MRI anatomy of schizophrenia. Biol Psychiatry 45:1099–1119, 1999

Meyerhoff DJ, MacKay S, Constans J-M, et al: Axonal injury and membrane alterations in Alzheimer's disease suggested by in vivo proton magnetic resonance spectroscopic imaging. Ann Neurol 36:40–47, 1994

Miatto O, Gonzalez RG, Buonanno F, et al: In vitro 31P NMR spectroscopy detects altered phospholipid metabolism in Alzheimer's disease. Can J Neurol Sci 13:535–539, 1986

Miller B, Moats R, Shonk T, et al: Alzheimer disease: depiction of increased cerebral myo-inositol with proton MR spectroscopy. Radiology 187:433–437, 1993

Miller BL, Chang L, Booth R, et al: In vivo 1H MRS choline: correlation with in vitro chemistry/histology. Life Sci 58:1929–1935, 1996

Moats RA, Ernst T, Shonk TK, et al: Abnormal cerebral metabolite concentrations in patients with probable Alzheimer disease. Magn Reson Med 32:110–115, 1994

Mohanakrishnan P, Fowler AH, Vonsattel JP, et al: An in vitro 1H nuclear magnetic resonance study of the temporoparietal cortex of Alzheimer brains. Exp Brain Res 102:503–510, 1995

Mohanakrishnan P, Fowler AH, Vonsattel JP, et al: Regional metabolic alterations in Alzheimer's disease: an in vitro 1H NMR study of the hippocampus and cerebellum. J Gerontol A Biol Sci Med Sci 52:B111–B117, 1997

Moonen CT, von Kienlin M, van Zijl PC, et al: Comparison of single-shot localization methods (STEAM and PRESS) for in vivo proton NMR spectroscopy. NMR Biomed 2:201–208, 1989

Moore CM, Christensen JD, Lafer B, et al: Lower levels of nucleoside triphosphate in the basal ganglia of depressed subjects: a phosphorus-31 magnetic resonance spectroscopy study. Am J Psychiatry 154:116–118, 1997

Murata T, Koshino Y, Omori M, et al: In vivo proton magnetic resonance spectroscopy study on premature aging in adult Down's syndrome. Biol Psychiatry 34:290–297, 1993

Murphy DG, Bottomley PA, Salerno JA, et al: An in vivo study of phosphorus and glucose metabolism in Alzheimer's disease using magnetic resonance spectroscopy and PET. Arch Gen Psychiatry 50:341–349, 1993

Nasrallah HA, Skinner TE, Schmalbrock P, et al: Proton magnetic resonance spectroscopy (1H MRS) of the hippocampal formation in schizophrenia: a pilot study. Br J Psychiatry 165:481–485, 1994

Nitsch R, Blusztajn J, Pittas A, et al: Evidence for a membrane defect in Alzheimer's disease brain. Proc Natl Acad Sci U S A 89:1671–1675, 1992

Ordidge RJ: Random noise selective excitation pulses. Magn Reson Med 5:93–98, 1987

Parnetti L, Lowenthal DT, Presciutti O, et al: 1H-MRS, MRI-based hippocampal volumetry, and 99mTc-HMPAO-SPECT innormal aging, age-associated memory impairment, and probable Alzheimer's disease. J Am Geriatr Soc 44:133–138, 1996

Parnetti L, Tarducci R, Presciutti O, et al: Proton magnetic resonance spectroscopy can differentiate Alzheimer's disease from normal aging. Mechanisms of Aging and Development 97:9–14, 1997

Pettegrew JW, Moossy J, Withers G, et al: 31P nuclear magnetic resonance study of the brain in Alzheimer's disease [published erratum appears in J Neuropathol Exp Neurol 48:118–119, 1989]. J Neuropathol Exp Neurol 47:235–248, 1988a

Pettegrew JW, Panchalingam K, Moossy J, et al: Correlation of phosphorus-31 magnetic resonance spectroscopy and morphologic findings in Alzheimer's disease. Arch Neurol 45:1093–1096, 1988b

Pettegrew JW, Keshavan MS, Panchalingam K, et al: Alterations in brain high-energy phosphate and membrane phospholipid metabolism in first-episode, drug-naive schizophrenics. Arch Gen Psychiatry 48:563–568, 1991a

Pettegrew JW, Panchalingam KS, Kaplan D, et al: Phosphorus 31 magnetic resonance spectroscopy detects altered brain metabolism before onset of schizophrenia. Arch Gen Psychiatry 48:1112–1113, 1991b

Pettegrew JW, Panchalingam K, Klunk WE, et al: Alterations of cerebral metabolism in probable Alzheimer's disease: a preliminary study. Neurobiol Aging 15:117–132, 1994

Pettegrew J, Klunk W, Kanal E, et al: Changes in brain membrane phospholipid and high-energy phosphate metabolism precede dementia. Neurobiol Aging 16:973–975, 1995

Pfefferbaum A, Adalsteinsson E, Spielman D, et al: In vivo brain concentrations of N-acetyl compounds, creatine, and choline in Alzheimer disease. Arch Gen Psychiatry 56:185–192, 1999

Podo F, Henriksen O, Bovee WM, et al: Absolute metabolite quantification by in vivo NMR spectroscopy, I: introduction, objectives and activities of a concerted action in biomedical research. Magn Reson Imaging 16:1085–1092, 1998

Prasad M, Lovell M, Yatin M, et al: Regional membrane phospholipid alterations in Alzheimer's disease. Neurochem Res 23:81–88, 1998

Renshaw PF, Haselgrove JC, Leigh JS, et al: In vivo nuclear magnetic resonance imaging of lithium. Magn Reson Med 2:512–516, 1985

Renshaw PF, Lafer B, Babb SM, et al: Basal ganglia choline levels in depression and response to fluoxetine treatment: an in vivo proton magnetic resonance spectroscopy study. Biol Psychiatry 41:837–843, 1997

Satlin A, Bodick N, Offen W, et al: Brain proton magnetic resonance spectroscopy (1H-MRS) in Alzheimer's disease: changes after treatment with xanomeline, an M1 selective cholinergic agonist. Am J Psychiatry 154:1459–1461, 1997

Schreier HA: Mania responsive to lecithin in a 13 year old girl. Am J Psychiatry 139: 108–110, 1982

Schuff N, Amend D, Ezekiel F, et al: Changes of hippocampal N-acetyl aspartate and volume in Alzheimer's disease: a proton MR spectroscopic imaging and MRI study. Neurology 49:1513–1521, 1997

Sharma R, Venkatasubramanian PN, Barany M, et al: Proton magnetic resonance spectroscopy of the brain in schizophrenic and affective patients. Schizophr Res 8: 43–49, 1992

Shiino A, Matsuda M, Morikawa S, et al: Proton magnetic resonance spectroscopy with dementia. Surg Neurol 39:143–147, 1993

Shioiri T, Kato T, Inubushi T, et al: Correlations of phosphomonoesters measured by phosphorus-31 magnetic resonance spectroscopy in the frontal lobes and negative symptoms in schizophrenia. Psychiatry Res 55:223–235, 1994

Shioiri T, Hamakawa H, Kato T, et al: Proton magnetic resonance spectroscopy of the basal ganglia in patients with schizophrenia: a preliminary report. Schizophr Res 22:19–26, 1996

Shioiri T, Someya T, Fujii K, et al: Differences in symptom structure between panic attack and limited symptom panic attack: a study using cluster analysis. Psychiatry Clin Neurosci 51:47–51, 1997

Shonk T, Moats R, Gifford P, et al: Probable Alzheimer disease: diagnosis with proton MR spectroscopy. Radiology 195:65–72, 1995

Siever LJ, Davis KL: Overview: toward a dysregulation hypothesis of depression. Am J Psychiatry 142:1017–1031, 1985

Simmons ML, Frondoza CG, Coyle JT: Immunocytochemical localization of N-acetyl-aspartate with monoclonal antibodies. Neuroscience 45:37–45, 1991

Smith CD, Gallenstein LG, Layton WJ, et al: 31P magnetic resonance spectroscopy in Alzheimer's and Pick's disease. Neurobiol Aging 14:85–92, 1993

Smith C, Pettegrew L, Avison M, et al: Frontal lobe phosphorus metabolism and neuropsychological function in aging and in Alzheimer's disease. Ann Neurol 38:194–201, 1995

Stokes C, Hawthorne J: Reduced phosphoinositide concentrations in anterior temporal cortex of Alzheimer-diseased brains. J Neurochem 48:1018–1021, 1987

Stoll AL, Cohen BM, Hanin I: Erythrocyte choline concentrations in psychiatric disorders. Biol Psychiatry 29:309–321, 1991

Stoll AL, Renshaw PF, De Micheli E, et al: Choline ingestion increases the resonance of choline-containing compounds in human brain: an in vivo proton magnetic resonance study. Biol Psychiatry 37:170–174, 1995

Stoll AL, Sachs GS, Cohen BM, et al: Choline in the treatment of rapid-cycling bipolar disorder: clinical and neurochemical findings in lithium treated patients. Biol Psychiatry 40:382–388, 1996

Tedeschi G, Bertolino A, Lundbom N, et al: Cortical and subcortical chemical pathology in Alzheimer's disease as assessed by multislice proton magnetic resonance spectroscopic imaging. Neurology 47:696–704, 1996

Volz HP, Rzanny R, May S, et al: 31P magnetic resonance spectroscopy in the dorsolateral prefrontal cortex of schizophrenics with a volume selective technique: preliminary findings. Biol Psychiatry 41:644–648, 1997

Volz HP, Hubner G, Rzanny R, et al: High-energy phosphates in the frontal lobe correlate with Wisconsin Card Sort Test performance in control subjects, not in schizophrenics: a 31phosphorus magnetic resonance spectroscopic and neuropsychological investigation. Schizophr Res 31:37–47, 1998

Volz HP, Rzanny R, Riechmann S, et al: 31P magnetic resonance spectroscopy in the frontal lobe of major depressed patients. Eur Arch Psychiatry Clin Neurosci 248: 289–295, 1999

Wu JC, Gillin JC, Buchsbaum MS, et al: Effect of sleep deprivation on brain metabolism of depressed patients. Am J Psychiatry 149:538–543, 1992

Yurgelun-Todd DA, Renshaw PF, Gruber SA, et al: Proton magnetic resonance spectroscopy of the temporal lobes in schizophrenics and normal controls. Schizophr Res 19:55–59, 1996

13

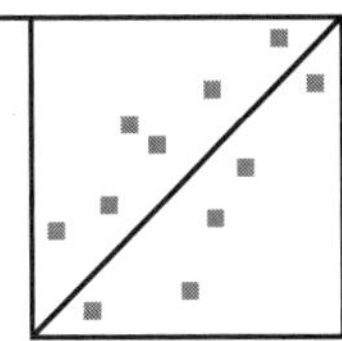

USE OF MAGNETIC RESONANCE IMAGING TO VISUALIZE CIRCUITS IMPLICATED IN DEVELOPMENTAL DISORDERS

The Examples of Attention-Deficit/ Hyperactivity Disorder and Anxiety

Daniel S. Pine, M.D.
Joseph Grun, B.S.
Bradley S. Peterson, M.D.

In this chapter, we review recent research on the use of magnetic resonance imaging (MRI) in the study of pediatric mental illnesses. We consider central issues in the design and implementation of MRI experiments involving children, through a review of paradigmatic models of pathophysiology, particularly in childhood psychiatric disorders. We first review neuroimaging approaches to the study of pediatric behavioral disorders, focusing on studies of attention-deficit/hyperactivity disorder (ADHD). In that section of the chapter, we illustrate the manner in which MRI can extend models of pediatric psychiatric disorder pathophysiology that are derived from research in the cognitive neurosciences. MRI research on ADHD provides a template for developing research

This research was supported by National Institute of Mental Health (NIMH) Scientist Development Awards for Clinicians (grant MH-01391 to D.S.P. and grants MH01232 and MH59139 to B.S.P.); NIMH center grant MH-43878 was awarded to the Center to Study Youth Depression, Anxiety and Suicide at New York State Psychiatric Institute.

programs focused on other less comprehensively studied conditions. In the second half of the chapter, we use this template to outline directions for imaging studies of pediatric anxiety disorders.

In MRI research involving children, neuroscientific and neuropsychological investigations can be integrated with the study of developmental psychopathology. We therefore review MRI research on pediatric anxiety and behavioral disorders in the context of prior neuroscientific investigations of these conditions. We begin with a summary of current neurobiologic models for a particular disorder, based largely on advances in neuroscience, coupled with imaging studies in adults. We emphasize the developmental aspects of each model. We then integrate this summary with a review of the neuropsychological literature, which extends findings in basic neuroscience and provides a rudimentary outline for neuroimaging paradigms. Existing neuroimaging data are then summarized. In the case of ADHD, we review relevant volumetric studies as well as functional paradigms that are designed to activate brain circuits that have been implicated in the pathophysiology of ADHD. In the case of anxiety disorders, we review current pathophysiologic models and efforts to extend these models by employing functional MRI (fMRI) paradigms that are suitable for children.

■ Attention-Deficit/Hyperactivity Disorder

Successful neuroimaging studies of specific pediatric psychiatric disorders depend on a unique set of advances in neuroscience, developmental psychopathology, and neuropsychology. The past 10 years have witnessed significant advances in research on the neural basis of attention, and these advances have coincided with advances in research on the neuropsychology and phenotypic features of ADHD. As a result, progress in neuroimaging research on ADHD has been relatively rapid compared with progress in pediatric mood or anxiety disorders. In this chapter, we focus on recent studies of ADHD, which shares possible pathophysiologic features with related conditions, including Tourette's syndrome and obsessive-compulsive disorder (Peterson and Klein 1997; Rosenberg and Keshavan 1998). We discuss MRI studies of such related conditions when the studies relate to a pathophysiology potentially shared with ADHD.

Pathophysiology

Neuroimaging experiments make it possible to weigh the advantages and disadvantages of specific models of pathophysiology in childhood disorders. A family of pathophysiologic models has emerged in ADHD, for example. In each model, the role of distinct brain circuitry in the disorder is emphasized, although the central role played by one or another area of the frontal cortex is emphasized in each model. Interestingly, the models derive from varying interpretations of similar experimental data generated in animal models or by indirect measures of attention in humans.

In one model, ADHD is attributed to a deficit in response inhibition (see, for example, Barkley 1997). The term *response inhibition* refers to the ability to suppress a prepotent (i.e., cognitively or behaviorally primed) response. Lesion experiments in animals as well as imaging studies in humans have implicated medial and ventral aspects of the frontal lobes, including components of both the orbitofrontal cortex and the cingulate gyrus (Barkley 1997; Fuster 1997; Posner and Raichle 1994), in behavioral inhibition. Deficient response inhibition in ADHD would therefore implicate a disturbance in orbitofrontal functioning. Furthermore, such a ventral defect is thought to disrupt more dorsal executive functions related to the regulation of behavior, cognition, and emotion. Therefore, ventral and medial prefrontal disturbances in ADHD are thought to contribute to the characteristic neuropsychological abnormalities and the clinical symptoms—impulsivity, distractibility, and hyperactivity—associated with the disorder.

In another model, ADHD is viewed as a heterogeneous group of syndromes resulting from disturbances in multiple related neural circuits (for example, see Swanson et al. 1998a, 1998b). In this model, as in the response inhibition model, a ventral prefrontal deficit is thought to produce the symptoms of impulsivity and hyperactivity. However, a greater emphasis is placed in this model on attentional deficits. These deficits include problems with "alerting" or maintaining attention—that is, focusing on a particular act, thought, or percept while excluding background stimuli (LaBerge 1995; Pashler 1998; Swanson et al. 1998a, 1998b). Lesion and imaging studies have implicated circuits that connect the right dorsolateral prefrontal and parietal cortices in this form of attention. In this model, therefore, an abnormality in right prefrontal and parietal cortices is posited as the basis for poor sustained effort in ADHD. Finally, a deficit in orienting, another aspect of attention, is thought to result from dysfunction in a third circuit involving the parietal lobes, superior colliculus, and pulvinar nucleus. Disturbances in this circuitry are thought to produce distractibility, another cardinal feature of ADHD.

Although these two models of ADHD are occasionally seen as competing theories, they can also be viewed as complementary. The activities of the dorsal and ventral aspects of the prefrontal cortex, for example, are tightly coupled (Fuster 1997). Different models may therefore account for distinct but equally important clinical features of ADHD. A primary ventral prefrontal abnormality, for instance, could impair executive functions regulated by the dorsolateral prefrontal cortex. Alternatively, a primary abnormality in dorsolateral prefrontal maturation may result in insufficient regulation of ventral prefrontal functioning (Arnsten et al. 1996; Barkley 1997; Fuster 1997). Moreover, from a developmental perspective, dorsal and ventral aspects of the prefrontal cortex play complementary roles in the response inhibition and maintenance functions of attention over time. For example, the effect of both dorsal and ventral lesions on delayed-response behavior in primates varies with age (Lewis 1997).

For each model of ADHD, deficits in prefrontal functioning represent a central aspect of disrupted functioning in larger and more distributed neural circuits. Emphasized in each model, from the input side of this circuitry, is a role for afferent monoamine tracts ascending from the midbrain to the prefrontal cortex in symptoms of ADHD, with the beneficial effects of stimulant medications being attributed to the agents' effects on prefrontal functioning (Arnsten 1997; Arnsten et al. 1996; Barkley 1997; Swanson et al. 1998a, 1998b). This view of the mechanism of stimulant action stands in contrast to earlier views in which successful treatment of ADHD was attributed to the restoration of "balance" among monoamine systems (Rogeness et al. 1992). In more current models, successful pharmacologic treatment involves modulation of disturbances in functioning of prefrontal circuits by the monoamine systems. Similarly, concerning the output side of this circuitry, the role of glutamatergic efferents from the prefrontal cortex to supplementary motor, premotor, and subcortical motor systems is emphasized in current models of ADHD. The disorder can therefore be viewed as a family of conditions resulting from an array of brain-based disturbances—in the afferents to the prefrontal cortex, in the prefrontal cortex itself, or in prefrontal efferents to the lower motor systems. This circuitry-based approach thereby provides a novel perspective on diagnostic heterogeneity. ADHD may represent a final common pathway resulting from defects in relatively complex but interrelated neural circuits, and distinct subtypes of the disorder may result from distinct abnormalities in particular portions of the underlying circuitry.

In summary, current theories suggest that ADHD is the clinical manifestation of a disturbance in one or more components of a complex neural circuit involving the prefrontal cortices and related premotor and subcortical motor systems. Existing brain imaging studies support these views, while providing clues for future clinical and neuroscientific investigations of attention and ADHD. As imaging technology progresses, the specific roles of circuits involving either the dorsal or ventral aspects of the frontal lobes will undoubtedly be investigated intensively. This work will require development of appropriate imaging paradigms, and such development will be aided by neuropsychological findings.

Neuropsychology

In current theories concerning the neural basis of ADHD, there is integration of extensive neuropsychological data on prefrontal and motor functioning. Numerous studies have implicated both dorsal and ventral prefrontal deficits in ADHD, as well as deficits in lower motor systems. We summarize these data only briefly, because recent reviews provide a more comprehensive summary of this vast literature (Barkley 1997; Oosterlaan and Sergeant 1996; Pennington and Ozonoff 1996; Swanson et al. 1998a, 1998b). In general, many of these reviews emphasize the findings from neuropsychological tests that probe frontal functions, regarded in general terms as tests of executive functioning. These functions also have been grouped at times into more narrowly defined classes of cognitive functioning, including functions with a predominant dorsal prefrontal, ventral prefrontal, or motor component. We describe characteristic tasks for each of these categories of executive functioning, emphasizing tasks that have been shown to differentiate children with ADHD from psychiatrically healthy children.

Classic tests of executive function that have a strong dorsal prefrontal component include working memory tasks (such as digit span recall or delayed-response tasks), language tasks (such as word generation), planning tasks (such as the Tower of London or Tower of Hanoi), and set-shifting tasks (such as the Wisconsin Card Sorting Test) (Pennington and Ozonoff 1996). In general, children with ADHD perform many of these tasks poorly, although the precise nature of the performance of a given task has varied across studies. Moreover, defects in some executive functions, particularly in attentional regulation, are implicated in many pediatric disorders, and the degree to which such abnormalities are specific to ADHD remains unclear.

Classic tests of executive function that have a strong ventral prefrontal component include tasks that require inhibition of prepotent responses. Such tasks include the Stroop Word-Color Test, go/no-go tasks, and continuous performance tasks (Barkley 1997; Oosterlaan and Sergeant 1996). Tasks developed from basic science studies of ventral prefrontal functioning have been used in more recent studies involving children with ADHD. Examples include time-estimation tasks, in which subjects must withhold a response until sufficient time has elapsed, and gambling tasks, in which subjects make choices after inferring different reward contingencies (Damasio 1994; White et al. 1994). With tasks having a ventral prefrontal focus, as with tasks with a dorsolateral prefrontal component, children with ADHD can be distinguished readily from psychiatrically healthy children. Moreover, children with ADHD have been distinguished, with tasks having a ventral prefrontal focus, from control subjects with anxiety disorders, although children with ADHD and children with other impulse control disorders tend to show similar deficits when they perform tasks that have a strong ventral prefrontal component (Oosterlaan and Sergeant 1996).

Finally, motor control tasks have also been used in studies involving children with ADHD. Typically rated with such tasks is a child's ability to perform motor manipulations, such as finger-to-finger opposition, tapping, or rapid-alternating movement. Although these tasks involve a prefrontal component, they depend heavily on the integrity of supplementary motor and premotor cortices as well as the basal ganglia and cerebellum. Children with ADHD generally perform these tasks poorly, but the degree to which motor control abnormalities characterize ADHD, as opposed to other disorders, remains unresolved (Carte et al. 1996; Pine et al. 1997; Rosenberg and Keshavan 1998; White et al. 1997).

MRI Research

ADHD neuroimaging studies have tested explicit hypotheses of ADHD-related circuitry derived from available neuropsychological data. In this section, we briefly summarize findings from volumetric and functional imaging studies.

Volumetric Studies

At least five research groups have compared the volumes of various central nervous system structures in children with ADHD and comparison children. Investigators have focused on a common set of neural structures, selected for analysis because they were implicated in ADHD pathophysiology by the neuropsychological and psychophysiologic studies described earlier. The most intensively studied structures include the prefrontal cortex; subcortical motor systems, including the basal ganglia and cerebellum; and the corpus callosum. The findings of these studies are summarized in Table 13–1.

As shown in Table 13–1, abnormalities have been found in every region thus far examined in patients with ADHD. However, the hypothesized between-group differences have not been noted in all studies, and when abnormalities have been noted, the effect sizes have been small. Rarely have chil-

TABLE 13–1. Structural magnetic resonance imaging studies of attention-deficit/hyperactivity disorder

Research group and reference	Findings			
	Prefrontal cortex	**Basal ganglia and cerebellum**	**Corpus callosum**	**Total cerebral volume**
NIMH (n=36–112)				
Castellanos et al. 1996	R frontal region volume reduction (4%) in ADHD pts (adjusted for total brain volume)	R > L caudate and L > R lenticular nucleus asymmetry in psychiatrically healthy control subjects, not in ADHD pts; caudate volume reduction on R R-sided globus pallidus volume reduction (10%) No difference in putamen volume		
Berquin et al. 1998		Cerebellar vermis and lobules VIII–X volume reduction (4%–6%)		2%–3% reduction
Giedd et al. 1994			Rostrum and rostral body volume reduction (7%–15%); not replicated in full sample	

TABLE 13–1. Structural magnetic resonance imaging studies of attention-deficit/hyperactivity disorder *(continued)*

Research group and reference	Findings			
	Prefrontal cortex	**Basal ganglia and cerebellum**	**Corpus callosum**	**Total cerebral volume**
MGH/HARVARD (*n*=30)				
Semrud-Clikeman et al. 1994			Plenium volume reduction (6%)	
Filipek et al. 1997	Frontal region volume reduction in ADHD pts, particularly on R (6%)	Caudate volume reduction in ADHD pts, particularly on L; L > R caudate asymmetry in psychiatrically healthy control subjects, not in ADHD pts		No statistically significant difference, although 5% reduction in ADHD pts
Univeristy of Georgia (*n*=22–30)				
Hynd et al. 1991, 1993		L > R caudate asymmetry in psychiatrically healthy control subjects; R > L caudate asymmetry in ADHD pts; L caudate volume reduction (11%) in ADHD pts	Genu and splenium volume reduction	No statistically significant difference
Hynd et al. 1990	Loss of R > L asymmetry in frontal region (on single slice)			

TABLE 13–1. Structural magnetic resonance imaging studies of attention-deficit/hyperactivity disorder *(continued)*

Research group and reference	Findings: Prefrontal cortex	Findings: Basal ganglia and cerebellum	Findings: Corpus callosum	Findings: Total cerebral volume
Johns Hopkins (n=37–55)				
Aylward et al. 1996		Globus pallidus volume reduction on L in ADHD pts No caudate asymmetry in psychiatrically healthy control subjects; slight L > R caudate asymmetry in ADHD pts		
Mostofsky et al. 1998		Superior cerebellar vermis and lobules VIII–X volume reduction		
Singer et al. 1993		R > L lenticular asymmetry in pts with both ADHD and Tourette's syndrome L > R putamen volume in control subjects but not in Tourette's syndrome pts		
Yale (n=28) (adults)				
Peterson et al. 1993		L > R asymmetry in lenticular nucleus in psychiatrically healthy control subjects but not in Tourette's syndrome pts		

Note. ADHD = attention-deficit/hyperactivity disorder; L = left; MGH = Massachusetts General Hospital; NIMH = National Institute of Mental Health; pts = patients; R = right.

dren with ADHD, for example, exhibited a consistent reduction in volume of more than 5% in any brain structure. Studies have focused on brain regions known to exhibit robust developmental changes, such as the prefrontal cortex or basal ganglia, and therefore the extent to which developmental differences between diagnostic groups influence findings remains unclear (Castellanos et al. 1996).

Prefrontal cortex All three studies that have compared cortical volumes in ADHD patients and psychiatrically healthy control subjects have found a reduction in the volume of the right prefrontal region (Table 13–1). Although this finding is consistent with current models of ADHD pathophysiology, the studies have yet to determine whether the volume of gray matter or white matter in the prefrontal cortex is reduced, nor have these studies examined the volumes of prefrontal subregions.

Subcortical motor systems Although two studies have found a reduction in cerebellar volumes in children with ADHD (Berquin et al. 1998; Mostofsky et al. 1998) (Table 13–1), abnormalities in basal ganglia volumes in ADHD remain among the most consistent findings in child psychiatry imaging research. At least five research groups have found some sign of an abnormality in the basal ganglia in children with ADHD; abnormal asymmetries of basal ganglia volumes are the most consistent finding. Nevertheless, there are inconsistencies in findings across studies (Table 13–1). First, reductions have been reported in different subregions of the basal ganglia. Second, although loss of asymmetry is the most consistent finding in ADHD, asymmetry has varied in psychiatrically healthy children; asymmetry findings also have involved differing basal ganglia subregions, with two studies finding greater right hemisphere volumes and three finding greater left hemisphere volumes. Finally, sample sizes in each study have been relatively small, and data from the largest study thus far suggest heterogeneity in the effect at least partially related to subject age (Castellanos et al. 1996).

The origin of reduced basal ganglia volumes in ADHD is unclear. Studies involving low-birth-weight children suggest a possible role for perinatal trauma (Whitaker et al. 1997), a theory consistent with the noted correlation between perinatal adversity and basal ganglia volume in ADHD (Castellanos et al. 1996). In contrast, studies involving patients with Tourette's syndrome raise the possibility that basal ganglia structure and function may be genetically determined (Hyde et al. 1995; Peterson et al. 1993; Singer et al. 1993; Wolf et al. 1996). Finally, basal ganglia abnormalities have been implicated in obsessive-compulsive disorder in children (Rosenberg and Keshavan 1998).

Some investigators have hypothesized that volume reductions in obsessive-compulsive disorder may result from immunological mechanisms related to infection with group A β-hemolytic streptococcus. Peterson et al. (1999) provided evidence that a comparable mechanism could play a role in ADHD.

Corpus callosum As shown in Table 13–1, a third consistent finding is reduced cross-sectional area of the corpus callosum. Like the findings relating to basal ganglia volumes, corpus callosum findings are highly variable across studies. Each study, for instance, has found reductions in distinct subregions of the corpus callosum, with some groups emphasizing reductions in the splenium and others emphasizing reductions in the genu. In general, investigators have attempted to place such findings in the context of basic neuroscience research on attention. Areas of association cortex, such as the prefrontal cortex, make a strong contribution to the white matter tracts in the corpus callosum, in accordance with the integrative function of this structure. Abnormalities in cortical association areas should be reflected in reduced volumes of projection fibers from these regions. Therefore, abnormalities in the prefrontal association cortex related to deficiencies in inhibitory functions would be expected to produce a reduction in genu size. Abnormalities in the parietal association cortex related to deficits in attention, on the other hand, would be expected to reduce the size of the splenium.

Integration of volumetric and neuropsychological data Whereas many initial MRI studies compared the volumes of specific brain regions of ADHD patients with those of psychiatrically healthy control subjects, subsequent studies began to examine group differences in brain-behavior associations, such as those between regional brain volumes and neuropsychological test performance. Castellanos et al. (1996), for instance, initially contrasted brain volumes in a relatively large sample of psychiatrically healthy children and children with ADHD. Casey et al. (1997a) then examined the associations between frontal and striatal volumes and measures of response inhibition across diagnostic groups in this sample. Associations were noted between ratings of performance of response inhibition tasks and prefrontal and basal ganglia volumes, consistent with response inhibition theories of ADHD (Barkley 1997). Other investigators have also related neuropsychological test performance to volumetric data. Reiss et al. (1996) and Castellanos et al. (1996), for example, noted an association between performance on an intelligence test and prefrontal volume. Similarly, Casey et al. (1995) noted an association between a measure of attention and cingulate volume. Each of these groups of researchers attempted to enhance the sensitivity for detecting brain-behavior associations by using neuropsychological tasks that had been previously linked to the functioning of specific brain regions.

Directions for future volumetric studies Although the ADHD findings are generally consistent with findings from neuropsychological and basic science studies, the ADHD studies have numerous limitations. Three issues appear particularly important.

First, none of the available studies took advantage of the sensitivity of current MRI methods to fully test hypotheses relating to ADHD circuitry. For example, with regard to hypotheses concerning the role of ventral prefrontal or cingulate cortices in inhibitory functions, it is possible to examine associations between specific volume reductions in these areas, particularly in cortical gray matter, with either the clinical phenotype of ADHD or performance on neuropsychological tests.

Second, current studies have generally used cross-sectional designs to model age-by-disorder interactions for brain volumes. Such studies have suggested that ADHD may be characterized by an abnormality in brain development, in that volume reductions in various brain regions can vary across groups as a function of age as well as of sex (Castellanos et al. 1996). Nevertheless, a longitudinal repeated-measures design, such as that recently used in a schizophrenia study (Rapoport et al. 1997), would provide greater sensitivity for detecting age-specific abnormalities in the brains of children with developmental disabilities.

Finally, reductions in brain volume are likely to play a role in the pathophysiology of ADHD by disrupting brain function. Schizophrenia studies have found that insights in this area can be gained by combining volumetric data with data obtained by fMRI or magnetic resonance spectroscopy. For example, schizophrenia is associated with a reduction in frontal lobe volume and a reduction in the viability of neurons in the frontal cortex as assessed with magnetic resonance spectroscopy (Lim et al. 1998). Similar advances could be made by integrating volumetric and functional imaging paradigms in children.

Current Functional Imaging Paradigms

To date, only one study exists in the literature in which fMRI was used to compare ADHD children with psychiatrically healthy control subjects (Vaidya et al. (1998). Moreover, the literature contains only a handful of studies in which fMRI was used to probe attentional and response inhibition circuitry in healthy volunteer children. Because of the paucity of research in this area, we briefly review findings from fMRI studies involving adults as well as children in this section, focusing on the neuropsychological tasks that are designed to activate components of ADHD-related neural circuitry. We emphasize paradigms that are currently being implemented in children. The study by Vaidya et al. (1998) is discussed within this context.

Tasks with a ventral prefrontal or striatal focus Several tasks seem to activate ventral prefrontal and related striatal regions consistently in adult subjects. Tasks that activate ventral frontal as well as related striatal regions and that also distinguish, in terms of behavior, psychiatrically healthy children from children with ADHD include go/no-go tasks, the Stroop task, and motor inhibition tasks (Peterson and Klein 1997). These tasks consistently activate components of the cingulate gyrus that seem to subserve inhibitory functions in animals (Devinsky et al. 1995). The tasks also activate areas of the ventral prefrontal cortex, including Brodmann's areas 11 and 12, with reasonable consistency. Finally, these tasks activate lower motor cortical regions and components of the basal ganglia, through which motor commands from the prefrontal cortex are channeled. Typically, these tasks require subjects to inhibit a prepotent response during the experimental phase of the task. The tasks also require subjects to perform related tasks without an inhibitory component during control phases of the task. For example, in a study by Peterson et al. (1999), subjects were required to inhibit the more automatic response (that of reading the text of colored word stimuli) during the experimental portion of the Stroop Word-Color Test. During control portions, subjects were required to perform the task that does not require response inhibition (i.e., the task of naming the color of the colored words). The anterior cingulate and ventral prefrontal cortices were shown to activate robustly during the response inhibition portions of the task. Shown in Figure 13–1 is the group average activation map for 34 subjects performing the Stroop task.

Vaidya et al. (1998) used fMRI to document the reduced capacity of ADHD children to activate the basal ganglia and ventral aspects of the frontal lobes when performing a go/no-go task. Stimulant medication increased basal ganglia activation in children who had ADHD but not in psychiatrically healthy children. This study exemplifies some of the ways in which future fMRI studies might provide key insights into the pathophysiology and therapeutics of ADHD.

Tasks with a dorsolateral prefrontal focus An extensive set of fMRI studies has mapped the role of the dorsolateral prefrontal cortex in working memory functions in adult subjects. Spatial working memory tasks, for instance, have

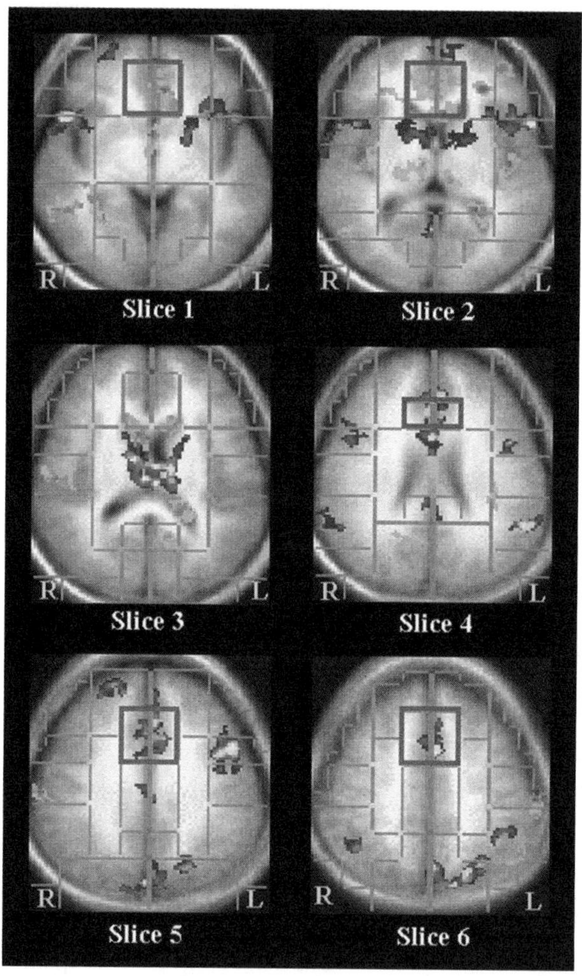

FIGURE 13–1. Composite activation map for 34 adult subjects (18 men and 16 women; ages 18–57 years [mean ± standard deviation, 29.3 ± 10.8 years]) performing the Stroop Color-Word Task. Slice 1 was the most ventral axial slice, Slice 6 the most dorsal. The green boxes correspond with Talairach-defined regions of interest. The box outlined in purple defines the anterior division of the cingulate gyrus. Decreases in activity are seen more ventrally and increases in activity are seen more dorsally in this region. Models of functional connectivity indicate that the functional activity in this region is tightly coupled with activity in most other regions that are activated during performance of the task (Peterson et al. 1999).

been used to activate superior aspects of the dorsolateral prefrontal cortex, and tests in which objects are employed as stimuli have been used to activate inferior aspects of this region. Casey et al. (1995) found that healthy children also activate the dorsolateral prefrontal cortex when performing similar tasks. Because this cortical region is implicated in the pathophysiology of ADHD, fMRI studies are currently using these tasks to compare prefrontal activation in children with and in those without ADHD. These studies may ultimately make it possible to test the competing hypotheses concerning the origin of dorsolateral prefrontal dysfunction in ADHD. As already noted, some investigators attribute dorsolateral prefrontal deficits to a primary ventral dysfunction (Barkley 1997), whereas others view dorsolateral prefrontal deficits as primary in some features of the ADHD symptom complex (Swanson et al. 1998a, 1998b).

Motor control paradigms In the earliest fMRI studies, efforts were made to map brain regions implicated in simple motor functions, such as finger movements. These studies spawned a second generation of fMRI studies, devoted to mapping brain regions implicated in the refinement of motor control. These studies included studies of short-term changes in brain regions during the implicit learning of a motor sequence and studies of slightly longer-term changes associated with learning motor control tasks over many days (Berns et al. 1998).

fMRI studies of motor performance are relevant to the pathophysiology of ADHD because the impulsivity and hyperactivity components of ADHD may relate to disturbances in the circuitry subserving motor control. For example, Peterson et al. (1998) examined activity in frontal and striatal regions during the suppression of motor tics. Significant activation of the inferior prefrontal region and inferior portions of all basal ganglia regions was associated with volitional tic suppression. More severe motor tics occurring outside the scanner predicted a reduced ability to activate these inhibitory circuits, suggesting that symptom severity in this hyperkinetic disorder is related at least in part to disturbances of inhibitory control.

Directions for future functional MRI studies Studies in adults have consistently shown activation in the appropriate brain regions using the tasks described. Activations have also been found in these regions in children in unpublished studies. The stage is set for studies that examine the neural circuitry underlying psychiatric disorders such as ADHD. At least three central methodological issues must be addressed in these studies: the need to develop methods that will permit quantification of the activity in distributed neural circuits; the importance of contrasting children with psychiatric illness and psychiatrically healthy children; and the importance of characterizing and adequately accounting for developmental changes in neural activity of the circuits of interest.

Discussion

Emphasized in current pathophysiologic models of ADHD is the role played by distributed neural circuits involving the prefrontal cortex, brain stem monoamine systems, and cortical and subcortical motor systems. These theories are largely derived from animal studies or human investigations that relied on indirect measures of brain function. With recent developments in MRI, both volumetric and functional imaging studies have begun to define a role for an aberrant frontostriatal circuitry in this condition. MRI therefore holds considerable promise for advancing research in ADHD. Assessment of the neural basis of this condition using MRI methods may make it possible to refine definitions for this syndrome, potentially clarifying controversial issues concerning diagnostic subtyping. Moreover, the insights obtained with MRI methods into the mechanisms underlying effective treatment may lead to major treatment advances. Finally, integration of serial MRI assessments performed early in life with studies of genetics and cognitive maturation may elucidate methods for early detection of ADHD, which could lead to major gains in disease prevention.

■ Anxiety

Whereas ADHD is one of the most studied childhood psychiatric disorders from the perspective of brain imaging, childhood anxiety disorders, particularly social phobia and generalized anxiety disorder, are among the least studied conditions. Neuroimaging studies in pediatric ADHD have benefited from extensive research using animal models, neuroimaging paradigms among adults, and neuropsychological paradigms among children. Imaging studies in ADHD represent the culmination of a systematic series of studies in these related fields.

Research on pediatric anxiety currently stands at the same juncture at which ADHD research stood only a few years ago. Animal studies have contributed to pathophysiologic models of adult anxiety disorders. Through neuropsychological and brain imaging research paradigms, these models are being applied successfully to the study of anxiety disorders in adults (Bechara et al. 1995; Bisaga et al. 1998; Bremner 1998). Efforts to apply these approaches in children have been stimulated by research on the course and familial nature of anxiety disorders, coupled with research on developmental plasticity in the neural circuitry that mediates anxiety in animals (Liu et al. 1997; Rosen and Schulkin 1998). Nevertheless, the literature contains no neuroimaging study to date that has examined children who have social phobia, generalized anxiety disorder, or even a related condition such as behavioral inhibition. In fact, to our knowledge, only one study has used fMRI to study emotion in children or adolescents (Baird et al. 1999).

Pathophysiology

Current pathophysiologic theories of human anxiety disorders draw heavily on basic science research that has contributed to animal models of anxiety. Much reliance has been placed on studies of fear conditioning, especially conditioning to explicit cues. When an animal is being conditioned to fear a stimulus, a discrete neutral conditioned stimulus (CS), such as a tone or a light, is paired with an aversive stimulus (unconditioned stimulus [UCS]) such as a shock or an aversive air-puff. The CS then acquires the ability to elicit behaviors that were formerly associated only with the UCS. Many converging lines of evidence suggest that information on the CS and UCS is transmitted from the relevant sensory organs to the basolateral nucleus of the amygdala, which in turn projects to the central nucleus of the amygdala (Davis 1997; LeDoux 1996, 1998). Fear responses are then mediated by output from the amygdala to motor and autonomic systems. Although various anxiety disorders are thought to involve these amygdala-based processes, phobias have been frequently linked to processes that subserve conditioned fear (LeDoux 1996). Over the past two decades, evidence implicating fear conditioning in the pathophysiology of phobias has included data from psychophysiologic, therapeutic, and brain imaging studies, discussed in detail later in this chapter.

When a more complicated stimulus serves as a CS, the process of fear conditioning is thought to involve the hippocampus (Berger and Orr 1983; Clark and Squire 1998; Gray and McNaughton 1996; McNaughton 1997). Hippocampal involvement in fear conditioning applies to phenomena such as trace conditioning, in which a temporal delay separates the CS from the UCS; hippocampal involvement may also apply to conditioning to context, in which an organism develops a fear response to the context in which the UCS was received. Involvement of the hippocampus may also relate to conscious processing of CS-UCS relationships with a complex CS. Recruitment of the hippocampus may be particularly important for the conscious, subjective state of "anxiety," a major source of suffering in anxiety disorders (Clark and Squire 1998). Given the possible role of the hippocampus in contextual conditioning and in the conscious experience of anxiety, there is a tendency in current anxiety theories to emphasize a role for hippocampus-dependent neural processes. Research on the hippocampus in anxiety disorders has appeared particularly relevant for three specific conditions: posttraumatic stress disorder, panic disorder with agoraphobia, and generalized anxiety disorder (Bremner 1998; Gray and McNaughton 1996; LeDoux 1996, 1998).

In the discussion that follows, we focus primarily on generalized anxiety disorder, because of previous intensive efforts to integrate the developmentally oriented clinical and basic science research on this condition (Gray and McNaughton 1996; Pine and Grun 1999). In addition to fear conditioning studies, studies of the effects of hippocampal lesions and pharmacologic agents on constructs related to generalized anxiety disorder have implicated the hippocampus in anxiety. Both manipulations reduce the bias that an organism faces in a conflict-laden situation (Gray and McNaughton 1996). Other evidence, summarized in the next section, derives from neuropsychological studies of fear-related bias in human anxiety disorder (Williams et al. 1996).

Neuropsychology and Psychophysiology

Social Phobia

Imaging studies of social phobia have extended earlier studies of the neuropsychology and psychophysiology of anxiety, the findings of which are in turn consistent with findings obtained with animal models of anxiety. Psychophysiologic and neuropsychological studies of the neural basis of fear in humans have in fact often adopted paradigms that were previously developed to elucidate the circuitry of fear in animals. For example, the fear-potentiated startle paradigm has been used to probe the circuitry of conditioned fear in humans, after observations regarding the central role of the amygdala in mediating fear-potentiated startle in animal models (Davis 1997; Grillon et al. 1997). In this paradigm, a CS enhances the startle reflex, a brain stem–based reaction that is modulated by higher circuits, including an amygdala-based circuit. Amygdala lesions in animals block this neuromodulation. Similarly, phobic individuals demonstrate potentiation of the startle reflex in the presence of a particularly feared object (Lang et al. 1990), a finding that suggests the presence of a similar amygdala-based influence of the startle response in phobic individuals.

Other investigators have manipulated perceptual features of conditioning tasks to examine the psychophysiology of fear. Öhman (1986), for example, developed the masking paradigm to examine the role of subcortical processing in phobias. He demonstrated the presence of conditioned responses to subliminally presented masked facial stimuli. Phobic individuals are thought to exhibit either enhanced conditioning or reduced habituation to these masked CSs. These psychophysiologic abnormalities in phobic persons may result from a preattentive bias for processing of fear-relevant stimuli.

Recent neuropsychological studies of anxiety have intensively examined fear-related bias in attentional tasks. Individuals with phobias show a preattentive bias for various phobia-relevant stimuli, including pictures or words (Williams et al. 1996). This bias is observable as a prolonged latency in performing a task such as the emotional Stroop, which requires color naming in the presence of emotionally laden written words. This preattentive bias for phobic and emotional stimuli may contribute to emotional memory, in which individuals exhibit memory-recall biases for stimuli that relate to fear-relevant stimuli (Cahill and McGaugh 1996; Lundh and Ost 1996). This recall bias might result from either amygdala-based or hippocampus-based processes (Gray and McNaughton 1996; Williams et al. 1996).

Generalized Anxiety Disorder

Findings from neuropsychological and psychophysiologic studies of generalized anxiety disorder overlap in part with findings from similar studies of phobias. Much like phobias, generalized anxiety disorder in adults is associated with a preattentive bias for aversive stimuli (Williams et al. 1996). In phobias, however, this bias relates to specific sensory cues, whereas in generalized anxiety disorder, the bias relates to more diffuse anxiety-provoking stimuli. Moreover, a preattentive bias in generalized anxiety disorder may arise in situations that involve an experimentally induced conflict between appetitive and aversive stimuli. The broader conceptualization of "anxiety," in fact, has been viewed as a bias for perceiving or recalling the aversive aspects of conflict situations that are inherent in many models of anxiety but are particularly prominent in models of generalized anxiety disorder (Gray and McNaughton 1996; McNaughton 1997). The frequent comorbidity between generalized anxiety and other anxiety disorders may in fact reflect the conflict between appetitive and aversive stimuli that accompanies many forms of human anxiety but that is most purely encountered in generalized anxiety disorder (Gray and McNaughton 1996).

Developmental Models of Anxiety

Paradigms used to study anxiety and phobias in adults have also been used in studies involving children, for the purpose of studying the developmental aspects of fear and anxiety. For example, Kagan (1995, 1997) documented an association between fearful or inhibited behavior in toddlers and psychophysiologic evidence of amygdala activity. Such findings are consistent with the finding of an association between inhibited behavior and clinical anxiety disorders in family-based and longitudinal studies (Pine et al. 1998).

More recently, other neuropsychological and psychophysiologic paradigms used to study adult anxiety have been used in the study of childhood populations. Such paradigms include perceptual bias, divided attention, fear-potentiated startle, and memory tasks (Chansky and Kendall 1997; Grillon et al. 1997; Pine et al. 1998, 1999; Vasey et al. 1996). In general, these studies have provided some evidence for an association between anxiety and cognitive functioning. However, the findings of these studies are quite heterogeneous, possibly because of individual variabilities in disease course and family history.

Discussion

Psychophysiologic and neuropsychological studies have implicated components of the fear-conditioning circuit in human anxiety, both in children and in adults. Findings in humans closely parallel findings in animal models of anxiety. Nevertheless, these data only indirectly implicate fear circuitry in human anxiety; in vivo imaging techniques are best suited for directly assessing the role of specific brain structures in basic human psychological processes.

Functional MRI Research

As already noted, very few neuroimaging studies have focused on childhood phobias or generalized anxiety disorder, and relatively few MRI studies of these conditions have been performed in adults. The majority of neuroimaging studies of anxiety have examined panic disorder, posttraumatic stress disorder, or obsessive-compulsive disorder, and most have been positron emission tomography (PET) studies. Despite the paucity of prior research, interest in imaging-based studies of childhood anxiety has grown considerably. Much of this interest has followed from observations in family-based and longitudinal studies that children at risk for chronic anxiety exhibit signs of anxiety disturbances early in life (Pine et al. 1998; Weissman et al. 1984). Interest has also been generated by the suggestions from adult imaging studies that the neural circuitry of fear states is similar across species. Extending developmental models of fear states from animals to humans is therefore important (Coplan et al. 1996; Liu al. 1997; Meaney et al. 1993).

fMRI has emerged as a particularly important method for extending these findings from animal models because this form of imaging combines safety and tolerability, with regard to children, and acquisition of functional data that have excellent spatial and good temporal resolution. Relative to structural MRI, fMRI is better suited for the study of state- as opposed to trait-related information, an aspect that may be critically important for the study of anxiety disorders. Although longitudinal studies have established an early age of onset for anxiety disorders, for instance, they also have documented the strong episodic nature of these disorders. In fact, in most children in these studies, anxiety disorders remit (Pine and Grun 1999). State-related information may therefore provide key insights into the neural basis on these conditions, particularly as it relates to natural history and to changes in symptom severity. We summarize here the recent fMRI studies that have examined the neural circuitry of fear and anxiety in adults, focusing on processes that are relevant to social phobia and generalized anxiety disorder. Recent findings in healthy adults have stimulated new research that is designed to probe the neural circuitry of pathological anxiety in both adults and children.

Social Phobia

As already noted, neuropsychological studies have demonstrated a bias in social phobia for socially relevant stimuli, and psychophysiologic data have indicated that this bias operates at a preattentive level of information processing. For example, persons with social phobia exhibit a bias for fearful faces that might relate to subcortical processing of fearful stimuli (Öhman 1986). Recent fMRI studies in adults have implicated the amygdala in the processing of fearful faces. In fact, at least four studies in adults have demonstrated amygdala activation during the processing of fearful faces (Breiter et al. 1996; Morris et al. 1996; Phillips and LeDoux 1992; Whalen et al. 1998b). A fifth study found amygdala activation in adolescents performing a facial recognition task (Baird et al. 1999).

Recent studies have focused on the role of conscious awareness in mediating amygdala activation during facial recognition tasks. Using PET, for instance, Morris et al. (1998, 1999) suggested that the right amygdala is active when facial stimuli are processed below the level of awareness; the left amygdala is active when faces are consciously perceived. Whalen and colleagues (1998b) used fMRI to demonstrate amygdala activation in response to subliminally presented masked faces, drawing on the masking procedures previously used by Öhman (1986). Following this lead, we used this task to contrast amygdala activity during the viewing of masked fearful faces with the activity during viewing of masked happy faces. An example of amygdala activation in response to fearful as opposed to happy faces is shown in Figure 13–2. Consistent with findings by Morris et al. (1999) and Whalen et al. (1998b), subliminally presented fearful faces produced right-sided amygdala activation.

More recent studies have explored the effect of other fear-inducing stimuli on the amygdala. Buchel et al. (1998), for example, used conditioned fearful faces to examine amygdala activation in an event-related imaging paradigm, noting amygdala activation during the viewing of formerly conditioned fearful faces. Similarly, LaBar et al. (1998) demonstrated amygdala activation in response to visual cues that had previously been conditioned with electric shock. In light of the relatively consistent amygdala activation seen in fMRI experiments using fear-relevant stimuli, ongoing studies are examining amygdala activity in child and adult patient groups. For example, Birbaumer et al. (1998) examined the extent of amygdala activation during a facial recognition task in socially phobic adults. These investigators noted increased amygdala activation in the patients with social phobia compared with psychiatrically healthy control subjects. Similarly, Baird et al. (1999) noted amygdala activation in response to fearful faces in volunteer children. These studies have set the stage for imaging research on pediatric social phobia.

Generalized Anxiety Disorder

The development of fMRI paradigms relevant to the study of generalized anxiety disorder has been slower. Nevertheless, recent fMRI studies have extensively considered the parameters that influence hippocampal activation, and these developments will be highly relevant for research on pediatric anxiety, given the abundant evidence for hippocampal involvement in generalized anxiety, panic, and posttraumatic stress disorders. Two experimental paradigms in particular have been designed to probe two different but essential aspects of hippocampal functioning, declarative and spatial memory (Buckner and Koutstaal 1998; Epstein and Kanwisher 1998).

Wagner et al. (1998) and Brewer et al. (1998) described methods for examining hippocampal involvement in declarative memory processes. With these methods, the hippocampus activates in response to viewed, successfully encoded mnemonic stimuli. Given that anxiety has been shown to affect memory in both children and adults (Pine et al. 1999; Williams et al. 1996), these methods can be used in patients with anxiety disorders to examine both hip-

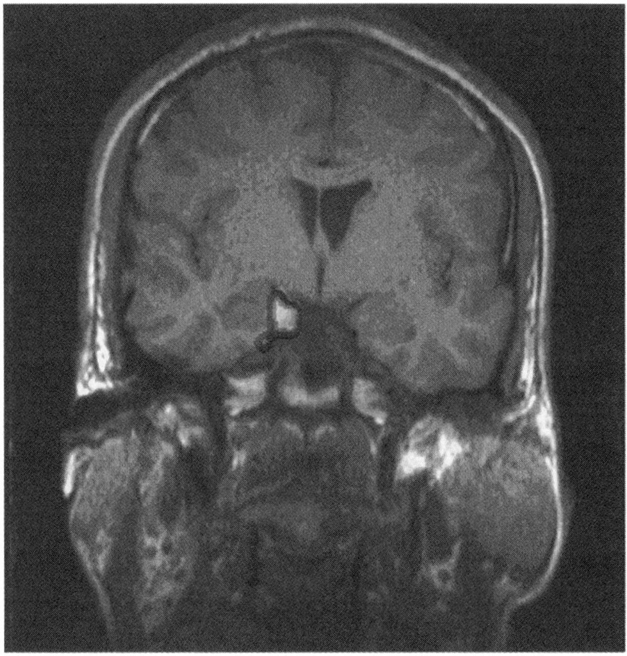

FIGURE 13–2. Contrast of blood oxygen level–dependent signal in one subject viewing masked fearful as opposed to happy faces. Subjects passively viewed a film described by Whalen et al. (1998b) and consisting of five epochs, with either masked fearful faces, masked happy faces, or a fixation cross. Images were acquired with a Siemens 1.5-tesla scanner (Erlangen, Germany), using single-shot echoplanar gradient-echo T2* weighting (repetition time, 2,800 milliseconds [ms]; echo time, 40 ms). Fourteen contiguous 7-mm coronal slices were acquired, with a 64 × 64 matrix and a 20-cm field of view. Data were realigned using AIR, smoothed with an 8-mm gaussian kernel, and analyzed using SPM 96 (Wellcome Department of Cognitive Neurology).

pocampal and amygdala activity during the encoding of disorder-relevant material. It may be possible, furthermore, to assess the specificity of amygdala and hippocampal involvement in anxiety disorders by contrasting their activity during encoding of disorder-relevant and disorder-irrelevant stimuli. Prior PET studies suggest a role for these structures in emotional memory, which may play a particularly central role in generalized anxiety as well as in panic disorder (Cahill and McGaugh 1996; Cahill et al. 1995; Hamann et al. 1999).

fMRI has also been used to study spatial memory. Epstein and Kanwisher (1998) and Wagner et al. (1998), for example, used fMRI to demonstrate hippocampal and parahippocampal activation when subjects viewed static visual scenes. Maguire and colleagues (Maguire 1997; Maguire et al. 1998), by contrast, used PET to document hippocampal activations when subjects traversed a taxi route in their imagination or when they directly traversed the route through a virtual-reality town. In collaboration with Maguire and her group, we used this virtual-reality task to document hippocampal activation with fMRI. Shown in Figure 13–3 is the increased hippocampal activity in an adult subject who used "internally guided" as opposed to "externally guided" navigation (Maguire et al. 1998).

Because hippocampal activation in these tasks can be demonstrated relatively consistently, it should be possible to adapt the tasks for use as functional imaging probes in the study of hippocampal involvement in fear states and anxiety disorders. For example, spatial coordinates can be conditioned to create an fMRI paradigm to study contextual fear in generalized anxiety disorder. Alternatively, intrinsically fearful stimuli, such as fearful faces, can be inserted into these spatial configurations, to examine hippocampal and amygdala activity in the perception of variously complex cues for fear. These designs could facilitate the testing of hypotheses concerning the role of various limbic structures in generalized anxiety disorder, as well as the mechanism of action for various anxiety medications (Gray and McNaughton 1996).

Directions for Future Functional MRI Studies of Pediatric Anxiety

Imaging research in pediatric anxiety is considerably less developed than is ADHD research. Although the obvious next step in imaging studies of pediatric anxiety is to apply to children the studies already used to investigate anxiety and anxiety-related circuitry in adults, these adult studies do raise a number of important methodological issues that are relevant to both adult and pediatric imaging. First, in contrast to the traitlike working memory or response inhibition functions based in the prefrontal cortex, emotions are transient and fluctuating. Consequently, the classic block design experiment that has typically been used to activate the prefontal cortex may not capture key aspects of emotional processing. Although Buchel et al. (1998) noted that event-related tasks can significantly enhance the temporal resolution required to study these transient events, the signal-to-noise limitations of current event-related tasks necessitate prohibitively long imaging times for children. Second, cognitive tasks in ADHD benefit from the availability of performance data relevant to the disorder. For example, brain activation patterns in children with ADHD can be referenced against the degree of speed or accuracy in performing the executive function of primary interest. The history of research on emotional processing in children has been plagued by a lack of performance-

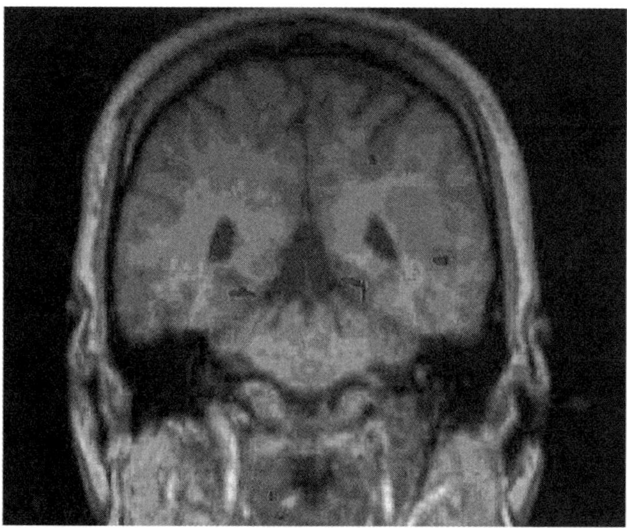

FIGURE 13–3. Contrast of blood oxygen level–dependent (BOLD) signal in one subject navigating through a virtual-reality town using internal as opposed to external cues. Subjects used a computer mouse to move through a virtual-reality town. Directions for navigation could be based either on a subject's memory for locations in the town acquired during a prescan training epoch (internal navigation) or on arrows located in the town (external navigation). Images were acquired with a Siemens 1.5-tesla scanner (Erlangen, Germany), using single-shot echoplanar gradient-echo T2* weighting (repetition time, 3,000 milliseconds [ms]; echo time, 40 ms). Fourteen contiguous 7-mm coronal slices were acquired, with a 64×64 matrix and a 20-cm field of view. Forty images were acquired in both the internal and external navigation epochs. Data were realigned using AIR, smoothed with an 8-mm gaussian kernel, and analyzed using SPM 96 (Wellcome Department of Cognitive Neurology), contrasting BOLD activity during internally versus externally guided navigation.

based data that reliably distinguish clinical groups. In addition to these significant hurdles, other major obstacles are likely to appear as imaging research on both ADHD and adult anxiety disorders continues.

■ CONCLUSION

We have attempted to indicate the tremendous promise of MRI research for the study of pediatric psychiatric disorders. Clearly, MRI has provided considerable insight in many areas of neuroscience. Nevertheless, the potential benefits for child psychiatry appear particularly important to realize. Child psychiatry has suffered from a relative absence of methodological tools for investigating the neurobiologic basis of individual conditions. MRI provides a unique means for testing competing models of human disease and for generating newer and more refined models of developmental psychopathology. The field is in great need of these tools. It is increasingly clear, moreover, that research on adult disorders would benefit from the application of these tools in the study of children's disorders, given the increasing appreciation of the importance of developmental psychopathology in adult disorders.

REFERENCES

Arnsten AF: Catecholamine regulation of the prefrontal cortex. J Psychopharmacol (Oxf) 11:151–162, 1997

Arnsten AF, Steere JC, Hunt RD: The contribution of alpha 2-noradrenergic mechanisms of prefrontal cortical cognitive function: potential significance for attention-deficit hyperactivity disorder. Arch Gen Psychiatry 53:448–455, 1996

Aylward EH, Reiss AL, Reader MJ, et al: Basal ganglia volumes in children with attention-deficit hyperactivity disorder. J Child Neurol 11:112–115, 1996

Baird AA, Gruber SA, Fein DA, et al: Functional magnetic resonance imaging of facial affect recognition in children and adolescents. J Am Acad Child Adolesc Psychiatry 38:195–199, 1999

Barkley RA: Behavioral inhibition, sustained attention, and executive functions: constructing a unifying theory of ADHD. Psychol Bull 121:65–94, 1997

Bechara A, Tranel D, Damasio H, et al: Double dissociation of conditioning and declarative knowledge relative to the amygdala and hippocampus in humans. Science 269:1115–1118, 1995

Berger TW, Orr WB: Hippocampectomy selectively disrupts discrimination reversal conditioning of the rabbit nictitating membrane response. Behav Brain Res 8:49–68, 1983

Berns GS, Cohen JD, Mintun MA: Brain regions responsive to novelty in the absence of awareness. Science 276:1272–1275, 1998

Berquin PC, Giedd JN, Jacobsen LK, et al: Cerebellum in attention-deficit hyperactivity disorder: a morphometric MRI study. Neurology 50:1087–1093, 1998

Birbaumer N, Grodd W, Diedrich O, et al: fMRI reveals amygdala activation to human faces in social phobics. Neuroreport 9:1223–1226, 1998

Bisaga A, Katz JL, Antonini A, et al: Cerebral glucose metabolism in women with panic disorder. Am J Psychiatry 155:1178–1183, 1998

Breiter HC, Etcoff NL, Whalen PJ, et al: Response and habituation of the human amygdala during visual processing of facial expression. Neuron 17:875–887, 1996

Bremner DJ: Neuroimaging of posttraumatic stress disorder. Psychiatric Annals 28: 445–450, 1998

Brewer JB, Zhao Z, Desmond JE, et al: Making memories: brain activity that predicts how well visual experience will be remembered. Science 281:1185–1187, 1998

Buchel C, Morris J, Dolan RJ, et al: Brain systems mediating aversive conditioning: an event-related fMRI study. Neuron 20:947–957, 1998

Buckner RL, Koutstaal W: Functional neuroimaging studies of encoding, priming, and explicit memory retrieval. Proc Natl Acad Sci U S A 95:891–898, 1998

Cahill L, McGaugh JL: Modulation of memory storage. Curr Opin Neurobiol 6:237–242, 1996

Cahill L, Babinsky R, Markowitsch H, et al: The amygdala and emotional memory. Nature 377:295–296, 1995

Carte ET, Nigg JT, Hinshaw SP: Neuropsychological functioning, motor speed, and language processing in boys with and without ADHD. J Abnorm Child Psychol 24:481–498, 1996

Casey BJ, Cohen JD, Jezzard P, et al: Activation of prefrontal cortex in children during a nonspatial working memory task with functional MRI. Neuroimage 2:221–229, 1995

Casey BJ, Castellanos FX, Giedd JN, et al: Implication of right frontostriatal circuitry in response inhibition and attention-deficit/hyperactivity disorder. J Am Acad Child Adolesc Psychiatry 36:374–383, 1997a

Castellanos FX, Giedd JN, Marsh WL, et al: Quantitative brain magnetic resonance imaging in attention-deficit hyperactivity disorder. Arch Gen Psychiatry 53:607–616, 1996

Chansky TE, Kendall PC: Social expectancies and self-perceptions in anxiety-disordered children. J Anxiety Disord 11:347–363, 1997

Clark RE, Squire LR: Classical conditioning and brain systems: the role of awareness. Science 280:77–81, 1998

Coplan JD, Andrews MW, Rosenblum LA, et al: Persistent elevations of cerebrospinal fluid concentrations of corticotropin-releasing factor in adult nonhuman primates exposed to early-life stressors: implications for the pathophysiology of mood and anxiety disorders. Proc Natl Acad Sci U S A 93:1619–1623, 1996

Damasio AR: Descartes' Error: Emotion, Reason, and the Human Brain. New York, Avon Books, 1994

Davis M: Neurobiology of fear responses: the role of the amygdala. J Neuropsychiatry Clin Neurosci 9:382–402, 1997

Devinsky O, Morrell MJ, Vogt BA: Contributions of anterior cingulate cortex to behaviour. Brain 118:279–306, 1995

Epstein R, Kanwisher N: A cortical representation of the local visual environment. Nature 392:598–601, 1998

Filipek PA, Semrud-Clikeman M, Steingard R, et al: Volumetric MRI analysis comparing subjects having attention-deficit hyperactivity disorder with normal controls. Neurology 48:589–601, 1997

Fuster JM: The Prefrontal Cortex: Anatomy, Physiology, and Neuropsychology of the Frontal Lobes. New York, Lippincott-Raven, 1997

Giedd JN, Castellanos FX, Casey BJ, et al: Quantitative morphology of the corpus callosum in attention deficit hyperactivity disorder. Am J Psychiatry 151:665–669, 1994

Gray JA, McNaughton N: The neuropsychology of anxiety: reprise, in Perspectives on Anxiety, Panic, and Fear, Vol 43. Edited by Hope DA. Omaha, NE, University of Nebraska Press, 1996, pp 61–134

Grillon C, Dierker L, Merikangas KR: Startle modulation in children at risk for anxiety disorders and/or alcoholism. J Am Acad Child Adolesc Psychiatry 36:925–932, 1997

Hamann SB, Ely TD, Grafton ST, et al: Amygdala activity related to enhanced memory for pleasant and aversive stimuli. Nat Neurosci 2:289–293, 1999

Hyde TM, Aaronson BA, Randolph C, et al: Cerebral morphometric abnormalities in Tourette's syndrome: a quantitative MRI study of monozygotic twins. Neurology 45:1176–1182, 1995

Hynd GW, Semrud-Clikeman M, Lorys AR, et al: Brain morphology in developmental dyslexia and attention deficit disorder/hyperactivity. Arch Neurology 47:919–926, 1990

Hynd GW, Semrud-Clikeman M, Lorys AR, et al: Corpus callosum morphology in attention deficit-hyperactivity disorder: morphometric analysis of MRI. J Learn Disabil 24:141–146, 1991

Hynd GW, Hern KL, Novey ES, et al: Attention deficit-hyperactivity disorder and asymmetry of the caudate nucleus. J Child Neurol 8:339–347, 1993

Kagan J: Galen's Prophecy. New York, Basic Books, 1995

Kagan J: Temperament and the reactions to unfamiliarity. Child Dev 68:139–143, 1997

LaBar KS, Gatenby JC, Gore JC, et al: Human amygdala activation during conditioned fear acquisition and extinction: a mixed-trial fMRI study. Neuron 20:937–945, 1998

LaBerge D: Attentional Processing: The Brain's Art of Mindfulness. Cambridge, MA, Harvard University Press, 1995

Lang PJ, Bradley MM, Cuthbert BN: Emotion, attention, and the startle reflex. Psychol Rev 97:1–19, 1990

Lang PJ, Bradley MM, Cuthbert BN: Emotion, motivation, and anxiety: brain mechanisms and psychophysiology. Biol Psychiatry 44:1248–1263, 1998

LeDoux J: The Emotional Brain: The Mysterious Underpinnings of Emotional Life. New York, Simon & Schuster, 1996

LeDoux J: Fear and the brain: where have we been and where are we going? Biol Psychiatry 44:1229–1238, 1998

Lewis DA: Development of the primate prefrontal cortex, in Neurodevelopment and Adult Psychopathology. Edited by Keshavan MS, Murray RM. Cambridge, UK, Cambridge University Press, 1997, pp 12–30

Lim KO, Adalsteinsson E, Spielman D, et al: Proton magnetic resonance spectroscopic imaging of cortical gray and white matter in schizophrenia. Arch Gen Psychiatry 55:346–352, 1998

Liu D, Diorio J, Tannenbaum B, et al: Maternal care, hippocampal glucocorticoid receptors, and hypothalamic-pituitary-adrenal responses to stress. Science 277: 1659–1662, 1997

Lundh LG, Ost LG: Recognition bias for critical faces in social phobics. Behav Res Ther 34:787–794, 1996

Maguire EA: Hippocampal involvement in human topographical memory: evidence from functional imaging. Philos Trans R Soc Lond B Biol Sci 352:1475–1480, 1997

Maguire EA, Burgess N, Donnett JG, et al: Knowing where and getting there: a human navigation network. Science 280:921–924, 1998

McNaughton N: Cognitive dysfunction resulting from hippocampal hyperactivity—a possible cause of anxiety disorder? Pharmacol Biochem Behav 56:603–611, 1997

Meaney MJ, Bhatnagar S, Diorio J, et al: Molecular basis for the development of individual differences in the hypothalamic pituitary-adrenal stress response. Cell Mol Neurobiol 13:321–347, 1993

Morris JS, Frith CD, Perret DI, et al: A differential neural response in the human amygdala to fearful and happy facial expression. Nature 383:115–118, 1996

Morris JS, Öhman A, Dolan RJ: Conscious and unconscious emotional learning in the human amygdala. Nature 398:467–470, 1998

Morris JS, Öhman A, Dolan RJ: A subcortical pathway to the right amygdala mediating "unseen" fear. Proc Natl Acad Sci U S A 96:1680–1685, 1999

Mostofsky SH, Reiss AL, Lockhart P, et al: Evaluation of cerebellar size in attention-deficit hyperactivity disorder. J Child Neurol 13:434–439, 1998

Öhman A: Face the beast and fear the face: animal and social fears as prototypes for evolutionary analyses of emotion. Psychophysiology 23:123–145, 1986

Oosterlaan J, Sergeant JA: Inhibition in ADHD, aggressive, and anxious children: a biologically based model of child psychopathology. J Abnorm Child Psychol 24:19–36, 1996

Pashler HE: The Psychology of Attention. Cambridge, MA, MIT Press, 1998

Pennington BF, Ozonoff S: Executive functions and developmental psychopathology. J Child Psychol Psychiatry 37:51–87, 1996

Peterson BS, Klein JE: Neuroimaging of Tourette's syndrome neurobiological substrate. Child Adolesc Psychiatr Clin N Am 6:343–364, 1997

Peterson B[S], Riddle MA, Cohen DJ, et al: Reduced basal ganglia volumes in Tourette's syndrome using three-dimensional reconstruction techniques from magnetic resonance images. Neurology 43:941–949, 1993

Peterson BS, Skudlarski P, Anderson AW, et al: A functional magnetic resonance imaging study of tic suppression in Tourette syndrome. Arch Gen Psychiatry 55:326–333, 1998

Peterson BS, Skudlarski P, Gatenby JC, et al: An fMRI study of Stroop word-color interference: evidence for cingulate subregions subserving multiple distributed attentional systems. Biol Psychiatry 45:1237–1258, 1999

Phillips RG, LeDoux JE: Differential contribution of amygdala and hippocampus to cued and contextual fear conditioning. Behav Neurosci 106:274–285, 1992

Pine DS, Grun J: Childhood anxiety: integrating developmental psychopathology and affective neuroscience. J Child Adolesc Psychopharmacol 9:1–12, 1999

Pine DS, Wasserman GA, Fried JE, et al: Neurological soft signs: one-year stability and relationship to psychiatric symptoms in boys. J Am Acad Child Adolesc Psychiatry 36:1579–1586, 1997

Pine DS, Cohen P, Gurley D, et al: The risk for early-adulthood anxiety and depressive disorders in adolescents with anxiety and depressive disorders. Arch Gen Psychiatry 55:56–64, 1998

Pine DS, Wasserman GA, Workman SB: Memory and anxiety in prepubertal boys at risk for delinquency. J Am Acad Child Adolesc Psychiatry 38:1024–1031, 1999

Posner MI, Raichle ME: Images of Mind.New York, NY, Scientific American Library, 1994

Rapoport JL, Giedd J, Kumra S, et al: Childhood-onset schizophrenia—progressive ventricular change during adolescence. Arch Gen Psychiatry 54:897–903, 1997

Reiss AL, Abrams MT, Singer HS, et al: Brain development, gender and IQ in children: a volumetric imaging study. Brain 119:1763–1774, 1996

Rogeness GA, Javors MA, Pliszka SR: Neurochemistry and child and adolescent psychiatry. J Am Acad Child Adolesc Psychiatry 31:765–781, 1992

Rosen JB, Schulkin J: From normal fear to pathological anxiety. Psychol Rev 105:325–350, 1998

Rosenberg DR, Keshavan MS: Toward a neurodevelopmental model of obsessive-compulsive disorder. Biol Psychiatry 43:623–640, 1998

Semrud-Clikeman M, Filipek PA, Biederman J, et al: Attention-deficit hyperactivity disorder: magnetic resonance imaging morphometric analysis of the corpus callosum. J Am Acad Child Adolesc Psychiatry 33:875–881, 1994

Singer HS, Reiss AL, Brown JE, et al: Volumetric MRI changes in basal ganglia of children with Tourette's syndrome. Neurology 43:950–956, 1993

Swanson J, Posner MI, Cantwell D, et al: Attention-deficit/hyperactivity disorder: symptom domains, cognitive processes, and neural networks, in The Attentive Brain. Edited by Parasuraman R. Cambridge, MA, MIT Press, 1998a, pp 445–460

Swanson J, Castellanos FX, Murias M, et al: Cognitive neuroscience of attention deficit hyperactivity disorder and hyperkinetic disorder. Curr Opin Neurobiol 8:263–271, 1998b

Vaidya CJ, Austin G, Kirkorian G, et al: Selective effects of methylphenidate in attention deficit hyperactivity disorder: a functional magnetic resonance imaging study. Proc Natl Acad Sci U S A 24:14494–14499, 1998

Vasey MW, el-Hag N, Daleiden EL: Anxiety and the processing of emotionally threatening stimuli: distinctive patterns of selective attention among high- and low-test-anxious children. Child Dev 67:1173–1185, 1996

Wagner AD, Schacter DL, Rotte M, et al: Building memories: remembering and forgetting of verbal experiences as predicted by brain activity. Science 281:1188–1191, 1998

Weissman MM, Leckman JF, Merikangas KR, et al: Depression and anxiety disorders in parents and children. Arch Gen Psychiatry 41:845–852, 1984

Whalen PJ, Bush G, McNally RJ, et al: The emotional counting Stroop paradigm: a functional magnetic resonance imaging probe of the anterior cingulate affective division. Biol Psychiatry 44:1219–1228, 1998a

Whitaker AH, Van Rossem R, Feldman JF, et al: Psychiatric outcomes in low-birth-weight children at age 6 years: relation to neonatal cranial ultrasound abnormalities. Arch Gen Psychiatry 54:847–856, 1997

White JL, Moffit TE, Caspi A, et al: Measuring impulsivity and examining its relationship to delinquency. J Abnorm Psychol 103:192–205, 1994

Williams JMG, Mathews A, MacLeod C: The emotional Stroop task and psychopathology. Psychol Bull 120:3–24, 1996

Wolf SS, Jones DW, Knable MB, et al: Tourette syndrome: prediction of phenotypic variation in monozygotic twins by caudate nucleus D2 receptor binding. Science 273:1225–1227, 1996

14

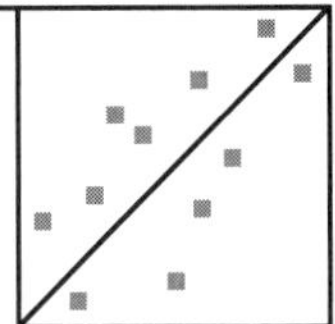

FUNCTIONAL MAGNETIC RESONANCE IMAGING IN ANIMALS

Applications in Psychiatric Research

Craig F. Ferris, Ph.D.
David P. Olson, M.D., Ph.D.
Jean A. King, Ph.D.

Functional magnetic resonance imaging (fMRI) has greater spatial and temporal resolution than do positron emission tomography and single photon emission computed tomography, and fMRI is more convenient because it does not require production of radioactive molecules (Neil 1993). With fMRI, subjects can be repeatedly studied within a single session and over time. This aspect has led to a rapid increase in fMRI methodology for use in neuroscience research pertaining to functional brain mapping in humans. However, animal work has not kept pace with human studies, which is unfortunate because fMRI in preclinical research would allow investigators to study animal models of neurological and psychiatric diseases—that is, to conduct studies that could not be performed in humans. In this chapter, we discuss the use of fMRI in anesthetized and awake animals, methodological considerations to be taken into account when imaging animals, and future applications that may help in elucidating and treating mental illness.

Use of Functional MRI in Anesthetized Animals

The primary focus of fMRI studies in anesthetized animals has been on evoked brain and spinal cord activity in response to peripheral sensory stimulation. Hyder and co-workers (1994), in collaboration with Robert Shulman at Yale University, were the first to report changes in blood oxygen level–dependent (BOLD) signal in the somatosensory cortex of chloralose-anesthetized rats with electrical stimulation of the forepaw. Using a 7.0-tesla (T) spectrometer (Bruker Medical, Billerica, Massachusetts), these investigators found signal changes of 17% in the frontal and parietal cortices, changes that agreed with the topographical representation of the forelimb sensory and motor systems. With the use of a gradient-echo pulse sequence and a surface coil, spatial and temporal resolutions were 300 × 300 × 500 μm and 18 seconds, respectively. Subsequent studies conducted at other laboratories and involving electrical stimulation of rat paws found BOLD signal changes of 1%–6% in a 2.0-T system with animals under propofol anesthesia (Lahti et al. 1999; Scanley et al. 1997) and 11% in a 4.7-T system with animals under chloralose anesthesia (Gyngell et al. 1996).

Porszasz et al. (1997) examined spinal cord activation in isoflurane-anesthetized rats after injection of formalin under the skin of the hindpaw. Injection of formalin is used to induce spinal hyperactivity associated with pain and hyperalgesia (Dickenson and Sullivan 1987). The experiments were run in a 4.7-T spectrometer (Bruker Medical, Karlsruhe, Germany) with a modified radiofrequency coil and restraining device for imaging the spinal cord. Spatial and temporal resolutions were 117 × 234 × 1,000 μm and 120 seconds, respectively. Susceptibility artifacts associated with imaging of the spinal cord necessitated the use of a spin-echo pulse sequence to compensate for magnetic field inhomogeneities that resulted in a suboptimal temporal resolution at this field strength. Injection of formalin into the hindpaw altered activity in the lumbar region of the spinal cord. There was an unexpected decrease in BOLD signal on the ipsilateral spinal cord, focused between lumbar segments L4 and L5. These researchers speculated that the negative BOLD signal might be due to an increase in perfusion rate or increased oxygen consumption in combination with constant or reduced blood flow.

The utility of fMRI in anesthetized animals and the sensitivity of such imaging to peripheral stimulation were best exemplified in two studies by Yang and co-workers (1996, 1998), performed with a 7.0-T spectrometer. In the first study, activation of a single whisker caused increases in BOLD signal of 2%–7% in discrete cortical barrels, a finding in keeping with expected neuroanatomical topography (Yang et al. 1996). The rat whisker is a sensitive tactile organ with a well-defined cortical representation characterized by cylindrical columns or barrels measuring 300–500 μm in diameter. This study demonstrated high spatial resolution and activation in the cortex in response to a discrete sensory stimulus—vibration of a single whisker. In the second, more recent study, Yang et al. (1998) mapped changes in BOLD signal in the olfactory bulb in response to the smell of isoamyl acetate. Activation maps overlaid on high-resolution MRI anatomical maps show increases in BOLD signal of more than 20% in the outer glomerular level. This outer layer has the highest density of synapses in the olfactory bulbs, suggesting that the robust change in BOLD signal reflects an odor-induced increase in synaptic activity, a notion consistent with findings of 2-deoxyglucose studies (Sharp et al. 1977). In these studies, a single image could be acquired in 36 seconds and fMRI data required no image averaging, attesting to the high temporal resolution and robust nature of odor-induced activation of the olfactory bulbs in the anesthetized rat.

■ Use of Functional MRI in Awake Animals

Until recently, awake animals were not used in fMRI studies, because of technical problems associated with movement of the animals in the magnetic resonance spectrometer. Any minor head movement can distort the image and may also create a change in signal intensity that can be mistaken for stimulus-associated changes in brain activity (Hajnal et al. 1994). In addition to head movement, motion outside the field of view can also obscure or mimic the signal from neuronal activation (Birm et al. 1996).

We published the first detailed description of fMRI in an awake animal (Lahti et al. 1998); our approach involved the use of a head and body holder (Insight Neuroimaging Systems, Inc., Worcester, Massachusetts) customized for adult male rats weighing 300–350 g. The technology was validated by showing changes in BOLD signal in the somatosensory cortex of the rat with electrical stimulation of the paw. Data were acquired with a 2.0-T spectrometer (GE NMR Instruments, Fremont, California). With a gradient-echo pulse sequence and a birdcage radiofrequency coil, spatial and temporal resolutions were $250 \times 250 \times 2{,}000$ μm and 60 seconds, respectively. In brief, rats were given a short-acting anesthetic and fitted into the restraining device. Gold-plated surface electrodes were attached to the skin of the hindpaw and connected to an electrical stimulator that provided 0.3-millisecond pulses at 3 Hz, with current intensity sufficient to cause contraction of the hindpaw (approximately 1–3 milliamperes, depending on skin resistance). Animals routinely recovered from the anesthesia within 30 minutes, as evidenced by tail withdrawal, hindlimb movement, and occasional vocalizations.

Multiple baseline data sets collected before stimulation and subtracted from one another reflected nominal motion artifacts or changes in signal intensity over time. Stimulation of the left or right hindpaw led to an increase in signal intensity in the contralateral somatosensory cortex, relative to baseline (Figure 14–1). The stimulation response in the somatosensory cortex was an increase in BOLD signal of 3.9%–18.8%. The enhanced BOLD signal was accompanied by a robust change in cerebral blood flow to the same area of the somatosensory cortex. The change in relative cerebral blood flow to the cortex after electrical stimulation of the paw ranged from 75% to 88%.

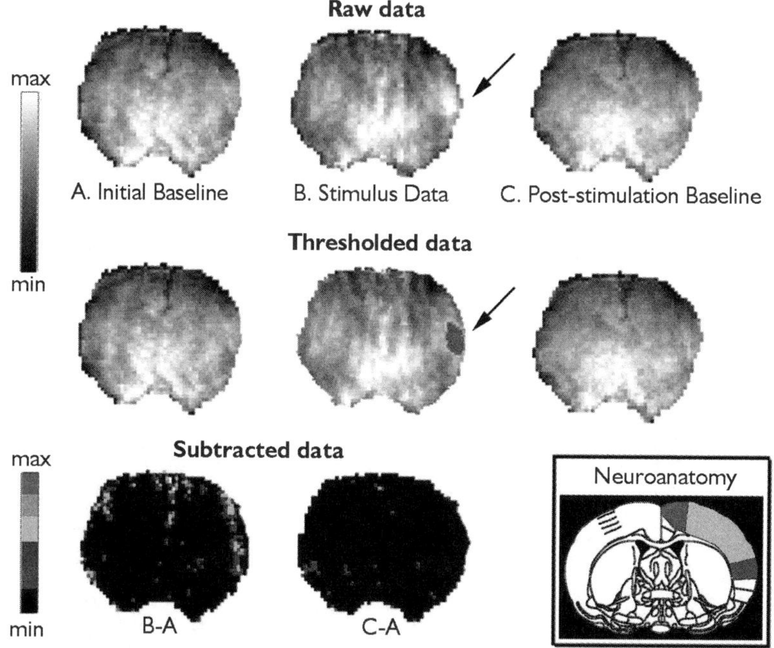

FIGURE 14–1. Evoked cortical activity in a concious rat. Arrows point to areas of activation. T2*-weighted blood oxygen level–dependent (BOLD)–based images of a rat brain were obtained under baseline and stimulated conditions. Imaging parameters were as follows: repetition time, 200 milliseconds (ms); echo time, 20 ms; and number of excitations, 1. Baseline images were acquired before (A) and after (C) electrical stimulation of the hindpaw. Changes were observed in the contralateral somatosensory cortex. The differences between stimulated and initial baseline conditions and between baseline conditions after and before stimulation are shown in the subtracted data sets. Linear scales represent the maximum and minimum signal intensities for their respective data sets. The neuroanatomy of the approximate slice is shown. The color region shows (from left to right) the motor cortices, the primary sensory cortex, and the secondary somatosensory cortex.

Source. Reprinted with permission from Lahti KM, Ferris CF, Li F, et al.: "Imaging Brain Activity in Conscious Animals Using Functional MRI." *Journal of Neuroscience Methods* 82:75–83, 1998.

In a subsequent study, we examined the differences in BOLD signal associated with electrical stimulation of paws of awake and anesthetized rats (Lahti et al. 1999). Animals were tested for evoked cortical activity while fully conscious as well as while under anesthesia induced with the short-acting anesthetic propofol. The greatest increases in signal intensity were observed in the contralateral somatosensory cortex in response to electric shock of the hindpaw in the conscious state (Figure 14–2). These increases in cortical signal ranged from 6% to 25%. In some of the animals studied, propofol depressed signal intensity by as much as tenfold.

Hagino et al. (1998) used fMRI in awake animals to examine the effects of dopamine D_2 receptor agonists and antagonists on brain activity. Rats fixed with cranioplastic caps were acclimated over 7–10 days to a restraining cage and a 21-hour water-deprivation regimen. Earbars inserted into the cranioplastic cap held the head motionless in the restraining cage. During acclimation to a daily episode of progressively longer durations of restraint (1–3 hours), each animal was rewarded by being given a solution of 5% glucose from a spout in front of its mouth. After this training period, the water-deprivation regimen was terminated, and animals were tested in a 4.7-T spectrometer (SMIS, Guildford, UK) before and after parenteral treatment with haloperidol or bromocriptine.

With a gradient-echo pulse sequence, spatial and temporal resolutions were $310 \times 310 \times 2{,}000$ μm and approximately 210 seconds, respectively. To improve the signal-to-noise ratio in this experimental paradigm, Hagino et al. (1998) ran eight excitations (i.e., sequences of phase-encoding steps), prolonging acquisition time and decreasing temporal resolution. However, temporal resolution was not critical in these studies, because the drugs were active over many hours. Activation of D_2 receptors with bromocriptine caused a slow but significant increase in BOLD signal in the hypothalamus, dorsomedial thalamus, and ventral posterior thalamus. Two hours after treatment, BOLD signal increased by 4%–8% in these regions. Blockade of D_2 receptors with haloperidol decreased BOLD signal in the caudate-putamen, hypothalamus, and perirhinal cortex by 3%–6% within the first 30 minutes; BOLD signal returned to baseline by 90 minutes after treatment. The thalamic nuclei showed depressed BOLD signal when animals were injected with a high dose of haloperidol after experiencing sustained drug levels for 2 weeks.

It was anticipated that areas with a high density of D_2 receptor (e.g., the caudate-putamen) would show the greatest changes in BOLD signal. However, the most robust response to acute activation and chronic blockade of D_2 receptors was in thalamic areas having few or no dopamine binding sites (Boyson et al. 1986; Dubois et al. 1986). This finding highlights one of the

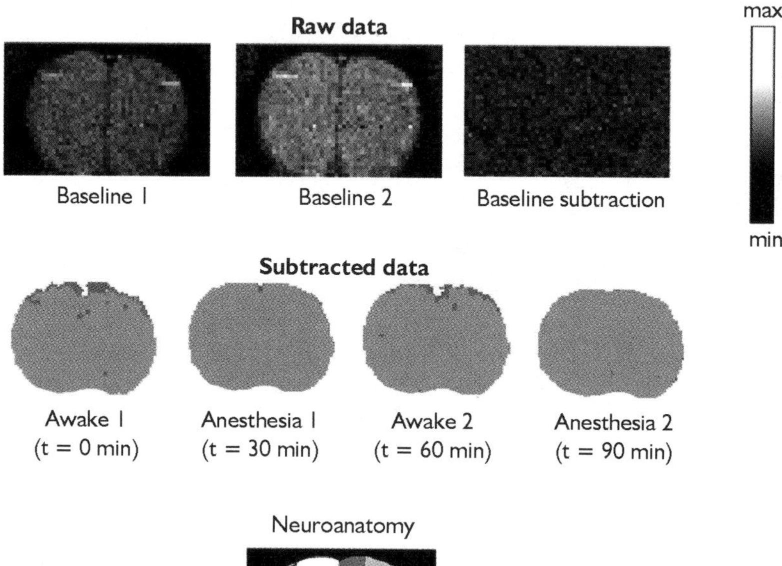

FIGURE 14–2. Effect of anesthetic on evoked cortical activity. Two blood oxygen level–dependent (BOLD)–based images of a rat brain (top) were obtained sequentially under baseline conditions, using a T2*-weighted sequence (repetition time, 200 milliseconds [ms]; echo time, 20 ms; number of excitations, 2). The differences in evoked cortical signal between awake and anesthetized conditions over sequential trials are shown in the subtracted data sets. The linear scale represents the maximum and minimum signal intensities for the respective data sets. The neuroanatomy of the approximate slice as described in Figure 14–1 is shown.
Source. Reprinted with permission from Lahti KM, Ferris CF, Li F, et al.: "Comparison of Evoked Cortical Activity in Conscious and Propofol-Anesthetized Rats Using Functional MRI." *Magnetic Resonance Medicine* 41:412–416, 1999.

advantages of fMRI as a noninvasive method, that of revealing activation in sites secondary to those of interest. These data on D_2 activation and blockade may aid efforts to understand the mechanisms of action of antipsychotic medications.

In a recently completed study, we used fMRI in awake rats to follow the initiation and propagation of general seizure caused by the administration of pentylenetetrazol (Ferris et al. 1998). Adult male rats were imaged in a 4.7-T spectrometer (Bruker Medical, Billerica, Massachusetts). With a multislice gradient-echo pulse sequence and a surface coil, we were able to scan four slices with a spatial resolution of 500 × 500 × 1,000 μm every 18 seconds over a 16-minute observation period before and after initiation of seizure activity. A body-and-shoulder restrainer was developed to isolate the intense muscular activity of the neck and body from the head restrainer and surface coil. Within 2 minutes of injection of pentylenetetrazol, seizure occurred, evidenced by a twisting convulsive movement of the hind end, usually preceded by Straub tail. It was not unexpected that the intense "electrical storm" characteristic of seizure was accompanied by robust changes in BOLD signal, which in some areas (e.g., the entorhinal and parietal cortices) exceeded 100%. The entorhinal cortex, hippocampus, and olfactory bulbs showed enhanced BOLD signal before the first convulsion. There was a striking lateralization of cortical activity during a convulsive episode.

Although fMRI in rodents has potential applications in psychiatric research, imaging fully conscious nonhuman primates would extend the field of preclinical research and yield data more relevant to humans. Dubowitz and co-workers (1998), conducting experiments on an adult male rhesus monkey, were the first to image changes in BOLD signal in the occipital cortex in response to a visual stimulus. This work was done with a conventional 1.5-T clinical spectrometer. With an echo-planar pulse sequence and a standard radiofrequency volume coil coadapted for the human knee, spatial and temporal resolutions were 3.13 × 3.13 × 3 mm and approximately 4 minutes, respectively. Ninety scans or data acquisitions at 2.5 seconds each were acquired for eight slices. The 2.6%–4.6% change in BOLD signal in the primary visual cortex was comparable to changes reported for visual stimulation in human subjects (Bandettini et al. 1993; Belliveau et al. 1991). Key to these studies was the cooperation of the monkey and the design of a head restrainer. The animal tested was trained to lie prone in a sphinx-like position. A custom-built head cap with a vertical post was secured to the skull anterior to the occipital cortex to avoid image artifact. The vertical post could be locked into a receptacle "head-cap locator" built into the radiofrequency volume coil. With the head held firmly and the animal trained to lie quietly in the bore of the magnet, it was possible to obtain BOLD images with little motion artifact.

At the Max Plank Institute for Biological Cybernetics in Tübingen, Germany, Logothetis and co-workers (1999) developed a technology for imaging brain activity in response to visual stimuli in awake rhesus monkeys in a custom-built 4.7-T spectrometer with a vertical bore (Bruker Medical, Ettlingen, Germany). An air-conditioned primate chair supporting radiofrequency filters, a head-restraining stereotaxic device, and a radiofrequency volume coil were constructed for these experiments. Once secured in the chair, the monkey to be studied is lowered and positioned within the magnet with a special transport system. A fiber optics system projects an LCD image to the animal's eyes. Over a 3-month period, four animals were adapted to the imaging procedure and primate chair in a simulated environment. Eye movement was detected with an infrared system. Animals were trained to respond to different colors or different visual objects by pressing buttons attached to the front of the primate chair. With a multislice, contrast-enhanced gradient-echo, echo planar technique, spatial and temporal resolutions were $1 \times 1 \times 2$ mm and 6 seconds, respectively. Activation maps overlaid on high-resolution MRI anatomical maps showed changes in BOLD signal in the primary visual cortex and extrastriate areas (Figure 14–3). The increases in BOLD signal ranged from 3.5% to 4.8% and were dependent on the size and position of the stimulus in the visual field.

■ METHODOLOGICAL CONSIDERATIONS

Enhanced Magnetic Resonance Signal in Awake Animals

Comparing changes in BOLD signal intensity in anesthetized and conscious animals across studies can be misleading, because of differences in experimental protocols, imaging parameters, or magnetic field strengths. In studies in anesthetized rats, electrical stimulation of the paw evokes changes in signal intensities in the somatosensory cortex that range from 3% at 2.0 T (Scanley et al. 1997) to 11% at 4.7 T (Gyngell et al. 1996) to 17% at 7.0 T (Hyder et al. 1994). Such differences in signal intensity in anesthetized rats are due in part to the different field strengths used in the studies. BOLD signal intensity increases linearly with magnetic field strength. In contrast, stimulation of the paw in unanesthetized rats at 2.0 T evokes BOLD signal changes in the cortex ranging from 4% to 25% (Lahti et al. 1998, 1999), equal to and in some cases exceeding those measured at 4.7 and 7.0 T in anesthetized rats. The enhanced signal in awake animals, relative to the signal in anesthetized animals, is not due to differences in experimental protocols; all of the studies mentioned involved low-frequency foot shock or median nerve stimulation in adult rats. Rather, the enhanced BOLD signal in awake animals is due to the absence of active anesthetic agents, as we demonstrated by measuring evoked cortical activity in animals that were awake and in the same animals under anesthesia (Figure 14–2).

The increased BOLD signal in awake animals is most likely due to enhanced cerebral blood flow to the area of activation. Laser Doppler studies

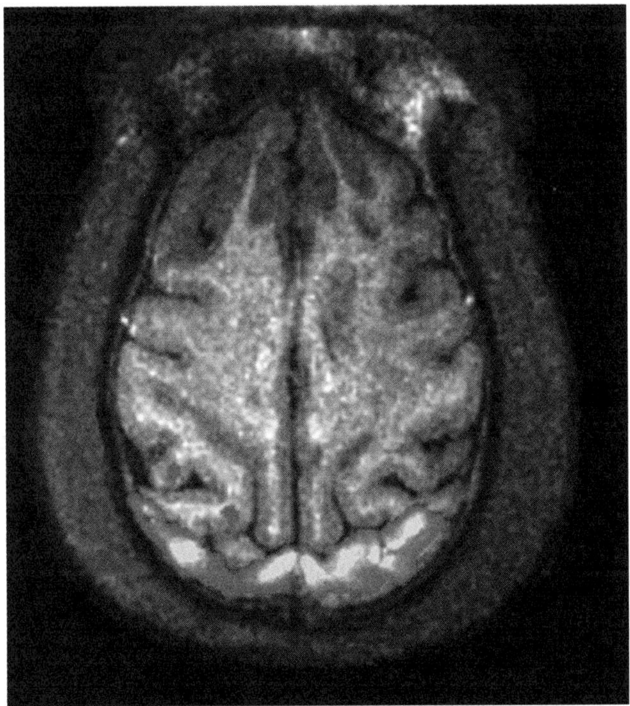

FIGURE 14–3. Horizontal slice showing blood oxygen level–dependent (BOLD) activation in the striate and extrastriate cortex in an alert monkey. The stimulus was a polar-transformed checkerboard extending 30 × 23 degrees of visual angle. The monkey fixated a centrally presented spot and reacted to small changes in the spot luminance by pressing buttons attached to the front side of the primate chair (the right button was pressed when intensity decreased, and the left button was pressed when intensity increased). While the monkey performed this task, the full-screen checkerboard was turned on and off. Each epoch lasted 48 seconds.
Source. N.K. Logothetis, personal communication, March 1999.

have demonstrated large increases in cerebral blood flow in conscious animals compared with anesthetized animals (Bonvento et al. 1994). Changes in BOLD signal intensity require prompt and robust changes in local hemodynamics in response to increases and decreases in neuronal activity (Ogawa et al. 1990). Given that all general anesthetics depress central nervous system metabolic activity and reduce basal cerebral blood flow (Ueki et al. 1992), it is not surprising that anesthetized animals have reduced BOLD signal compared with awake animals.

Enhanced BOLD signal in the absence of anesthesia makes fMRI possible in animals using magnetic resonance spectrometers with magnetic field strengths between 1.0 and 2.0 T. Indeed, there are many 1.5-T clinical spectrometers that can be used for functional imaging in awake animals. This advantage was pointed out by Dubowitz and co-workers (1998), who obtained high-resolution images of the visual cortex in an awake monkey with a conventional 1.5-T clinical spectrometer.

With greater BOLD signal, the temporal and spatial resolution in any particular experiment can be increased. As noted earlier, we have used gradient-echo imaging to obtain multiple slices of rat brain every 18 seconds before and after drug-induced general seizure. Individual voxel analysis revealed changes in BOLD signal in excess of 100% above control values. Given the robust nature of these signals, it is possible to perform echo-planar imaging over multiple slices every 3–4 seconds with a single acquisition. This level of temporal resolution may allow researchers to follow the global activity of neural networks associated with the initiation and propagation of seizure or any behavioral response that elicits intense neuronal activity.

Acclimation of Animals to Immobilization Stress

The stress caused by immobilization and noise from the magnetic resonance scanner during functional imaging in awake animals is a major concern. Although motion artifact is eliminated or minimized with animal restraining devices, stress can limit the number of experimental applications and cloud interpretation of data. If animals can adapt to the imaging procedure, as evidenced by measured basal levels of stress hormones and resting levels of autonomic activity, investigators can isolate the stress-mediated changes in brain activity from those of interest.

Work with monkeys has indicated that these animals can readily adapt to the imaging procedure. In our laboratory, we have begun studies in the common marmoset *(Callithrix jacchus)*, a South American primate of the family Callithricidae. We have successfully imaged conscious male marmosets, obtaining T1-weighted anatomy and T2*-weighted BOLD images, with a 2.0-T spectrometer. Concerned about the stress of the imaging procedure, we subjected adult male marmosets to repeated episodes of immobilization and measured changes in salivary cortisol levels. Animals showed high cortisol levels on the first day of testing. Levels ranged between 220 and 340 mg/dL. However, by the third day of testing, all animals showed basal levels of cortisol (approximately 50 mg/dL) in response to the immobilization and imaging procedure (C.F. Ferris and J.A. King, unpublished data, June 1998).

Rhesus monkeys are also adequate subjects for fMRI, because they can be trained to relax quietly in a sphinx-like position in a horizontal bore (Dubowitz et al. 1998) or sit upright in a vertical bore (Logothetis et al. 1999). However, these studies with rhesus monkeys are designed to examine functional activity associated with visual stimuli and cognitive tasks. The visual stimuli carry minimal emotional valence that might elicit an autonomic response such as fear or rage and increase the possibility of motion artifact.

Endocrine studies measuring norepinephrine, epinephrine, and corticosterone levels have indicated that it may be difficult to adapt rats to daily episodes of immobilization stress. There is little or no acclimatization to immobilization stress with 2 weeks of daily immobilization (Hauger et al. 1990; Ma et al. 1997). The method of Hagino et al. (1998) of using a water-deprivation regimen to coax immobilized animals to focus on drinking a 5% glucose solution instead of their desire to escape may be one way of acclimating rodents to a variety of fMRI procedures. However, it will be necessary to study the endocrinology of these animals to determine the level of activation of the stress axis.

Eliciting of Complex Behavioral Responses in the Magnet

As discussed previously, studies examining cortical responses to peripheral sensory stimulation in the form of olfactory, visual, or sensorimotor activation are technically feasible and amenable to fMRI. These behavioral responses might be classified as simple responses, measured by a priori changes in activity in discrete brain areas in response to neutral stimuli. However, fMRI can be used to study more complex behaviors, consisting of multiple components exciting many brain areas in response to external and internal stimuli.

What complex behaviors can be studied in the magnet, and how are they elicited? Obviously, any behavior that requires a consummatory act would be difficult to study with fMRI, because immobilization alone may prevent the motor response that defines the behavior. Fear, anger, and hunger are examples of internal states of arousal and motivation. These types of behavioral conditions are fertile areas of investigation using fMRI. An investigator can collect a library of vocalizations, smells, and visual images that have proven ethological significance in the animal's natural habitat and in the seminatural environment of the laboratory. These vocalizations, smells, and images can be used to communicate with the animal in the magnet. For example, if acclimatization to the stress of immobilization is achieved in rodents, a male rat might be presented with the stimuli of a predator to elicit fear.

Identification of Discrete Behavioral Responses

The brain activity identified with fMRI in awake animals may be harder to interpret than the signal obtained from anesthetized animals, because the quality of the stimulus is more complex. For example, a fully conscious animal's perception of foot shock combined with the stress of the immobilization and the imaging procedure, mild pain, and heightened arousal will collectively contribute to the quality of the stimulus and enhanced cortical activity. Sensory modalities with committed neural pathways may be spread over larger cortical areas. Dubowitz and co-workers (1998) suggested that the appearance of unexpected asymmetrical functional activation in the visual cortex of their monkey might have been due to a global physiological response to the visual stimulus. Indeed, we discovered that the area of activation during unilateral foot shock in the awake condition appeared in both somatosensory cortices but with greater signal intensity and spread on the side contralateral to the stimulus (Lahti et al. 1999). In the same animal, the cortical activity was greatly reduced in the anesthetized condition and was primarily restricted to a small area of somatosensory cortex contralateral to the stimulus. In such instances, measures of simple behavior (i.e., mapping of cortical activity in response to peripheral sensory stimulation) may be better done in the anesthetized animal than in the awake animal. However, for more complex behaviors related to motivational, emotional, and cognitive processes, studies must be performed when the animal is awake.

How does one tease apart the elements of a complex behavior and correlate these changes with brain activity using fMRI? With careful attention to the temporal pattern of behavioral activation, it may be possible to identify and correlate nuances in a complex behavior with changes in BOLD signal. For example, the presentation of olfactory and visual stimuli of a predator to elicit a fear response in an animal would be expected to activate olfactory and visual pathways and limbic and cortical structures mixed with motor pathways involved in initiating freezing or escape behavior. Outside the magnet, this stimulus-evoked behavior could be videotaped, time-coded, and analyzed to yield a record of the sequence and chronology of the behavioral response in the form of a time-event table (van Hooff 1982). With lag sequence analysis, the contingency and timing between subtle behavioral events can be predicted. The fMRI parameters can be set to provide the temporal resolution necessary to match this time-event table. When experiments on fear, anger, etc., are combined with well-designed control studies, it may be possible to correlate the spatial and temporal pattern of brain activity with discrete events in the complex behavior.

Applications in Psychiatric Research

Examining Brain-Environment Interactions During Development

Myriad animal studies have shown that an early emotional or environmental insult can affect brain development, with long-term neurobiologic and behavioral consequences. Insights into the etiology of mental illness may be gleaned in longitudinal studies of interactions between vulnerable animal populations and stressful environments at critical times in development. fMRI is noninvasive and can be used to study the same animal over the course of its life. Magnetic resonance systems with higher field strengths (9.4 and 11 T and beyond), some of which are already in operation, will provide the increased spatial and temporal resolution to observe developmental changes in neuroanatomy, brain activity, and brain chemistry in animals, even in animals as small as mice.

Investigating Effects of Drug Treatments

The study by Hagino et al. (1998), who examined changes in brain activity after acute and prolonged exposure to dopamine receptor agonists and antagonists, is an obvious example of application of fMRI in animal studies. Use of animal studies to investigate the effects of treatment with serotonin reuptake inhibitors can also be helpful. Serotonin reuptake inhibitors cause a prompt increase in brain levels of serotonin in animals (Guan and McBride 1988). Accompanying the increase in serotonin are observable changes in behavior (Ferris et al. 1997). Nonetheless, patients treated for depression or obsessive-compulsive disorder with serotonin reuptake blockers require weeks of treatment before they can report an improvement in their condition. This fact suggests that drug efficacy with regard to mental illness is due to secondary changes in the serotonin system or other interrelated neurochemical signals and pathways, which are slowly affected by the continuous exposure, through chronic drug treatment, to increased serotonin levels. With fMRI, the same animal can be imaged over long periods to determine progressive changes in brain activity associated with continuous drug treatment.

Testing Cognitive Performance

Deficits in learning and memory are symptoms of several psychiatric disorders, including attention-deficit/hyperactivity disorder (Gansler et al. 1998) and schizophrenia (Curtis et al. 1998). Many learning paradigms do not require any signs of overt behavior and are therefore amenable to testing with fMRI. Because animals readily respond to peripheral stimulation while in the magnet during fMRI, they may be used in studies of classical conditioning. For example, foot shock can be used as an unconditioned response that, when coupled with a conditioned stimulus such as light, can be used in learning studies examining discrimination and perception. Operant conditioning would be more difficult because a behavioral action (e.g., bar pressing, eliciting rewarding or punishing stimuli) would be necessary. However, Logothetis and co-workers (1999) demonstrated that awake rhesus monkeys can be trained to press buttons during MRI protocols. These advances in awake animals open the area of cognitive neuroscience to investigation with fMRI.

■ REFERENCES

Bandettini PA, Jesmanowicz A, Wong EC, et al: Processing strategies for time-course data sets in functional MRI of the human brain. Magn Reson Med 30:161–173, 1993

Belliveau JW, Kennedy DN Jr, McKinstry RC, et al: Functional mapping of the human visual cortex by magnetic resonance imaging. Science 254:716–719, 1991

Birm RM, Yetkin FZ, Hyde JS: Artifact in fMRI caused by motion outside the FOV (abstract). 4th Scientific Meeting of the ISMRM, New York, NY, April 27–May 3. Berkely, CA, Publishers Society of Magnetic Resonance, 1996, p 1770

Bonvento G, Charbonne R, Correze JL, et al: Is alpha-chloralose plus halothane induction a suitable anesthetic regimen for cerebrovascular research? Brain Res 665:213–221, 1994

Boyson SJ, McGonigle P, Molinoff PB: Quantitative autoradiographic localization of the D_1 and D_2 subtypes of dopamine receptors in rat brain. J Neurosci 6:3177–3188, 1986

Curtis VA, Bullmore ET, Brammer MJ, et al: Attenuated frontal activation during a verbal fluency task in patients with schizophrenia. Am J Psychiatry 155:1056–1063, 1998

Dickenson AH, Sullivan AF: Subcutaneous formalin-induced activity of dorsal horn neurones in the rat: differential response to an intrathecal opiate administered pre or post formalin. Pain 30:349–360, 1987

Dubois A, Savasta M, Curet O, et al: Autoradiographic distribution of the D_1 agonist [^{3}H]SKF 38393 in the rat brain and spinal cord: comparison with the distribution of D_2 dopamine receptors. Neuroscience 19:125–137, 1986

Dubowitz DJ, Chen DY, Atkinson DJ, et al: Functional magnetic resonance imaging in macaque cortex. Neuroreport 9:2213–2218, 1998

Ferris CF, Melloni RH Jr, Koppel G, et al: Vasopressin/serotonin interactions in the anterior hypothalamus control aggressive behavior in golden hamsters. J Neurosci 17:4331–4340, 1997

Ferris CF, Mattingly M, Lahti KM, et al: Visualizing brain activation associated with kindling and propagation of epileptic seizure in awake animals using fMRI (abstract). Society for Neuroscience 24:719, 1998

Gansler DA, Fucetola R, Krengel M, et al: Are there cognitive subtypes in adult attention deficit/hyperactivity disorder? J Nerv Ment Dis 186:776–781, 1998

Guan XM, McBride WJ: Fluoxetine increases the extracellular levels of serotonin in the nucleus accumbens. Brain Res Bull 21:43–46, 1988

Gyngell ML, Bock C, Schmitz B, et al: Variation of functional MRI signal in response to frequency of somatosensory stimulation in α-chloralose anesthetized rats. Magn Reson Med 36:13–15, 1996

Hagino H, Tabuchi E, Kurachi M, et al: Effects of D_2 dopamine receptor agonist and antagonist on brain activity in the rat assessed by functional magnetic resonance imaging. Brain Res 813:367–373, 1998

Hajnal JV, Myers R, Oatridge A, et al: Artifacts due to stimulus correlated motion in functional imaging of the brain. Magn Reson Med 31:283–291, 1994

Hauger RL, Lorang M, Irwin M, et al: CRF receptor regulation and sensitization of ACTH responses to acute ether stress during chronic intermittent immobilization stress. Brain Res 532:34–40, 1990

Hyder F, Behar KL, Martin M, et al: Dynamic magnetic resonance imaging of the rat brain during forepaw stimulation. J Cereb Blood Flow Metab 14:649–655, 1994

Lahti KM, Ferris CF, Li F, et al: Imaging brain activity in conscious animals using functional MRI. J Neurosci Methods 82:75–83, 1998

Lahti KM, Ferris CF, Li F, et al: Comparison of evoked cortical activity in conscious and propofol-anesthetized rats using functional MRI. Magn Reson Med 41:412–416, 1999

Logothetis NK, Guggenberger H, Peled S, et al: Functional imaging of the monkey brain. Nat Neurosci 2:555–562, 1999

Ma X-M, Levy A, Lightman SL: Emergence of an isolated arginine vasopressin (AVP) response to stress after repeated restraint: a study of both AVP and corticotropin-releasing hormone messenger ribonucleic acid (RNA) and heteronuclear RNA. Endocrinology 138:4351–4357, 1997

Neil JJ: Functional imaging of the central nervous system using magnetic resonance imaging and positron emission tomography. Curr Opin Neurol 6:927–933, 1993

Ogawa S, Lee TM, Nayak AS, et al: Oxygenation-sensitive contrast in magnetic resonance image of rodent brain at high magnetic fields. Magn Reson Med 14:68–78, 1990

Porszasz R, Beckmann N, Bruttel K, et al: Signal changes in the spinal cord of the rat after injection of formalin into the hindpaw: characterization using functional magnetic resonance imaging. Proc Natl Acad Sci U S A 94:5034–5039, 1997

Scanley BE, Kennan RP, Cannan S, et al: Functional magnetic resonance imaging of median nerve stimulation in rats at 2.0 T. Magn Reson Med 37:969–972, 1997

Sharp FR, Kauer JS, Shepherd GM: Laminar analysis of 2-deoxyglucose uptake in olfactory bulb and olfactory cortex of rabbit and rat. J Neurophysiol 40:800–813, 1977

Ueki M, Mies G, Hossmann KA: Effect of alpha-chloralose, halothane, pentobarbital and nitrous oxide anesthesia on metabolic coupling in somatosensory cortex of rat. Acta Anaesthesiol Scand 36:318–322, 1992

van Hooff JARAM: Categories and sequences of behavior: methods of description and analysis, in Handbook of Methods in Nonverbal Behavior Research. Edited by Scherer KR, Ekman P. New York, Cambridge University Press, 1982, pp 362–439

Yang X, Hyder F, Shulman RG: Activation of single whisker barrel in rat brain localized by functional magnetic resonance imaging. Proc Natl Acad Sci U S A 93:475–478, 1996

Yang X, Renken R, Hyder F, et al: Dynamic mapping at the laminar level of odor-elicited responses in rat olfactory bulb by functional MRI. Proc Natl Acad Sci U S A 95: 7715–7720, 1998

15

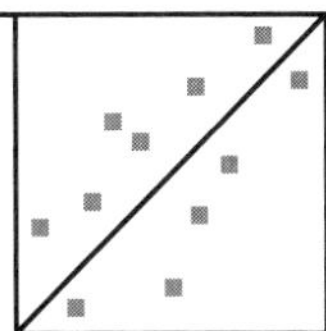

TOWARD A NEUROCOGNITIVE GENETICS

Goals and Issues

Stephen M. Kosslyn, Ph.D.
Robert Plomin, Ph.D.

The 1990s were christened the Decade of the Brain for good reason; an enormous amount was learned about the brain in those 10 years. However, this knowledge is primarily in two areas. On the one hand, the molecular basis of neural activity, including genetics, is understood far better today than one could have hoped a decade ago. On the other hand, dramatic developments in neuroimaging technologies have led to elucidation of the functions of the specific areas in the human brain. However, an enormous gulf exists between these two domains of vigorous activity and rapid progress. Although there has been an increase in understanding how simple genetic abnormalities underlie various types of diseases and cognitive disorders, little is known about the links between genetic mechanisms and the neural mechanisms that underlie normal human cognition. The time is rapidly approaching when it will be possible to bridge this gulf. In this chapter, we focus not on studies of the genetics or functional anatomy of disease or disorders but rather on ways to extrapolate from such studies to studies of normal "cognition" (i.e., mental events, such as memory and imagery) and "behavior" (i.e., observable actions). The ultimate goal of this new enterprise would be to discover how genes and environment interact

Preparation of this chapter was supported by Air Force Office of Scientific Research grant F49620-98-1-0334 (to S.M.K.), National Institute on Aging grant R01 AG12675-02 (to S.M.K.), and National Institute of Child Health and Human Development grant HD27694 (to R.P.).

to affect the efficacy of brain circuits that underlie normal human cognition, which in turn produces behavior and, presumably, behavioral disorders. In this chapter, we outline some of the ways in which this goal can begin to be approached and point out some issues that must be resolved along the way.

■ BEHAVIORAL GENETICS

At present, behavioral genetics offers the only viable approach to connecting genes to normal human behavior (see, for example, Plomin et al. 2001). As its name implies, behavioral genetics involves the genetic analysis of behavior, which includes both quantitative genetic quasi-experimental approaches, such as twin and adoption designs, and molecular genetic approaches that seek to identify specific genes responsible for genetic influence. However, the term does not adequately convey the important role of behavioral genetics in investigating environmental influences while controlling for genetic influences. A more informative term is *genetic-environmental analysis of behavior.* This distinction is important because behavioral genetic research has shown that environmental influences are at least as important as genetic factors for all complex dimensions and disorders. Moreover, given the importance of both genetics and environment for complex behavior, understanding environmental influences requires the use of genetically sensitive designs to untangle the roles of nature and nurture.

Behavioral genetics has a long history, and the most progress has been made in quantitative genetic analyses comparing the resemblance of family members who differ in their genetic relatedness. Most studies in this domain examine cognitive abilities, personality, and psychopathology by comparing identical and fraternal twins (the former have identical sets of genes, and the latter share only half their genes), with the most dramatic studies involving twins who were raised together and those who were raised apart. The methods have become increasingly sophisticated and subtle and may involve complex mathematical models. Quantitative genetic research studies are in agreement that all "specific" cognitive abilities investigated to date, such as verbal ability, spatial ability, memory, and the ability to process information quickly (assessed psychometrically or with information-processing response-time measures), show substantial genetic influence. These diverse measures of cognitive functioning covary considerably, and this overlap of diverse cognitive abilities is known as *general cognitive ability* (*g*) or *general intelligence* (Jensen 1998). *g* is even more heritable than specific cognitive abilities and shows increasingly greater genetic influence throughout life (McClearn et al. 1997; McGue et al.

1993). Multivariate analyses of the genetic links between specific cognitive abilities and *g* indicate that genetic influences on cognitive abilities are general to a surprising extent. That is, once genetic effects on *g* are taken into account, it is evident that genetic effects on specific cognitive abilities—at least as measured heretofore—are modest. Nonetheless, some genetic effects directly affect elementary cognitive processes (assessed by response-time measures), and some genetic effects are specific to certain cognitive abilities but not others (Neubauer et al., in press; Plomin and Petrill 1997). Quantitative genetic findings such as these will help chart the course for exploring the etiological relationships between neurocognitive processes and behavioral measures of cognitive performance.

In addition, researchers have begun to harness the power of new molecular genetic methods to identify specific genes that influence behavior for even complex traits, which are influenced by multiple genes as well as multiple environmental factors (Plomin et al. 1994). Such genes in multiple-gene systems are called *quantitative trait loci* (QTLs) because traits influenced by multiple genes are likely to be distributed quantitatively as dimensions rather than qualitatively as dichotomous disorders. The first replicated QTL linkage for human cognitive disability involved reading disability (Cardon et al. 1994; S. E. Fisher et al. 1999; Gayán et al. 1999; Grigorenko et al. 1997). QTL associations with *g* have been reported as well (Chorney et al. 1998; P. J. Fisher et al. 1999). Considerable progress has also been made in demonstrating genetic influence on nonhuman learning and memory; more powerful methods can be used because both genotype and environment can be manipulated.

The focus of human behavioral genetics is on behavioral differences within the human species and the extent to which genetic and environmental differences can account for these observed differences in behavior. The human genome contains about 3 billion steps in the spiral staircase of DNA, and some 3 million of these DNA base pairs differ from one person to the next. The 99.9% of DNA bases that is identical for all individuals includes DNA that makes people humans, primates, and mammals. The 0.1% of DNA that differs is what makes individuals unique, and the effects of such genetic differences on cognition and behavior is one subject of behavioral genetics. In contrast, the vast bulk of what has been learned from research in cognitive neuroscience relates to universals of the human species, rather than variations on these universal themes. For example, humans are natural language users in the sense that nearly all humans readily use language. At this level of analysis, language is so important that natural selection tolerates no genetic variation. However, individuals differ greatly in terms of rate of language acquisition during development and ultimate ability to use language. These individual differences may or may not be due to genetic differences, because the causes of universals (i.e., means) are not necessarily related to the causes of individual differences (i.e., variance). Means and variances represent different levels of analysis. One level of analysis is not more important than the other, but it is important to note that human genetic methods address individual differences whereas cognitive neuroscience research tends to focus on species universals. However, as we discuss later in this chapter, there is a strand of research in cognitive neuroscience that does examine the relationship between individual differences in characteristics of the brain and behavior.

■ PUTTING THE BRAIN BETWEEN THE GENES AND BEHAVIOR

Although behavioral genetic research using quantitative genetic techniques has found evidence for strong genetic influence in most behaviors, initial findings of links between specific genes and behavior are weak and complex, and thus they are often difficult to replicate. Complex traits are likely to have complex origins, including multiple genes and multiple environmental influences. The greater the number of intervening processes between the genes and the phenotype, the more likely it is that multiple genetic systems affect the phenotype, increasing its heritability but also increasing its complexity. There may be a better way to relate genes to behavior by tapping into the system prior to the production of the observable behavior per se.

One can begin by drawing a historical parallel: Behaviorism attempted to forge direct connections between stimulus and response. In contrast, cognitivism interposed information processing between the stimulus and the response (see, for example, Gardner 1985). This paradigm turned out to have much more power for explaining behavior because it allowed generalizations to be based on inferred internal events rather than solely on directly observed stimulus characteristics and behavior.

An example of these two approaches is shown in Figure 15–1. In the stimulus-response paradigm, one would need to posit many distinct relations between each stimulus and response. Not only is this mapping complex, but it also is not clear why that particular set of stimuli all produce that set of responses—why the patterns of stimulus generalization occur as they do. The situation becomes simpler if an "intervening variable" (in Figure 15–1, thirst) is posited (Miller 1959). If all of those stimuli produce the same internal state, and that state leads to the same set of responses, then the mapping from stimulus to response becomes simpler and it is clear why those stimuli all produce those responses.

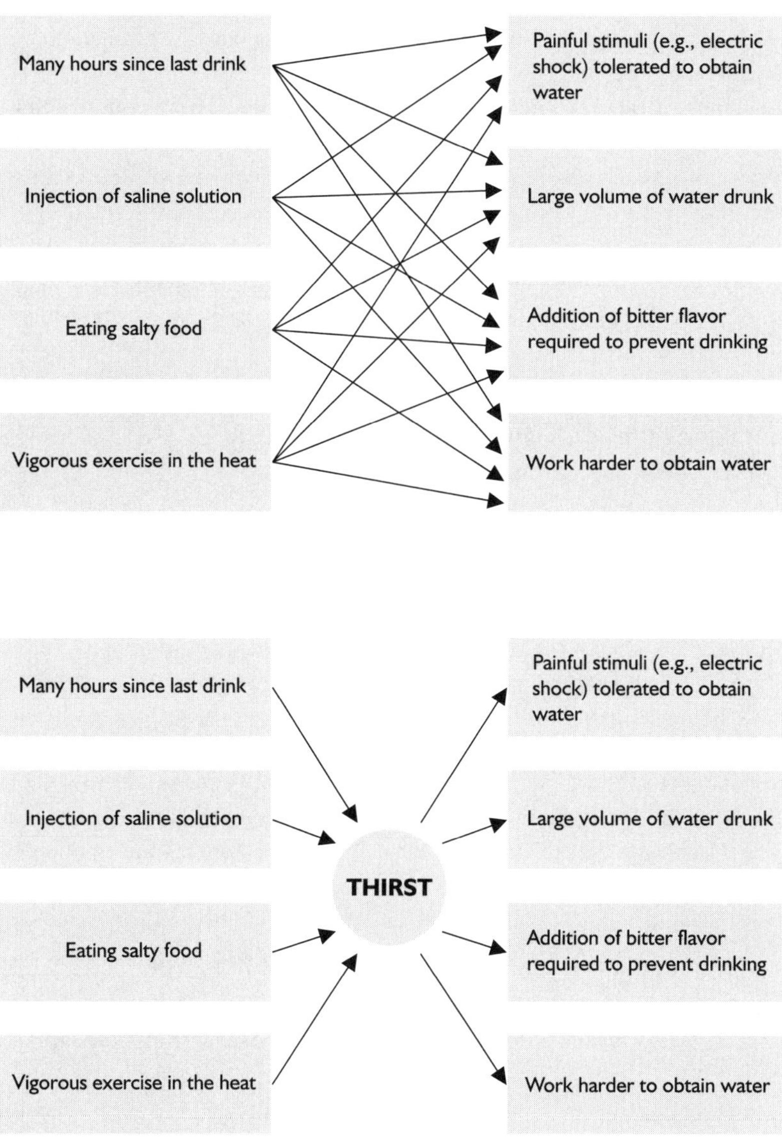

FIGURE 15–1. Two conceptions of the relationship between stimuli and responses. Mapping is simpler and patterns of generalization are more transparent if an "intervening construct" is posited.
Source. Adapted from Anderson and Bower 1973.

In short, we suggest that another paradigm would afford greater power for linking genes to behavior, a paradigm that recognizes that brain intervenes between the genes and behavior.

This general idea is not a new one to researchers who study the genetics of fruit flies, knockout mice, and other genetic preparations. Three aspects of the present proposal make it novel: 1) the focus is on the human brain, 2) neuroimaging techniques are used to discover which aspects of the anatomy and physiology of the human brain predict specific types of behavior, and 3) findings from the Human Genome Project are used to link the genes to the appropriate morphology (i.e., neuroanatomy) and function (i.e., neurophysiology) of the human brain, as assessed by neuroimaging.

■ Using Neuroimaging to Link Neuroanatomy and Neurophysiology to Behavior

The present proposal is to break one step (genes to behavior) into two steps (genes to brain and brain to behavior). In this section, we consider the second step, relating human behavior to the brain, with a focus on individual differences.

Researchers use neuroimaging technologies to chart both the neuroanatomy and neurophysiology of the brain. Both sorts of information may provide links to behavior. We first consider examples in which individual differences in regional cerebral blood flow (rCBF) in specific brain areas were used to predict behavior. Then we briefly consider how pharmacologic variations can predict behavior. Finally, we consider how neuroanatomical information can also be used to predict behavior.

Linking Regional Brain Activation Levels and Behavior

Most contemporary neuroimaging studies, using positron emission tomography (PET) or functional magnetic resonance imaging (fMRI), are designed to answer a different kind of question than the one being considered here. In most studies, researchers are interested in determining which brain areas are activated across subjects during a particular task, relative to a baseline condition. The goal, ultimately, is to discover the set of brain areas and their interactions that allow the brain, on average across individuals, to produce specific behavior, such as uttering grammatically correct sentences (see, for example, Stromswold et al. 1996) or recognizing objects (for instance, see Sergent et al. 1992). Research of this sort focuses on intraindividual changes from baseline to the time of performance of the task of interest but does not consider interindividual differences.

The approach we propose has a different focus. Differences in rCBF between people are not treated as "noise" and simply averaged over; rather, such variations are studied directly. With such direct study, investigators can also circumvent a major conceptual and methodological difficulty associated with standard neuroimaging research, that of comparing a "test task" condition with a specific baseline. The brain is never truly at rest, so using rest as a baseline is problematic; not only is it unclear what the brain does when one rests, but different people may engage in different sorts of cognitive activity (e.g., daydreaming, fantasizing, planning, or worrying), which would introduce variability. Thus, many researchers have attempted to compare a test condition with a "minimally different" baseline. For example, Kosslyn et al. (1994) compared recognition of objects seen from a canonical (typical) point of view with recognition of objects seen from a noncanonical (atypical) point of view, keeping all other aspects of the task identical (e.g., counterbalancing the stimuli over groups of subjects). A problem with this approach, however, is that a minimal difference in the features of a task does not necessarily imply that there is a minimal difference in how the brain performs the task. This problem was well understood at the turn of the last century, when researchers began comparing response times in different conditions (for a brief review, see Kosslyn et al. 1994). Such difficulties can be eliminated if the question is changed, and changed in a way that makes it more useful for ultimately linking brain function to the genes.

Instead of asking which brain areas underlie performance of a task, investigators can ask which areas underlie interindividual differences in performance of the task. In other words, for which processes (implemented in specific brain areas) would more affective operation allow a person to perform the task better? If "Variations in which processes lead one person to perform better than another?" is the question asked, then the logic of the neuroimaging experiment is different. Most critically, only one condition is needed; comparison of a test task and a baseline task is not required. Naturally occurring variation in rCBF is studied and related to variation in task performance.

The key to this approach is to design the tasks in advance so that they tap specific aspects of information processing. Any given task necessarily draws on numerous underlying processes (if only because of input and output requirements for performance). Thus, it is important to sort processes into two categories. The first category, which typically includes most of the processes used to perform a given task, encompasses processes that are not taxed by the task. That is, for many processes, simply being able to perform above a minimal threshold of efficiency may be enough to perform one aspect of a particular task, and variations in the efficacy of the process would not affect performance in that task. For example, when one is attempting to recognize objects under optimal viewing conditions (e.g., in the presence of good lighting), variations in the efficacy of the processes that perform figure-ground segregation probably do not affect how well one recognizes objects.

In contrast, processes in the second category are taxed by the task. Because the efficacy of these processes determines how well the task itself is performed, it may be useful to think of them as the *rate-limiting steps* for performance of a given task. A rate-limiting step occurs when variation in the efficacy of the process will affect performance of the task. Thus, interindividual differences emerge only when these processes are taxed by a task.

The following mental rotation task serves to illustrate this concept. A subject is shown the letter *L*, which is either facing normally or mirror-reversed. The letter is presented tilted at various orientations about a circle, and the task is to decide in each case whether it faces normally or is mirror-reversed. If the letter is in the usual upright position, the decision is easy; however, the time required to make a judgment increases as the letter is rotated greater amounts (for example, see Shepard and Cooper 1982). Such findings have been taken to reflect a process of mental rotation, in which one mentally reorients the letter before making a judgment (for example, see Kosslyn 1980, 1994). Because the judgment itself is so simple, when the letter is presented at a great tilt it is the difficulty of mentally rotating the letter that accounts for most of the time taken to perform the task. Thus, interindividual differences in the overall time to perform the task when the letter is tilted typically reflect (assuming that the subjects are neurologically healthy and literate) variations in the ease of performing this one aspect of the task—the rate-limiting step.

According to the logic of this approach, then, neuroimaging studies of interindividual differences would have three steps: First, a task with a small number of rate-limiting steps is designed. Second, subjects are tested on the task while measures of performance (typically response times and error rates) and measures of rCBF are recorded. Third, for each person the measures of task performance are regressed onto measures of rCBF in different brain areas (delineated as *regions of interest* [ROIs]). The results will indicate for which ROIs interindividual differences in rCBF are related to differences in performance. Variations in rCBF in areas that implement rate-limiting steps should correlate with variations in performance, if it is assumed that greater rCBF reflects greater activation level. (This assumption will be discussed shortly.)

Three illustrations are presented here. First, Kosslyn et al. (1996) were interested in whether the amount of rCBF in Brodmann's Area 17 (the first cortical area that receives input from the eyes during visual perception) predicts how quickly participants perform a visual mental imagery task when their eyes are closed. Sixteen subjects performed a task that was like those previously shown to evoke imagery (see Kosslyn 1980). On each trial, these people heard the name of a letter and, 4 seconds later, the description of a characteristic (e.g., "curved lines"). On hearing the letter, they were to visualize an uppercase version of it and to hold the image; on hearing the characteristic, they were to decide as quickly as possible whether the letter had that characteristic (curved lines, for example, are present in *B* and *C* but not *A* and *E*). While the subjects performed the task, PET was used to assess rCBF throughout the brain (see Kosslyn et al. 1996). For analysis, each brain was normalized to the same mean value, and then response times were regressed onto a set of ROIs; these ROIs were defined a priori on the basis of results from previous studies of imagery. Three results are of interest: First, the slowest subjects had the least amount of blood flow in Area 17 (r=–0.65); indeed, a significant correlation between rCBF in Area 17 and response time persisted even after factoring out the contributions of two other ROIs in which rCBF was correlated with response times. Second, rCBF in a total of three areas was correlated with response time. The multiple correlation between rCBF and response time was remarkable (R=0.94). Third, in two of the areas the correlation was negative (i.e., less rCBF in the areas was related to slower times), but in the other area the correlation was positive (i.e., less rCBF was related to faster times). We will return to the interpretation of positive versus negative correlations shortly.

A study by Nyberg et al. (1996) serves as a second illustration of the use of neuroimaging to study interindividual differences. These investigators used interindividual differences in brain activation to predict recognition memory for words. They included three visual recognition conditions: 1) recognition of words after subjects had encoded them using a "semantic" strategy, 2) recognition of words after subjects had encoded them using a perceptual strategy, and 3) recognition of words that were not in fact studied at the outset of the experiment. They also included a baseline condition in which subjects read words. The researchers used PET to measure rCBF in each condition and then correlated rCBF measures and recognition measures in each condition. They found that activation in the left medial temporal lobe (the parahippocampal gyrus, in particular) was correlated with recognition (r=0.80 for the first scan and r=0.83 for a replication scan). In addition, two other areas had correlations larger than r=0.7. Data from an additional set of subjects demonstrated a correlation between memory and left medial temporal lobe activation. These subjects studied 20 nouns and then were scanned while they decided whether they had studied each of a set of words (i.e., while they participated in a yes/no recognition test). Again, activation in the left hippocampus was strongly correlated ($r=0.82$) with the number of words recognized. Positive correlations with memory performance are equivalent to negative correlations with response time (where longer times indicate worse performance, in contrast to higher recall indicating better performance).

In a study by Cahill et al. (1996), the third illustration, researchers asked subjects to view emotionally arousing film clips or emotionally neutral film clips while radioactively tagged glucose was administered; more of such glucose is taken up in brain areas that are more active while one performs a task. PET was then used to assess which brain areas had been most active while subjects were viewing the films (these scans assessed regional cerebral metabolic rate [rCMR]). Each subject participated in two sessions, one with each type of film clip. Three weeks later, subjects were asked to recall all they could about the films. As expected, given previous findings, subjects recalled more of the emotionally arousing films. Moreover, metabolic rate in the right amygdaloid complex was correlated ($r=0.93$) with accuracy of memory for the emotionally arousing films but was not correlated with accuracy of memory for the emotionally neutral films ($r=0.33$). These researchers focused specifically on the amygdaloid complex, which is known to play a crucial role in emotion (see, for example LeDoux 1994); however, they also reported correlations between recall and rCMR in another area in the emotionally arousing film condition but not in the neutral film condition, and another correlation was present in both conditions (the magnitudes of these correlations were not provided).

In short, these results illustrate three general points: First, interindividual variations in the activation of brain areas do indeed predict variation in task performance. Second, variation in the activation of different brain areas predicts variations in the performance of different tasks. Third, the correlations typically indicate that more activation (in terms of blood flow or metabolic rate) is related to better performance.

In one case, however, more blood flow reflected poorer performance. At first glance, this result is easily interpreted as indicating that subjects who were not as good at performing a particular process had to try harder, which engendered more blood flow. Thus, increased rCBF can be interpreted as indicating either more effective processing or less effective processing! The situation may simply reflect differences in skill level. If a subject is unpracticed and can perform a process effectively, more blood flow may reflect better performance. On the other hand, a subject who is highly practiced and good at performing the process should require less blood flow; more blood flow would reflect poorer performance. The direction of the correlation thus may depend on how adept the subjects are at a particular kind of processing. One way to address this problem is to require subjects to practice the task in advance until their performance approaches their personal asymptotes (interindividual differences are still expected). It is worth noting, however, that people often change strategies as they practice more (for instance, see Kosslyn 1999; Raichle et al. 1994); thus, the processes used after much practice may not be the same as those used at the outset. However, this problem does not necessarily relate to the present goal of discovering possible genetic bases of interindividual differences in variations in rCBF and in genetic links between rCBF and cognitive processing. The tasks must be designed with the effects of practice in mind from the start.

Linking Pharmacology and Behavior

Blood flow, metabolic rate, and oxygen consumption are not the only possible measures of brain function. PET and MRI can be used to assess other measures, which in turn can be related to behavior. It is possible to use PET to chart the density of specific types of receptors in the brain and to observe how they are upregulated or downregulated by specific types of performance. With production of radioactive molecules that mimic specific neurotransmitters or neuromodulators (i.e., ligands), one can use PET to observe where in the brain these molecules are concentrated during a task. These maps in some ways are analogous to the measures of brain activation obtained by assessing rCBF or rCMR using PET or activation level using functional MRI.

In addition to such measures, one can obtain more global measures of the amount of specific pharmacologic agents in the brain by using magnetic resonance spectroscopy (MRS). This technique relies on the fact that atoms in different molecules resonate to different frequencies of magnetic pulses. Magnetic resonance spectroscopy allows one to determine how performing different types of tasks affects global measures of specific agents in the brain. Again, measures of task performance can be regressed onto such measures of brain function. Refinements of this type of imaging will make it possible to examine such variations in specific parts of the brain (see also Bottomley et al. 1983; Y. Cohen et al. 1991) and to correlate individual differences in such variations with behavior.

Linking Brain Structure and Behavior

In addition to relating brain function to behavior, one can also relate morphological properties of brain structures to behavior. Merzenich and colleagues (for example, Merzenich et al. 1983) showed that the size of a cortical area reflects the use of that area in a particular kind of processing. In their work with monkeys, for example, they showed that removing a digit results in larger cortical areas for the remaining digits. It is possible that this larger area is in turn related to increased sensitivity. This conjecture is plausible in light of findings such as those by Schlaug et al. (1995; see also Elbert et al. 1995). These researchers used MRI to measure the size of different anatomical regions. They found that in professional musicians who play string instruments, compared with control subjects, the right motor strip has larger regions for controlling the fingers of the left hand (see also Karni et al. 1995). In addition, Pascual-Leone and colleagues (Pascual-Leone and Torres 1993; Pascual-Leone et al. 1995; for a review, see Hamilton and Pascual-Leone 1998) used transcranial magnetic stimulation to show that, as people learn to read braille, larger parts of motor cortex are recruited; these researchers did not, however, correlate behavior with the relative size of the appropriate brain areas. Nevertheless, this method in principle clearly can be applied to this question.

All of the examples just noted rely on differences in the amount of practice that lead to variations in the size of a brain area. It is possible that practice has different effects on people with different genetic endowments, just as the effects of lifting weights on muscle mass are different for people with different genes. Another approach would be to correlate the sizes of brain areas that are not likely to be affected by practice with behavior. For example, Rademacher et al. (1993) showed enormous individual differences in various structural features of the brain. The length of the calcarine fissure (the central landmark of Area 17 in the human brain), for example, varies by a factor of two to one over people. Does this structural variation correlate with visual sensitivity? With the ease of forming certain types of mental images? Such research has yet to be done but is clearly feasible with current technologies.

Discussion

In summary, both the function of specific areas (assessed by measuring rCBF, rCMR, activation level, or relative concentrations of pharmacologic substances) and structural differences can be correlated with measures of specific types of behavior. Such a simple and straightforward approach will relate properties of the brain to properties of cognition and behavior. Genetic research is needed to elucidate the genetic and environmental contributions to interindividual differences in such properties of the brain (which cannot be assumed to be completely genetic in origin [Hyman and Nestler 1993]) and to the relationships between properties of the brain and cognition and behavior. Multivariate genetic research mentioned earlier has shown that much genetic influence on behavioral measures of cognitive performance is general or diffuse but that some genetic effects also operate independently at the level of specific cognitive abilities and even specific tasks. Thus, two overarching hypotheses may be presented: First, some genetic differences affect the functioning of many brain areas, perhaps by affecting the operation or efficacy of neuromodulators that affect overall speed, the density of neurons, the efficacy of the vasculature, and so on. Second, depending on the task, different areas of the brain are engaged, and hence the genetics of those areas become relevant. Genes that are related to performance of a particular task per se should be those that affect the efficacy of the brain areas used in that task.

■ Linking Genetics to Neuroanatomy and Neurophysiology

As described earlier, the evidence is strong for links between genetics and behavior. The premise of the present proposal is to break one step into two steps: genes to brain and brain to behavior. In the previous section, we showed that the second step is promising when brain neuroanatomy and neurophysiology are assessed by neuroimaging. In this section, we consider the first step, the genetics of neuroanatomy and neurophysiology.

Little is known about the genetic and environmental influences on interindividual differences in neuroanatomy and neurophysiology in humans. However, studies investigating such influences have begun to be reported. For example, electroencephalographic studies involving twins suggest substantial genetic influence (Deary and Caryl 1993). In addition, a study involving 213 twin pairs assessed peripheral nerve conduction velocity (PNCV) as well as general cognitive ability and information-processing measures of reaction times (Rijsdijk 1997). However, even though high heritability (77%) was found for PNCV, PNCV was not related to cognitive ability.

We are not aware of human quantitative genetic research on neuroimaging measures of brain functioning. Most valuable would be a multivariate analysis of the genetic and environmental links between neuroimaging measures and behavior. Such a project is certainly feasible in terms of the availability of twins: More than 1 in 100 births are twin births, and registers of twins are available in several states in the United States and in other countries. Moreover, twins are renowned for their willingness to participate in research, presumably because twins believe that they are special. For this reason, twins would be especially suitable subjects for this type of neuroimaging research.

However, the large sample needed for a twin study is likely to be a deterrent. At least 50 pairs of identical twins and 50 pairs of fraternal twins are needed if heritability is moderate. Moreover, adequate power to compare one heritability estimate with another requires much larger samples. Because twin analyses are based on the difference between correlations for identical and fraternal twins, studies of 20 pairs of each type of twin could detect heritability only if heritability were greater than 100% (that is, if the assumptions of the twin model were violated). Nonetheless, if the need for large samples could be satisfied, perhaps by a multisite collaboration, the rewards would be great.

The fruits of molecular genetic research also may be used to investigate links between specific genes and brain function. Again, however, sample size requirements will deter attempts to find genes associated with brain function. Most gene-hunting studies use several hundred individuals or sibling pairs. But it is not necessary to try to identify new genes in the course of the present project; instead, reliance can be placed on previously identified genes. Much smaller samples can be used in studies of the effects of a specific, previously identified gene. For example, candidate genes involved in a particular brain function—genes involved in hippocampal function, for instance—could be studied by comparing "phenotypic" trait scores of relatively small groups of individuals who differ genotypically for the gene or by comparing genotypic frequencies among groups of individuals at the extremes of the phenotypic dimension. However, because tens of thousands of genes are expressed in the brain and a case could be made for nominating many of these genes as candidate genes for cognitive functioning, the candidate gene approach could be criticized as a fishing expedition.

More likely, the impact of molecular genetics on cognitive neuroscience will come as genes are identified that are known to be linked to behavioral measures of cognitive function or dysfunction (Plomin and Rutter 1998). These genes will become targets in studies of brain function as an intervening variable between genes and behavior. For example, as noted earlier, linkage between reading disability and DNA markers on the short arm of chromosome 6 has been replicated in several studies—the first replicated QTL for human cognition. There is reason to believe that the gene responsible for this linkage may have a relatively large effect on normal reading. One strategy is to study reading-disabled subjects who have the "increasing" alleles and those who do not. This strategy is possible because any allele associated with a complex disorder such as reading disability is more frequent in individuals with reading disability but many reading-disabled individuals do not have the allele.

However, the QTL perspective—which, as explained earlier, assumes that complex traits are quantitatively distributed because they are influenced by multiple genes—also makes it possible to study interindividual differences in reading ability throughout the normal range. The QTL perspective assumes that complex dimensions and disorders are influenced by multiple genes that act as probabilistic risk factors rather than as necessary and sufficient causes of a disorder. For this reason, the QTL perspective suggests that there may be no genes for a disorder, only genes that contribute quantitatively to dimensions (Plomin et al. 1994). That is, the gene on chromosome 6 for reading disability may be a gene that makes good readers poorer at reading and makes poor readers even poorer. In some cases the decrement in reading results in an individual's performing below an arbitrary diagnostic cutoff point of poor reading. This QTL perspective makes it possible to use the gene on chromosome 6 to go beyond the investigation of cognitive dysfunction involved in reading disability, to study normal cognitive processing involved in reading, although it remains to be seen whether the "reading gene" has an effect throughout the distribution of reading ability as predicted by the QTL perspective. If such were the case, researchers could study subjects who were not reading disabled, in order to focus on the effects of this particular reading gene by randomizing the effects of other genes that affect reading disability. Subjects could be selected for this reading gene on the basis of whether they had two increasing alleles or two decreasing alleles for the gene. Alternatively, phenotypic selection rather than genotypic selection could be used to select subjects. That is, subjects could be selected at the extreme of the trait distribution, as explained later in this section.

These genotypically selected or phenotypically selected groups could then be compared on multiple neuroimaging measures of neuroanatomy and neurophysiology in order to trace the brain processes intervening between QTLs and behavioral measures of reading performance. It is more likely that several genes are associated with most complex disorders and dimensions. Even if each of these genes accounts for only a small amount of variance, together they might account for a sufficiently large portion of variance to warrant their investigation in neurocognitive studies. Genotypic selection could be based on selection of one group with increasing alleles for several of these genes and another group with decreasing alleles.

Sample sizes would depend on the size of the expected effect of the gene. Reading ability and reading disability both yield heritabilities of about 50%, as do most cognitive abilities and disabilities. If the reading gene accounts for 10% of this heritability (a large effect by QTL standards), it would account for 5% of the variance in the population. An effect of this size represents a mean difference between the genotypically or phenotypically selected groups that is half their standard deviation. To attain 80% power to detect a mean difference between two groups that accounts for 5% of the variance, investigators would need to enroll 65 subjects in each group (J. Cohen 1988) (P=0.05; one-tailed test, because the direction of the expected effect is known). If the effect size accounts for 2% of the heritability (1% of the population variance, a mean difference that represents one-fifth of the standard deviation), 300 subjects in each group would be needed to attain the same power.

It is an understatement to say that these numbers are discouraging to neuroimaging researchers, who find samples of 16 large. However, at least one general strategy might allow neuroimaging to be used in this enterprise in a practical way. This approach involves five steps: The first is to develop the tasks that are believed to tap the process of interest. The second step is to perform a relatively small neuroimaging study in which interindividual differences in the activation of the appropriate ROIs (or, for example, in the variations in the size of specific brain areas, or in the amounts of a pharmacologic agent) are shown to predict interindividual differences in performance. The third step is to administer the task (which has been "neurally validated" in the second phase) off-line to a large number of potential subjects. The fourth step is to select the phenotypic extremes from the off-line testing to be tested in a neuroimaging study; the results from this study can then be used to screen links to genetic variations. That is, the high and low extremes on the proxy neurally validated phenotype can be used to investigate genotypic frequency differences for any relevant genes. (The advantage of phenotypic selection for extremes is that the same samples can be used to screen all genes.) The final step, undertaken when this screen with the proxy phenotype indicates an association with a gene, is to collect additional neuroimaging data for a more in-depth investigation of the gene's effects by selecting the phenotypic extremes genotypically. That is, individuals with decreasing alleles would be selected from the low extreme and individuals with increasing alleles would be selected from the high extreme in order to examine the gene's effects on, for example, different ROIs. Because this fifth step involves a type of replication, smaller samples than those just described would be more acceptable, although the neuroimaging study itself would still be subject to the same power constraints.

Even if the presence or absence of specific alleles or combinations thereof is shown to be related to a brain characteristic, the following question remains unanswered: What is it about those genes that ultimately leads them to be related to the observed brain characteristics? Three more steps are necessary: First, the proteins expressed by the genes are determined. Second, this information is used to narrow down the range of possible mechanisms. For example, interindividual differences in activation of a certain brain area could arise because of the sheer number of neurons, the number of glial cells, differences in the density of receptors of specific types, the richness of the vasculature, the density of axonal arborization from distant neuromodulatory areas, and so on. It is necessary to consider as many brain features that could be affected by the genes as possible. If a certain protein is known to play a key role in building a particular type of receptor but no role in defining the vasculature, for example, the range of possible mechanisms is restricted.

The third step is to evaluate empirically the hypothesized mechanisms. Animal models will play a crucial role in this enterprise for the foreseeable future. After development of a hypothesis regarding the molecular mechanism whereby the genes produce the brain differences, it will be necessary to modify the corresponding gene in a lower mammal and determine whether it has the predicted effects on neurons. This last step will be fraught with difficulty, given that there are no obvious animal models for many of the functions of interest in the human brain (language being the most obvious example). Nevertheless, if the hypothesis is cast at the right level of precision, it may be possible to document the cascade of events that are produced by specific genes that in turn affect specific aspects of neural function. Mouse models will become increasingly valuable not just for identifying genes but also for characterizing developmental mechanisms in the pathways between genes and behavior (Battey et al. 1999). In such research, it is possible to create genetic variation experimentally in genes that do not naturally vary among individuals, through techniques known as *gene targeting* and *gene knockouts* (see, for instance, Capecchi 1994). For example, one of the first knockout experiments concerning behavior involved a gene for a protein, α-calcium-calmodulin kinase II, which is found in the hippocampus and thought to be involved in long-term memory. Mutant mice homozygous for this knockout gene were slower in performing a water-maze task than were control mice, even though their behavior seemed otherwise normal (Silva et al. 1992a, 1992b). Knockout alleles of several other genes have also been shown to affect learning and memory in mice (Wehner et al. 1996) and fruit flies (Tully et al. 1994).

This enterprise will necessarily involve collaboration between researchers in a number of different disciplines, in some cases disciplines whose members currently have virtually no contact (e.g., neuroimaging and behavioral genetics).

■ Conclusion

The project that we envision arises from the following considerations: 1) Cognitive psychologists have developed theories that lead to the design of tasks that tap very specific processes. 2) There are interindividual differences in the performance of all these tasks. 3) These interindividual differences are reflected by individual differences in aspects of brain function and structure. 4) Behavioral geneticists have developed ways to assess the genetic and environmental contributions to interindividual differences in performance. 5) The brain stands between the genes and behavior; therefore, the genes and environment must affect the brain, which in turn affects behavior. Therefore, why not try to discover how the genes and environment affect the brain to produce individual differences in the tasks designed by cognitive psychologists?

■ REFERENCES

Anderson JR, Bower GH: Human Associative Memory. New York, Wiley, 1973

Battey J, Jordan E, Cox D, et al: An action plan for mouse genomics. Nat Genet 21:73–75, 1999

Bottomley PA, Hart HR, Edelstein WA, et al: NMR imaging/spectroscopy system to study both anatomy and metabolism. Lancet 2:273–274, 1983

Cahill L, Haier RJ, Fallon J, et al: Amygdala activity at encoding correlated with long-term, free recall of emotional information. Proc Natl Acad Sci U S A 93:8016–8021, 1996

Capecchi MR: Targeted gene replacement. Sci Am 270:52–59, 1994

Cardon LR, Smith SD, Fulker DW, et al: Quantitative trait locus for reading disability on chromosome 6. Science 266:276–279, 1994

Chorney MJ, Chorney K, Seese N, et al: A quantitative trait locus (QTL) associated with cognitive ability in children. Psychological Science 9:1–8, 1998

Cohen J: Statistical Power Analysis for the Behavioral Sciences. Hillsdale, NJ, Erlbaum, 1988

Cohen Y, Sanada T, Pitts LH, et al: Surface coil spectroscopic imaging: time and spatial evolution of lactate production following fluid percussion brain injury. Magn Reson Med 17:225–236, 1991

Deary IJ, Caryl PG: Intelligence, EEG, and evoked potentials, in Biological Approaches to the Study of Human Intelligence. Edited by Vernon PA. Norwood, NJ, Ablex, 1993, pp 259–315

Elbert T, Pantev C, Wienbruch C, et al: Increased cortical representation of the fingers of the left hand in string players. Science 270:305–306, 1995

Fisher PJ, Turic D, Williams NM, et al: DNA pooling identifies QTLs on chromosome 4for general cognitive ability in children. Hum Mol Genet 8:915–922, 1999

Fisher SE, Marlow AJ, Lamb J, et al: A quantitative-trait locus on chromosome 6p influences different aspects of developmental dyslexia. Am J Hum Genet 64:146–156, 1999

Gardner H: The Mind's New Science: A History of the Cognitive Revolution. New York, Basic Books, 1985

Gayán J, Smith SD, Chereny SS, et al: Quantitative-trait locus for specific language and reading deficits on chromosome 6p. Am J Hum Genet 64:157–164, 1999

Grigorenko EL, Wood FB, Meyer MS, et al: Susceptibility loci for distinct components of dyslexia on chromosomes 6 and 15. Am J Hum Genet 60:27–39, 1997

Hamilton RH, Pascual-Leone A: Cortical plasticity associated with braille learning. Trends in Cognitive Neuroscience 2:168–174, 1998

Hyman SE, Nestler EJ: The Molecular Foundations of Psychiatry. Washington, DC, American Psychiatric Press, 1993

Jensen AR: The *g* Factor: The Science of Mental Ability. London, Praeger, 1998

Karni A, Meyer G, Jezzard P, et al: Functional MRI evidence for adult motor cortex plasticity during motor skill learning. Nature 377:155–158, 1995

Kosslyn SM: Image and Mind. Cambridge, MA, Harvard University Press, 1980

Kosslyn SM: Image and Brain. Cambridge, MA, MIT Press, 1994

Kosslyn SM: If neuroimaging is the answer, what is the question? Philos Trans R Soc Lond B Biol Sci 354:1283–1294, 1999

Kosslyn SM, Alpert NM, Thompson WL, et al: Identifying objects seen from different viewpoints: a PET investigation. Brain 117:1055–1071, 1994

Kosslyn SM, Thompson WL, Kim IJ, et al: Individual differences in cerebral blood flow in area 17 predict the time to evaluate visualized letters. J Cogn Neurosci 8:78–82, 1996

LeDoux JE: The Emotional Brain. New York, Simon & Schuster, 1994

McClearn GE, Johansson B, Berg S, et al: Substantial genetic influence on cognitive abilities in twins 80+ years old. Science 276:1560–1563, 1997

McGue M, Bouchard TJ Jr, Iacono WG, et al: Behavioral genetics of cognitive ability: a life-span perspective, in Nature, Nurture, and Psychology. Edited by Plomin R, McClearn GE. Washington, DC, American Psychological Association, 1993, pp 59–76

Merzenich MM, Kaas JH, Wall JT, et al: Progression of change following nerve section in the cortical representation of the hand in areas 3b and 1 in adult owl and squirrel monkeys. Neuroscience 10:639–665, 1983

Miller NE: Liberalization of basic S-R concepts: extensions to conflict behavior, motivation, and social learning, in Psychology: A Study of a Science, Vol 2. Edited by Koch S. New York, McGraw-Hill, 1959, pp 196–292

Neubauer AC, Spinath FM, Riemann R, et al: Genetic (and environmental) influence on two measures of speed of information processing and their relation to psychometric intelligence: evidence from the German Observational Study of Adult Twins. Intelligence (in press)

Nyberg L, McIntosh AR, Houle S, et al: Activation of medial temporal structures during episodic memory retrieval. Nature 380:715–717, 1996

Pascual-Leone A, Torres F: Sensorimotor cortex representation of the reading finger of braille readers: an example of activity-induced cerebral plasticity in humans. Brain 116:39–52, 1993

Pascual-Leone A, Wassermann EM, Sandato N, et al: The role of reading activity on the modulation of motor cortical outputs to the reading hand in braille readers. Ann Neurol 38:910–915, 1995

Plomin R, Petrill SA: Genetics and intelligence: what's new? Intelligence 24:53–77, 1997

Plomin R, Rutter M: Child development, molecular genetics, and what to do with genes once they are found. Child Dev 69:1221–1240, 1998

Plomin R, Owen MJ, McGuffin P: The genetic basis of complex human behaviors. Science 264:1733–1739, 1994

Plomin R, DeFries JC, McClearn GE, et al: Behavioral Genetics, 4th Edition. New York, Worth Publishers, 2001

Rademacher J, Galaburda AM, Kennedy DN, et al: Topographic variation of the human primary cortices: implications for neuroimaging, brain mapping, and neurobiology. Cereb Cortex 3/4:313–329, 1993

Raichle ME, Fiez JA, Videnn TO, et al: Practice-related changes in human brain functional anatomy during non-motor learning. Cereb Cortex 4:8–26, 1994

Rijsdijk F: The Genetics of Neural Speed: A Genetic Study on Nerve Conduction Velocity, Reaction Times and Psychometric Abilities. Enschede, The Netherlands: PrintPartners Ipskamp, 1997

Schlaug G, Jancke L, Huang Y, et al: In vivo evidence of structural brain asymmetry in musicians. Science 267:699–701, 1995

Sergent J, Ohta S, MacDonald B: Functional neuroanatomy of face and object processing: a positron emission tomography study. Brain 115:15–36, 1992

Shepard RN, Cooper LA: Mental Images and Their Transformations. Cambridge, MA, MIT Press, 1982

Silva AJ, Paylor R, Wehner JM, et al: Deficient hippocampal long-term potentiation in α-calcium-calmodulin kinase II mutant mice. Science 257:201–206, 1992a

Silva AJ, Paylor R, Wehner JM, et al: Impaired spatial learning in α-calcium-calmodulin kinase II mutant mice. Science 257:206–211, 1992b

Stromswold K, Caplan D, Alpert N, et al: Localization of syntactic comprehension by positron emission tomography. Brain Lang 52:452–473, 1996

Tully T, Preat T, Boynton SC, et al: Genetic dissection of consolidated memory in *Drosophila.* Cell 79:35–47, 1994

Wehner JM, Bowers BJ, Paylor R: The use of null mutant mice to study complex learning and memory processes. Behav Genet 26:301–312, 1996

INDEX

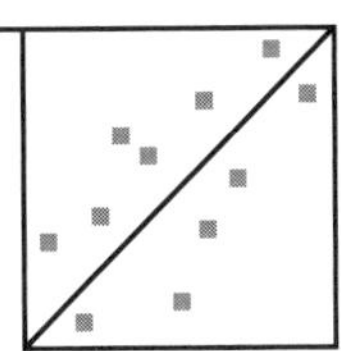

Page numbers printed in **boldface** *type refer to tables or figures.*